ACSM's Behavioral Aspects of Physical Activity and Exercise

ACSM's Behavioral Aspects of Physical Activity and Exercise

EDITOR

Claudio R. Nigg, PhD

Director: Health Behavior Change Research Workgroup
Department of Public Health Sciences, John A. Burns School of Medicine
University of Hawaii at Manoa
Honolulu, Hawaii

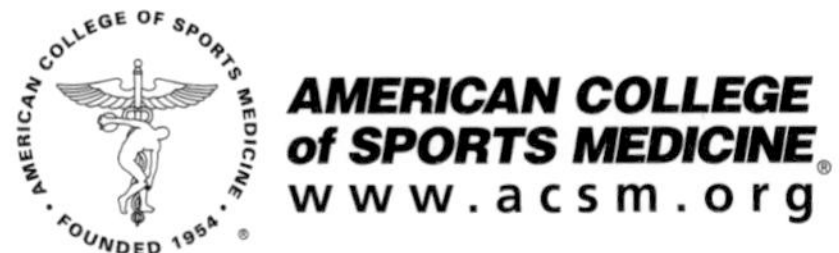

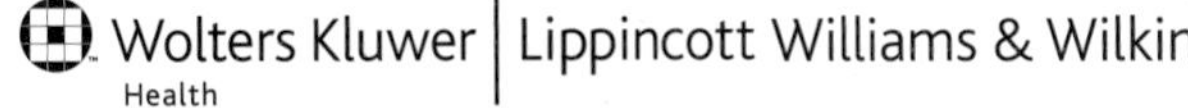

Philadelphia • Baltimore • New York • London
Buenos Aires • Hong Kong • Sydney • Tokyo

Acquisitions Editor: Emily Lupash
Managing Editor: Meredith L. Brittain
Marketing Manager: Shauna Kelley
Vendor Manager: Alicia Jackson
Manufacturing Coordinator: Margie Orzech
Designer: Holly McLaughlin
Compositor: S4Carlisle Publishing Services
ACSM Publication Committee Chair: Walter R. Thompson, PhD, FACSM, FAACVPR
ACSM Group Publisher: Katie Feltman
Umbrella Editor: Jonathan K. Ehrman, PhD, FACSM

Printed in China

9 8 7 6 5 4 3

Library of Congress Cataloging-in-Publication Data

ACSM's behavioral aspects of physical activity and exercise / editor, Claudio R. Nigg.
p. ; cm.
Behavioral aspects of physical activity and exercise
Includes bibliographical references and index.
ISBN 978-1-4511-3211-3 (alk. paper)—ISBN 1-4511-3211-5 (alk. paper)
I. Nigg, Claudio R., editor of compilation. II. American College of Sports Medicine, issuing body. III. Title: Behavioral aspects of physical activity and exercise.
[DNLM: 1. Exercise—psychology. 2. Health Behavior. 3. Motivation. 4. Patient Compliance—psychology. QT 255]
RA781
613.7'1—dc23

2013012305

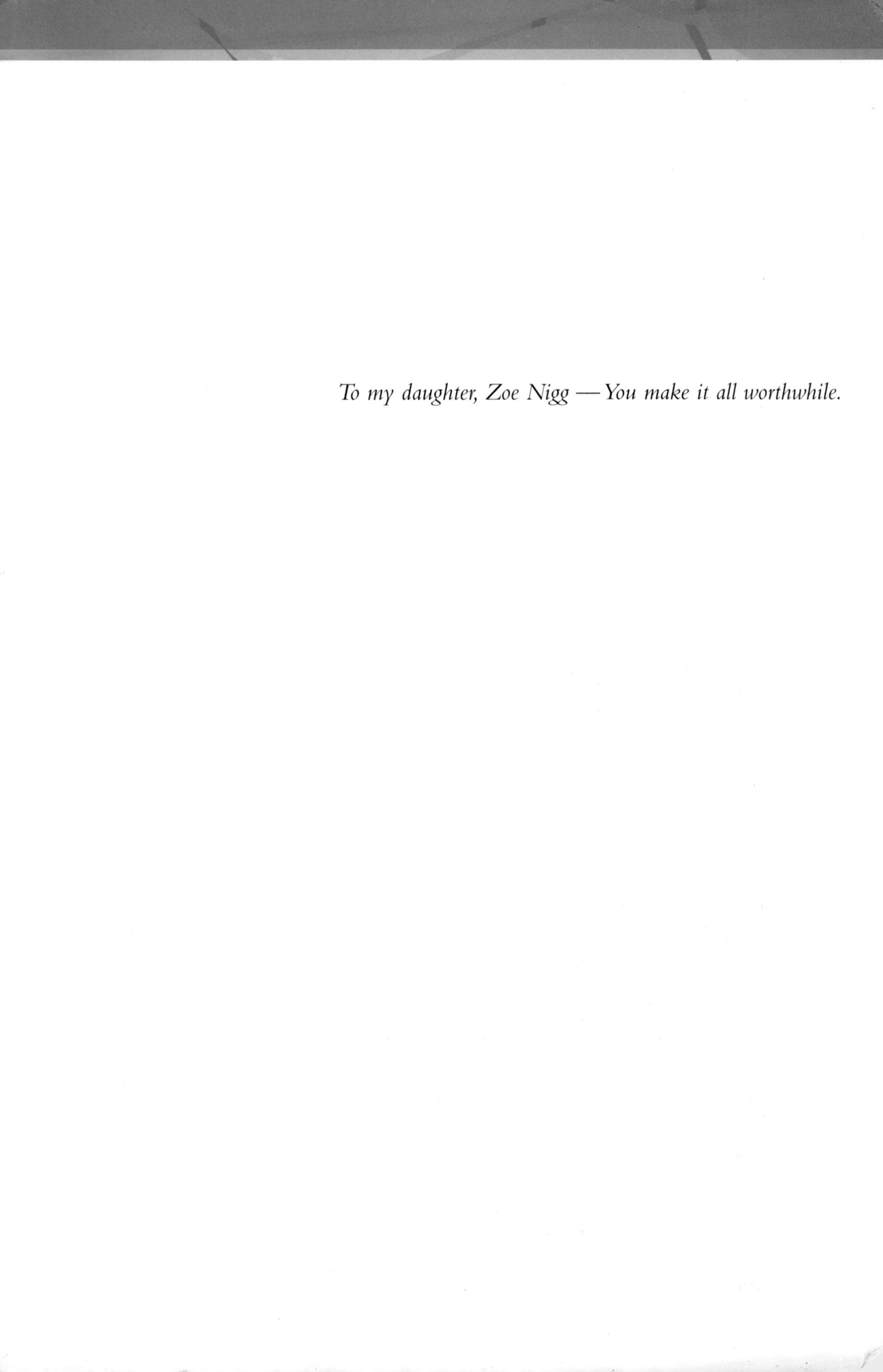

To my daughter, Zoe Nigg — You make it all worthwhile.

Preface

Our understanding of *why* people change their physical activity has grown substantially in the past century. But much less is written or known about *how* people change their physical activity, or what people do or use to become physically active on a regular basis. (If physical activity were available as a pill, it would be the most often prescribed pill!)

ACSM's Behavioral Aspects of Physical Activity and Exercise was written to fill this gap for the practitioner and student alike. For practitioners, the book provides information for use in the field for trying to motivate individuals to become more active. For students, the text shows how to change and promote physical activity. Whether you are a practitioner or a student, you will find useful the tools, tricks, techniques, how-to's, and strategies for the promotion of physical activity provided by our expert authors.

ORGANIZATIONAL PHILOSOPHY

The book is organized as follows:

First, Chapter 1 provides a theoretical foundation — the leading theories of physical activity behavior change, in the belief that practical applications are based on good theories.

Second, Chapter 2 addresses the idea that we cannot change what we cannot measure by providing know-how to assess the relevant aspects of physical activity (*i.e.,* what you need to know about the people you are trying to motivate).

Third, the main body of the book addresses how to change physical activity behavior. These chapters contain the majority of the tools, tricks, techniques, how-to's, and strategies that you can use to help people get active and stay active. This part of the book covers a broad range of topics, from how you can help clients acquire the necessary skills (Chapter 3), to addressing how ready the client is (Chapter 4), to how to communicate with the client (Chapter 5), to delivering physical activity messages using different media (Chapter 6).

Fourth, we provide the broader picture. This includes chapters about how to influence the environment and policy to help motivate people (Chapter 7), how to approach different populations (Chapter 8), and how to practically evaluate physical activity programs (Chapter 9).

Finally, the last chapter (Chapter 10) focuses on the practical applications of professional skills, behaviors, and other factors that can facilitate or impede behavior change.

FEATURES

The book is intended to be engaging, easily applied, and useful in your efforts to help people become more physically active. To this end, most of the chapters include each of the following features:

- **Concept Overview** briefly sets the stage for the chapter.
- **From the Practical Toolbox** sections contain forms, checklists, charts, worksheets, and other resources that can be used immediately. (A collection of all the tools in the book is available on the book's companion Web site; see the "Additional Resources" section that follows for more information.)
- **Evidence** sections include explanations of the latest research that support concrete recommendations.
- **Step-by-Step** applications are specific, user-friendly instructions that explain client-motivation techniques.

- **Case Scenarios** emphasize real-world application of the material.
- **Take-Home Messages** highlight the most important parts of the chapter.

In addition, for those of you who are instructors, several resources are included on the book's companion Web site, such as a Brownstone test generator, PowerPoint presentations, an image bank, and Learning Management System cartridges. See the "Additional Resources" section that follows for more information.

All the people involved in this project sincerely hope that it will help you to help people become physically active. Thank you for what you do and enjoy the book.

ACKNOWLEDGMENTS

I would like to thank the following people for their valuable contributions, without which this book would not have happened: the chapter authors for buying into this approach and writing to make a difference; Katie Amato and Ashley Tsumoto for editorial support for the chapters; Angie Chastain for keeping me organized (and on top of e-mails); Amanda Whittal for her support in copyediting Chapter 2; Phoebe Hwang for creation of the PowerPoint slides and test generator questions; and the ACSM and Wolters Kluwer editorial team for their professionalism and their expertise. Finally, I would like to acknowledge ACSM for their vision in asking me to put this book together.

Claudio R. Nigg, PhD
Editor

ADDITIONAL RESOURCES

ACSM's Behavioral Aspects of Physical Activity and Exercise includes additional resources for both instructors and students that are available on the book's companion Web site at http://thepoint.lww.com/ACSMBehav.

Instructors

Approved adopting instructors will be given access to the following additional resources:

- Brownstone test generator
- PowerPoint presentations
- Image bank
- Learning Management System cartridges

Students

Students who have purchased *ACSM's Behavioral Aspects of Physical Activity and Exercise* have access to the following additional resources:

- A collection of all the practical tools in the book, such as forms, checklists, charts, worksheets, and other resources

In addition, purchasers of the text can access the searchable full text on-line by going to the *ACSM's Behavioral Aspects of Physical Activity and Exercise* Web site at http://thePoint.lww.com/ACSMBehav. See the inside front cover of this text for more details, including the passcode you will need to gain access to the Web site.

Contributors

Kacie Allen, BS
Virginia Tech
Blacksburg, Virginia
Chapter 9: Evaluating Physical Activity Behavior Change Programs and Practices

Adrian Bauman, MD, MPH, PhD
University of Sydney
Sydney, New South Wales, Australia
Chapter 7: Influencing Policy and Environments to Promote Physical Activity Behavior Change

Ute Bültmann, PhD
University Medical Center Groningen
Groningen, The Netherlands
Chapter 2: Assessing Your Client's Physical Activity Behavior, Motivation, and Individual Resources

Lauren Capozzi, BSc
University of Calgary
Alberta, Canada
Chapter 8: Promoting Physical Activity Behavior Change: Population Considerations

Brian Cook, PhD
University of Kentucky
Lexington, Kentucky
Chapter 4: Building Motivation: How Ready Are You?

S. Nicole Culos-Reed, PhD
University of Calgary
Alberta, Canada
Chapter 8: Promoting Physical Activity Behavior Change: Population Considerations

Danielle Symons Downs, PhD
The Pennsylvania State University
State College, Pennsylvania
Chapter 1: Why Do People Change Physical Activity Behavior?

Paul Estabrooks, PhD
Virginia Tech
Blacksburg, Virginia
Chapter 9: Evaluating Physical Activity Behavior Change Programs and Practices

Carol Ewing Garber, PhD, ACSM-PD, ACSM-RCEP, ACSM-HFS
Columbia University
New York, New York
Chapter 10: Professional Practice and Practical Tips for the Application of Behavioral Strategies for the Physical Activity Practitioner

Klaus Gebel, PhD
University of Sydney
Sydney, New South Wales, Australia
Chapter 7: Influencing Policy and Environments to Promote Physical Activity Behavior Change

Heather Hausenblas, PhD
Jackson University
Jacksonville, Florida
Chapter 1: Why Do People Change Physical Activity Behavior?

Eric Hekler, PhD
Arizona State University
Phoenix, Arizona
Chapter 6: How to Deliver Physical Activity Messages

Sara Johnson, PhD
Pro-Change Behavior Systems, Inc.
West Kingston, Rhode Island
Chapter 4: Building Motivation: How Ready Are You?

Julia Kolodziejczyk, MS
San Diego State University
University of California, San Diego
Chapter 6: How to Deliver Physical Activity Messages

Kristina Kowalski, BSc, MSc, PhD(c)
University of Victoria
British Columbia, Canada
Chapter 3: Building Skills to Promote Physical Activity

Blake Krippendorf, BS
Virginia Tech
Blacksburg, Virginia
Chapter 9: Evaluating Physical Activity Behavior Change Programs and Practices

Sonia Lippke, PhD
Jacobs University
Bremen, Germany
Chapter 2: Assessing your Client's Physical Activity Behavior, Motivation, and Individual Resources

Rona Macniven, MSc, BSc
University of Sydney
Sydney, New South Wales, Australia
Chapter 7: Influencing Policy and Environments to Promote Physical Activity Behavior Change

Greg Norman, PhD
University of California - San Diego
San Diego, California
Chapter 6: How to Deliver Physical Activity Messages

Serena Parks, PhD
Virginia Tech
Blacksburg, Virginia
Chapter 9: Evaluating Physical Activity Behavior Change Programs and Practices

Heather Patrick, PhD
National Cancer Institute, National Institutes of Health
Bethesda, Maryland
Chapter 5: Communication Skills to Elicit Physical Activity Behavior Change: How to Talk to the Client

Kimberly Perez, MA, ACSM-HFS
Focus Personal Training Institute
New York, New York
Chapter 10: Professional Practice and Practical Tips for the Application of Behavioral Strategies for the Physical Activity Practitioner

Ernesto Ramirez, MS
University of California - San Diego
San Diego, California
Chapter 6: How to Deliver Physical Activity Messages

Erica Rauff, MS
The Pennsylvania State University
State College, Pennsylvania
Chapter 1: Why Do People Change Physical Activity Behavior?

Ken Resnicow, PhD
University of Michigan
Ann Arbor, Michigan
Chapter 5: Communication Skills to Elicit Physical Activity Behavior Change: How to Talk to the Client

Ryan Rhodes, PhD
University of Victoria
British Columbia, Canada
Chapter 3: Building Skills to Promote Physical Activity

Erin Smith, MA
Virginia Tech
Blacksburg, Virginia
Chapter 9: Evaluating Physical Activity Behavior Change Programs and Practices

Pedro J. Teixeira, PhD
Technical University of Lisbon
Cruz Quebrada, Portugal
Chapter 5: Communication Skills to Elicit Physical Activity Behavior Change: How to Talk to the Client

Claudia Voelcker-Rehage, PhD
Jacobs University
Bremen, Germany
Chapter 2: Assessing your Client's Physical Activity Behavior, Motivation, and Individual Resources

Geoffrey Williams, MD, PhD
University of Rochester
Rochester, New York
Chapter 5: Communication Skills to Elicit Physical Activity Behavior Change: How to Talk to the Client

Reviewers

Sherry Barkley, PhD, ACSM-RCEP
Augustana College
Sioux Falls, South Dakota

Beth Bock, PhD
Brown University and the Miriam Hospital
Providence, Rhode Island

Shane Callahan, MS, EdD
Lewis and Clark Community College
Godfrey, Illinois

Cynthia M. Castro, PhD
Stanford University
Stanford, California

Nickles I. Chittester, PhD
Concordia University Texas
Austin, Texas

Joseph T. Ciccolo, PhD
Columbia University
New York, New York

Bhibha M. Das, PhD, MPH
University of Georgia
Athens, Georgia

Kelliann K. Davis, PhD, ACSM-CES
University of Pittsburgh
Pittsburgh, Pennsylvania

Rebecca Ellis, PhD
Georgia State University
Atlanta, Georgia

Christy Greenleaf, PhD, ACSM/NPAS-PAPHS
University of Wisconsin - Milwaukee
Milwaukee, Wisconsin

Katie M. Heinrich, PhD
Kansas State University
Manhattan, Kansas

Patricia J. Jordan, PhD
Pacific Health Research and Education Institute
Honolulu, Hawaii

Mary Ann Kluge, PhD
University of Colorado - Colorado Springs
Colorado Springs, Colorado

Emily Mailey, PhD
Kansas State University
Manhattan, Kansas

Kathleen A. Martin Ginis, PhD
McMasters University
Hamilton, Ontario

Kristen McAlexander, PhD
Southern Methodist University
Dallas, Texas

Melissa Moore, PhD
Victoria University
Melbourne, Australia

Charles F. Morgan, PhD
University of Hawaii at Manoa
Honolulu, Hawaii

Terra Murray, PhD
Athabasca University
Athabasca, Canada

Neville Owen, PhD
Baker IDI Heart and Diabetes Institute
Melbourne, Australia

Ron Plotnikoff, PhD
University of Newcastle
Newcastle, Australia

Sarah Pomp, PhD
Free University of Berlin
Berlin, Germany

Deborah Riebe, PhD, FACSM, ACSM-HFS
University of Rhode Island
Kingston, Rhode Island

Carrie Safron, MA
Teachers College, Columbia University
New York, New York

David Seigneur, MS, ACSM-CES, FAACVPR
UPMC Mercy
Pittsburgh, Pennsylvania

Sarah A. Slattery, MA
Columbia University
New York, New York

John C. Spence, PhD
University of Alberta
Alberta, Canada

Takemi Sugiyama, PhD
Baker IDI Heart and Diabetes Institute
Melbourne, Australia

Sara Wilcox, PhD, FACSM
University of South Carolina
Columbia, South Carolina

Catherine B. Woods, PhD
Dublin City University
Dublin, Ireland

Julie A. Wright, PhD
University of Massachusetts
Amherst, Massachusetts

Contents

CHAPTER 1

Why Do People Change Physical Activity Behavior?

Danielle Symons Downs, Claudio R. Nigg, Heather A. Hausenblas, and Erica L. Rauff

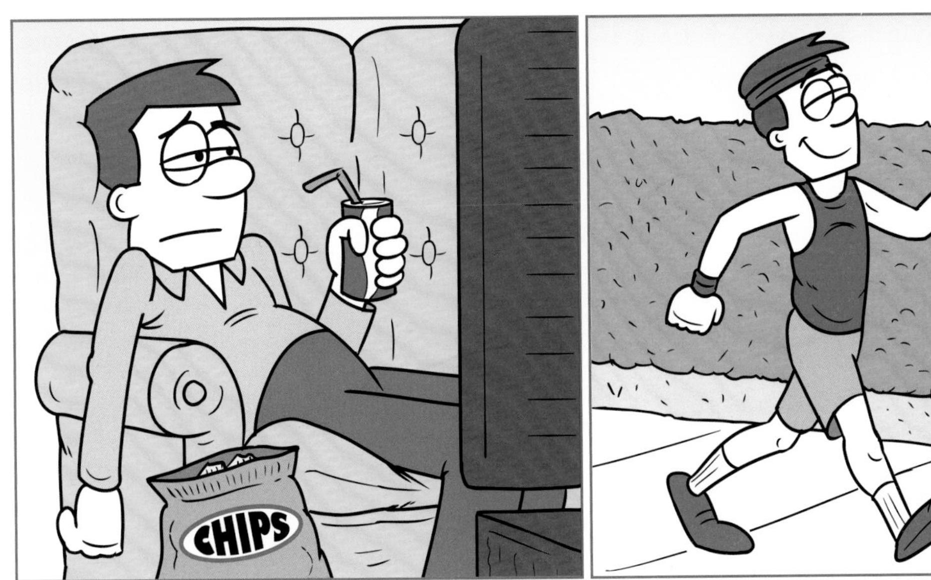

UNDERSTANDING THE PRINCIPLES OF BEHAVIOR CHANGE

CONCEPT OVERVIEW

WHAT IS BEHAVIOR?

Behavior is broadly defined as anything an organism or living being does, which includes actions, words, and manifestations of emotions and thoughts (17). Behavior must be observable, measurable, and operationally defined in order to determine how to modify or change it. Behaviors have important antecedents (cues or triggers that stimulate the behavior), as well as consequences (the positive and/or negative outcomes that follow the behavior). However, behavior is operationally defined differently across contexts. For example, physical activity behavior is often defined as a bodily movement, produced by skeletal muscles, that uses more energy than when a person is at rest (67). Physical activity has also been conceptualized as the "umbrella term" that includes several dimensions such as exercise, sport, leisure activities, dance, etc. (14). However, people generally also view physical activity as a behavior that is more like a habit, particularly when a person is regularly physically active. On the other hand, exercise is often defined as a behavior that is a planned and uses structured movement of the body that is designed with the goal of enhancing physical fitness (6). As a practitioner, you need to define the target behavior first before developing a plan for behavior change. Elements of behavior change are presented in more detail in the next section.

Behavior Change

Changing behavior is difficult. Why? Because people are creatures of habit and the things they do are the behaviors they really *want* to do. These are the actions that "work best" or "are easy to do." So to conceptualize behavior change, you need to understand that many behaviors, particularly physical activity and its related health behaviors, fall on a continuum from an undesired or health-risk behavior to a desired or healthy behavior. Changing an undesired or health-risk behavior involves making a conscious decision to repeatedly do something new or different or "not doing" something bad such as smoking or drinking excessive alcohol. Similarly, changing a desired behavior such as being physically active or eating healthy involves the same conscious decisions to repeatedly do the new behavior, until over time it becomes part of your regular routine. So why then is it so difficult to make positive behavior changes? Because it is common nature to actively seek out activities that you enjoy and avoid activities that you dislike. Unfortunately, many positive health behaviors involve doing things you may not "like." For example, although physical activity has numerous health benefits, it also requires time, effort, and energy; thus, you need to make a conscious decision to incorporate it into everyday life. Understanding the principles of reinforcement will further emphasize this idea.

Principles of Reinforcement

"The way positive reinforcement is carried out is more important than the amount." (*BF Skinner*)

Reinforcement is anything that increases the probability that a behavior will occur again, and the use of rewards and punishments will increase or decrease the likelihood of a similar response happening in the future. Skinner (62) argued that teaching rests entirely on the principles of reinforcement. Today, these principles are among the most widely accepted and practiced in psychology and are the foundation for changing behavior. The most basic assumption of reinforcement is if doing something results in a good consequence (being praised or rewarded), a person will try to repeat the behavior, whereas if doing something results in a bad consequence (being criticized or punished), a person will usually try not to repeat the behavior. For example, if you start jogging and within a few weeks, you see a friend who says "Wow, that jogging is really paying off. You look fantastic!" you will likely try to repeat the behavior in the future to receive more positive praise from friends and family. In contrast, if you receive negative feedback from an important other such as a family member who says "That running is only going to cause you to hurt yourself; I don't know why you even bother" you may stop jogging altogether in an effort to avoid this type of shame and criticism. However, reinforcement in the "real world" is not always this straightforward. The same reinforcer may affect people differently. For example, some people are motivated when a fitness instructor says "Come on, you need to work harder! You're just relaxing back there!" But other people may view this as negative feedback and stop the activity altogether. The reinforcer needs to be tailored to the individual for it to be effective, particularly when the behavior is as complex as physical activity. Thus, it is extremely important to understand the individual and the value he or she places on different reinforcers. What works for one person may not work for another!

The general consensus from most behaviorists is that the positive approach to reinforcement is most appropriate because it increases the likelihood that desirable behaviors will be repeated in the future. From a practical perspective, a positive approach to reinforcement also has a greater chance of strengthening important determinants of physical activity such as attitude, motivation, and self-efficacy. While there is not one set of guidelines for using positive reinforcement, researchers in the sport and exercise psychology domain (71) have recommended the following strategies for using positive reinforcement for behavior change:

- **Choose effective rewards:** Rewards should be important and relevant to the person who is doing the behavior. That is, you should like the reward, otherwise it will not be effective! Some of these rewards may be intrinsic, such as you taking pride in your accomplishment or working harder to learn more and perform better. Some of these rewards may be extrinsic, such as social (praise, public acknowledgement, clapping), material (clothing, trophies, certificates of achievement), and/or monetary (cash or gift cards) incentives.
- **Schedule reinforcers effectively:** Researchers (42,58,71) have demonstrated that continuous and immediate reinforcement is desirable when a behavior is new or the person is in the early stages of learning the behavior. Reinforcement should be immediate to maximize the likelihood of making a link or connection between the desired behavior and a positive response. However, once the behavior has become more routine, intermittent (sporadic or not expected) reinforcement is preferred because the reinforcement otherwise becomes monotonous and loses its impact or value.
- **Reward appropriate behaviors:** As with scheduling reinforcers effectively, it is also important to be selective about the behaviors that are rewarded. If you get

rewarded for every behavior you do, the impact of the reward structure is lost. Thus, you should know which are the most important behaviors or outcomes to reward for a target person and when to consider rewarding close approximations to this behavior. This is called *shaping*, which is when behaviors that are close to the desired behavior are rewarded in an effort to gradually change an existing behavior over time (50,62).

- **Reward performance and effort; not just the outcome:** Similar to the goal-setting literature, it is important to reward process or procedural determinants of behavior such as hard work, effort, and dedication in addition to the actual performance or behavior. This will increase the likelihood you are able to repeat the behavior in the face of adversity or barriers because you learn the value of the process and will be less likely to give up when it is challenging to achieve the behavior.
- **Positive motivational climate:** Using positive reinforcers within a positive and supportive environment can maximize the likelihood of behavior change. Feedback on the behavior should be given with instruction and encouragement, patience, and an opportunity for discussion and additional feedback with the target person or group.

However, behavior change is frequently determined by more than the principles of reinforcement. Thus, it is important to consider theories that incorporate a more comprehensive approach to behavior change. The following sections will provide an overview of why using theories and models to guide behavior change is important and will also describe several frequently used behavioral theories to explain and predict physical activity behaviors. Case example illustrations are also included to demonstrate how to apply these theories.

THEORIES OF BEHAVIOR CHANGE

The Importance of Theories and Models

"There is nothing more practical than a good theory." (Lewin, K. (1952). Field theory in social science: Selected theoretical papers by Kurt Lewin. London: Tavistock.)

Theories and models of behavior change can at first seem overwhelming to understand. However, once the initial sense of apprehension for using theory passes, a practitioner often quickly sees the underlying value and added benefits of using a theoretical approach. A simple way to view a theory or model is to see it as a structured logical explanation or way of describing a certain phenomenon. A *theory* allows you to understand, explain, and predict behavior. They provide the "how and/or why" a behavior occurs and offer an empirically-based framework or "blueprint" from which to develop interventions to promote healthy behaviors such as physical activity. A *model* provides a visual representation of a phenomenon—or an illustration of how certain parts, known as the components, are related within a structure (10). Many theories have models but not all models are based on a theory. From a practical perspective, a good theory often uses a model to demonstrate how the components of the theory are related and predict behavior. Health promotion experts may choose to use theories and/or models for many different reasons, including to better explain the factors that facilitate or inhibit behavior change at the individual, community, and societal levels and/or to guide the selection and development of appropriate health promotion strategies. It is important to note that theories should never be applied without a good understanding of the "big picture"—that is, without a thorough insight and awareness of the individuals, groups, organizations, and communities you are working with to promote healthy behavior changes. Remember, a theory isn't the solution, but rather the foundation.

To change or promote physical activity behavior, it is important to recognize the critical elements of the most commonly used, evidence-based theories and models of behavior change. To this end, this section provides an overview of several widely used theories/models applied to physical activity behavior, reviews evidence from the literature with summaries of the research in the physical activity domain, offers a step-by-step description of how to use the theory in practice, and presents example scenarios for illustration.

SELF-EFFICACY THEORY

CONCEPT OVERVIEW

WHAT IT IS AND WHY IT WORKS

Self-efficacy is a person's situation-specific belief in his or her capabilities to perform a behavior (7,8). Whether you realize it or not, self-efficacy influences just about every choice you make—from deciding to drive a car on a freeway to choosing to walk or jog today. Self-efficacy beliefs determine how you think, feel, and behave (7). A belief that you have the capability to successfully carry out any or all of the activities that you have thought about today will influence your decision to do or not do these actions. Also, the amount of effort you invest in these activities will be influenced by the value of the belief. If you have a weak belief in your personal capability to carry out a behavior successfully (*i.e.,* low self-efficacy), you will be uncertain and likely not invest much effort. On the other hand, if you have a strong belief in your ability to do a specific task (*i.e.,* high self-efficacy), you will undertake it with confidence and conviction. A strong sense of efficacy enhances personal well-being and facilitates motivation and effort. Higher assurances in your personal abilities also lead you to approach difficult tasks as challenges to be mastered rather than threats to be avoided (7).

Self-efficacy is an integrated component of Social Cognitive Theory (8) and stems from the assumption of Social Learning Theory (46) that if you are motivated to learn a behavior, the behavior would be learned by observation and reinforced with positive reinforcement. Self-efficacy is thought to be influenced by several main sources (see Figure 1.1). The first and most important source is *mastery (performance) experience*. When you successfully carry out a task, you believe that you have the capabilities necessary to repeat the behavior. Past successes have the most important influence on self-efficacy and confidence in doing a behavior in the future. However, self-efficacy is fragile and therefore, your past failures can also undermine your efficacy beliefs.

Another source of self-efficacy is *vicarious experience* or observational learning. The behaviors of others (both successes and failures) can influence your self-efficacy. That is, observing a friend or family member achieve success on a similar task can increase self-efficacy, whereas watching him/her fail in a similar circumstance can diminish it.

A third but weaker source of self-efficacy is *verbal persuasion*. When you receive verbal praises such as "Great job!" or "Keep going. You can do it!" from important others

continued

(friends, family members, coaches/trainers), these praises generally have an immediate increase in efficacy beliefs. In contrast, negative comments can damage or weaken efficacy beliefs—particularly under circumstances when there is already doubt about your abilities. Generally, verbal persuasion has its greatest impact on self-efficacy if you have some reason to believe that you could be successful if you persist.

Your *physiological state* can also impact self-efficacy. Factors such as rapid heart rate, elevated respiratory rate, and increased sweating can provide a signal or cue to you about your current level of self-efficacy. Your appraisal of the situation and these physiological cues is critical. When you are calm and confident, these physiological cues are generally interpreted as being a part of the activity and are usually in control. In contrast, if you interpret these physical signals as evidence of not being prepared, they can serve to undermine efficacy and make you question your abilities.

A final source, *emotional (mood) states*, influences self-efficacy because of the association between your past successes and failures and the moods associated with these events. When you are successful, these experiences are stored in memory along with positive feelings (*e.g.*, accomplishment, pride) that are associated with the event. However, failed experiences are also stored in memory and linked with negative feelings (*e.g.*, frustration, shame). Mood states before a future event can trigger events from memory and thus, the presence of a positive mood state prior to an action can prime memories of accomplishment and joy and thereby serve to improve self-efficacy.

Because self-efficacy is a situation-specific construct, different operational definitions have evolved over time. The following concepts are aspects of self-efficacy that have evolved in the research (45) as key factors related to physical activity behaviors:

- **Exercise efficacy:** Beliefs about your ability to successfully engage in incremental bouts of physical activity—varying across mode, intensity, and duration of the activity.
- **Barriers efficacy:** Belief about overcoming obstacles or barriers to physical activity participation. Barriers can be social (lack of spousal support), personal (lack of motivation, feeling lazy), and/or environmental (bad weather, unsafe neighborhood).
- **Scheduling efficacy:** Confidence in your ability to plan physical activity behaviors into a daily or weekly routine.
- **Health-behavior efficacy:** Beliefs about your capability to engage in health-promoting behaviors such as meeting the physical activity guidelines.

EVIDENCE

As mentioned earlier, the strongest source of self-efficacy is mastery (performance) experiences. It is thus not surprising that the relationship between self-efficacy and physical activity participation is reciprocal. That is, efficacy beliefs are associated with the initiation and maintenance of physical activity and in turn, short- and long-term physical activity participation leads to significant increases in self-efficacy (44). Studies have confirmed the important role of self-efficacy for exercise promotion. For example, a review of 27 self-efficacy and exercise studies revealed a positive relationship between self-efficacy and

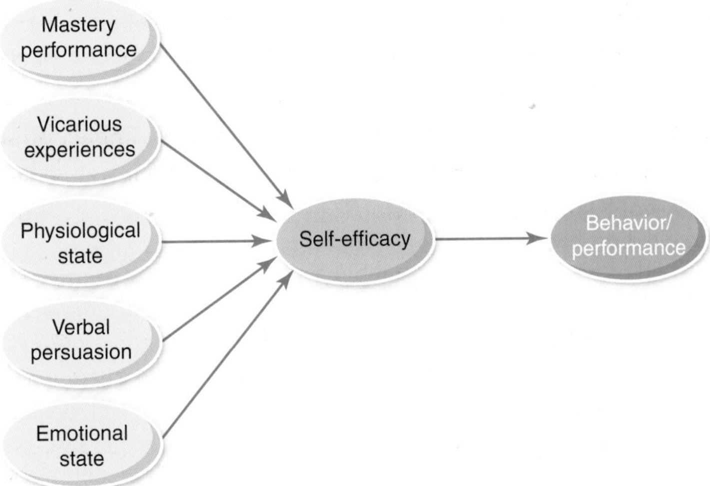

FIGURE 1.1. The Self-Efficacy Theory. (Adapted with permission from Bandura A. *Social foundations of thought and action.* Englewood Cliffs (NJ): Prentice Hall: 1986.)

exercise participation, and specifically among intervention studies, participation in an exercise program promoted exercise self-efficacy beliefs (35). The positive effects of self-efficacy on exercise participation appear to extend across a variety of populations including cardiac rehabilitation patients (64), people with developmental disabilities (11), adolescents with elevated diabetes and obesity risk factors (22), cancer survivors (47), and new mothers (23). Although there is an abundance of evidence that improving self-efficacy beliefs can promote physical activity behaviors, the important question is "How?" The next section provides a step-by-step description of how to apply self-efficacy theory to promote physical activity behaviors.

STEP-BY-STEP: HOW TO APPLY SELF-EFFICACY THEORY TO PHYSICAL ACTIVITY BEHAVIORS

Edward McAuley (43), an authority on the correlates of self-efficacy in physical activity, stated: "It is vitally important for practitioners and programs to provide experiences that maximize individuals' beliefs in their sense of personal capabilities with respect to exercise and physical activity. If practitioners fail to [do so], participants are likely to perceive the activity negatively, become disenchanted and discouraged, and discontinue." Thus, he proposed a series of strategies within each of the main sources to promote self-efficacy:

Step 1: Mastery Experiences

Set up the opportunity for mastery experiences by increasing the frequency of positive physical activity experiences. For example, gradually increase the frequency and intensity of the activity—do not start out with the maximum dosage from the start (*e.g.,* a max fitness test); integrate activities of daily life that provide a sense of accomplishment such as walking to work, taking the stairs instead of the elevator, and parking the car farther from the store; find activities that people enjoy and maximize their chances of engaging in these activities (*e.g.,* joining a community facility, identifying an exercise buddy).

Step 2: Vicarious Experiences

Maximize the exposure to positive modeling experiences. For example, showing videotapes of successful models of similar age, gender, physical characteristics, and capabilities; providing frequent participation in modeling or expert demonstrations to learn the activity form, improve the sense of comfort or ease with the activity, and repeat the actions; and facilitating group activities in a supportive and cooperative environment to increase peer-to-peer modeling.

Step 3: Verbal Persuasion

Augment opportunities for feedback with positive and encouraging feedback. For example, developing social support networks and "buddy systems" to provide multiple opportunities for encouragement, providing a telephone number for a contact person to provide emotional support and assist with overcoming barriers, tapping into social media (*e.g.,* Facebook, Twitter, online support groups), and using video/audio tape recordings or Internet podcasts of positive feedback received from supportive others (personnel, family, friends).

Step 4: Physiological States

Facilitate learning experiences to understand and interpret physical symptoms. For example, teach people how to accurately and positively infer symptoms such as heart rate, respiratory rate, perspiration, muscle soreness, weight changes, and general fatigue; explain how these symptoms are also positive cues for effective exercise participation.

Step 5: Emotional States

Increase opportunities to discuss emotions and maximize opportunities for positive emotional states prior to exercise participation. For example, provide supportive communication about feelings, thoughts, and moods as they relate to physical activity participation; use strategies such as positive imagery and muscle relaxation to promote feelings of calmness, control, and happiness prior to physical activity participation; assist a person with "making the connection" between positive mood states and positive physical activity experiences (*i.e.,* feeling better before exercise leads to feeling better during and after exercise).

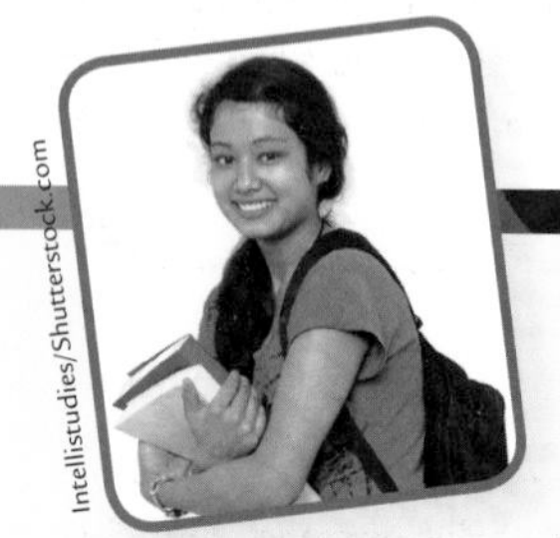
Intellistudies/Shutterstock.com

Case Scenario 1.1

Julie is entering her senior year of high school and about to begin preseason for her last year of high school soccer. Julie has been the team's star midfielder leading the team in goals and helping carry the team to the state playoffs. Julie is optimistic about the team this year; however, she is lacking the self-efficacy to perform well due to an anterior cruciate ligament (ACL) tear that occurred during the winter indoor soccer season. She was forced to have surgery to repair the ACL and missed out on the rest of her indoor soccer season and all of the elite spring traveling team that she usually played on due to the rehab therapy she was required to do. She is afraid that if she puts forth all of her efforts as she has done in the past, she might re-tear her ACL since the doctor told her that re-tears are more likely after an initial tear. She is also worried that the knee brace she must wear will inhibit her range of motion and that she won't be able to perform at the level she once did. She has dreams of playing collegiate soccer but fears these things might ruin her goal of playing soccer in college.

In order to help Julie, a practitioner should consider the following strategies:

1. **Past performance accomplishments:** Have Julie make a list of her accomplishments (particularly those she has achieved in the sport of soccer) and also include the barriers and challenges she experienced along the way so she can relate to those times and remember how she handled those challenges and what she did to overcome them.

Case Scenario 1.1 *continued*

2. **Vicarious experiences:** Show Julie pictures of videos of other elite athletes with a former ACL repair surgery so she can see that it is possible to still perform well after surgery.
3. **Verbal persuasion:** Enlist the help of her family, teammates, and coaches to provide a positive and supportive environment for her so she continues to gain confidence. These individuals should not focus on the fact that she is just recovering from a serious injury (*i.e.*, "Wow, you're really playing great considering the injury you just had" or her coach going easier on her due to her injury), but rather, they should treat her the same as before so that she doesn't feel isolated as a result of her injury.
4. **Physiological and affective states:** Julie needs to be taught to learn to listen to her body. She needs to start slowly. If her knee starts to feel sore, she may need to reduce her training or cut back on intensity or duration. The more in tune she is with her body, the less likely she will be to reinjure herself. She also should maximize opportunities for positive mood states prior to her training (*e.g.*, listening to music to get her excited, using imagery to visualize doing the activities correctly as she rehabilitates her knee, etc.).

TAKE-HOME MESSAGES

Self-efficacy is a powerful belief that you are capable of organizing and executing the behavior that is needed to produce a specific outcome. Self-efficacy is influenced by a variety of factors that include mastery (performance) experiences, vicarious experiences, verbal persuasion, physiological states, and emotional states. Specific to physical activity behaviors, self-efficacy plays an important role. When you are more efficacious, you are more likely to sustain motivation, participation, and adherence, and you are also more likely to report more positive and less negative effects after physical activity participation. As a result, you also enjoy physical activity more! Finally, efficacy beliefs are driven by the individual; therefore, understanding your sources of efficacy is essential for promoting positive efficacy beliefs.

TRANSTHEORETICAL MODEL

Note: This theory is presented here for chapter completeness. A more comprehensive approach for using this theory is presented in Chapter 4.

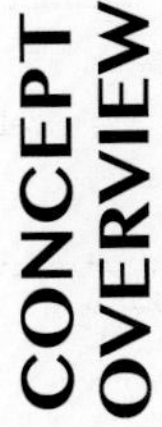

WHAT IT IS AND WHY IT WORKS

For most people, changing unhealthy behaviors (*e.g.*, physically inactive) to healthy behaviors (*e.g.*, physically active) is often challenging. Change usually does not occur all at once; it is a lengthy process that involves progressing through several stages. At each stage, your cognitions and behaviors are different, and so one approach to facilitating behavioral change is not appropriate. The concept of stages—or a "one size does not fit all" philosophy (39)—forms the basis for the Transtheoretical Model (TTM) of behavior change developed by James Prochaska and his colleagues (53).

continued

This model emerged from a comparative analysis of leading theories of psychotherapy and behavior change (56). The TTM includes the following four constructs:

1. stages of change
2. decisional balance
3. processes of change
4. self-efficacy

Each of these constructs is described briefly below and in detail in Chapter 4.

STAGES OF CHANGE

Stages of Change recognizes that behavior change unfolds slowly over time through a series of stages. Prochaska and DiClemente (54) hypothesized that as you change from an unhealthy to a healthy behavior—for example, from a sedentary to an active lifestyle—you move through a number of stages at varying rates and in a cyclical fashion with periods of progression and relapse. If you are sedentary, you may begin to think about the benefits (*e.g.*, more energy) and costs (*e.g.*, time away from watching television) of physical activity. Then, a few months later, you may buy a pair of walking shoes. Six months later, you may start walking 3 times a week. After a year of walking, however, you may become overwhelmed with the stress of work and stop it altogether. The cessation of physical activity would represent a regression to an earlier stage (*i.e.*, relapse). In short, as you go through the process of behavioral change, you typically cycle, or progress and relapse, as you recognize the need to change, contemplate making a change, make the change, and finally, sustain the new behavior. There are five main stages through which you pass in attempting any health behavior change: precontemplation, contemplation, preparation, action, and maintenance (57). Figure 1.2 provides a graphic illustration of the stages of change. A brief description of each stage is provided next. For a more comprehensive description, see Chapter 4.

Precontemplation ("I won't or I can't")

If you are in the precontemplation stage, you are either not considering or do not want to change your behavior. The so-called "couch potato" is an example of someone who would fall into the precontemplation stage for physical activity. As adopting physical activity is concerned, you may be in precontemplation because you do not think it's valuable, or think

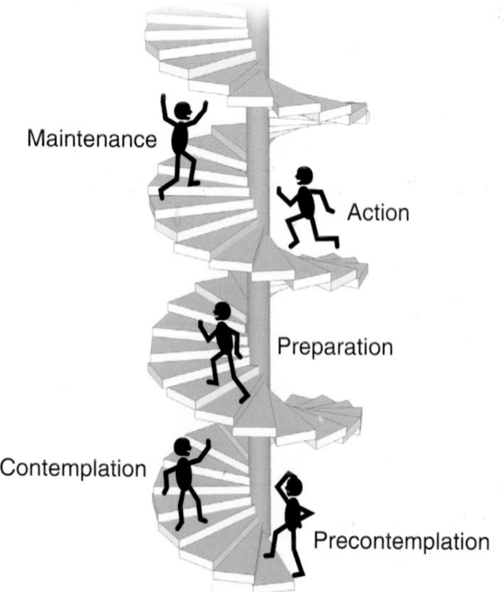

FIGURE 1.2. The Stages of Change Model.

it's valuable but may be overwhelmed by barriers such as lack of time. Precontemplators are the most difficult people to stimulate into behavioral change. They often think that change is not even a possibility.

Contemplation ("I might")

If you are in the contemplation stage, you acknowledge that you have a problem (*e.g.*, "I know I need to be more physically active") and are thinking about changing your behavior sometime within the next 6 months. You see a need for change because you are aware of the costs and benefits of changing your behavior (55).

Preparation ("I will")

In the preparation stage, you are planning to change your activity level in the near future, usually within the next month. Preparation is an unstable stage because when you are in this stage, you are more likely than precontemplators or contemplators to progress over the next 6 months (55).

Action ("I am")

When you have recently changed your behavior (*i.e.*, within the last 6 months), you are in the action stage. This is the stage that requires the greatest commitment of time and energy. Because you have just recently established the new habit, attentiveness is necessary to avoid relapse (*i.e.*, reduce or stopping physical activity).

Maintenance ("I have")

Once you have been regularly active for 6 consecutive months, you are deemed to have made it to the maintenance stage. Although the new behavior has become better established, boredom and a loss of focus can become a danger for inactivity. It is at this time that you work to reinforce the gains made through the various stages of change and strive to prevent a relapse.

DECISIONAL BALANCE

Decisional balance assesses the importance that you place on the potential advantages or *pros* and disadvantages or *cons* of a behavior (31). The balance between the pros and cons varies depending on which stage of change you are in. When the cons of exercise (*e.g.*, takes time away from other activities) are of greater importance than the pros of exercise (*e.g.*, improves psychological well-being), motivation to change behavior (*i.e.*, move from being sedentary to engaging in physical activity) is low. Thus, for example, in the precontemplation and contemplation stages, the cons are assumed to outweigh the pros. In the preparation stage, the pros and cons are believed to be relatively equal. Finally, in the action and maintenance stages, the pros are thought to outweigh the cons.

PROCESSES OF CHANGE

Processes of Change are the 10 processes of change that represent the behaviors, cognitions, and emotions that people engage in to change a behavior. They are defined in more detail in Chapter 4 and include:

- **Consciousness Raising** (gathering information)
- **Counterconditioning** (making substitutions)
- **Dramatic Relief** (being moved emotionally)
- **Environmental Reevaluation** (being a role model)
- **Helping Relationships** (getting social support)
- **Reinforcement Management** (being rewarded)
- **Self-Liberation** (making a commitment)
- **Self-Reevaluation** (developing a healthy self-image)
- **Social-Liberation** (taking advantage of social mores)
- **Stimulus Control** (using cues)

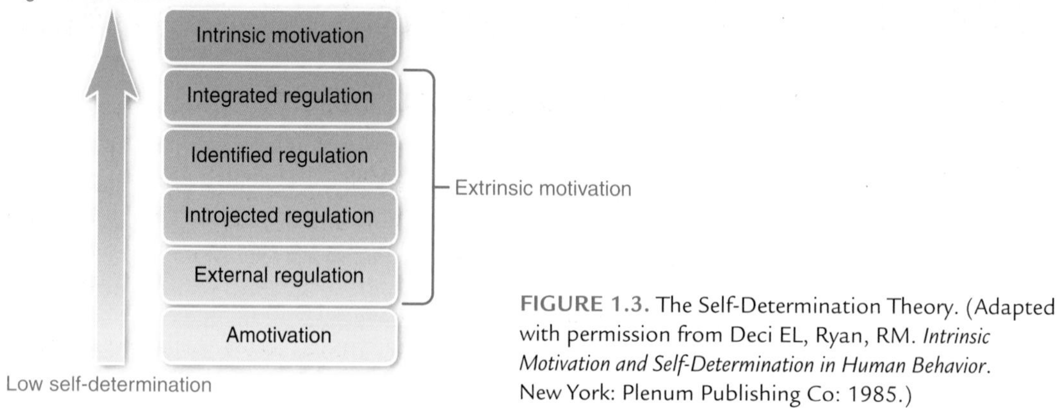

FIGURE 1.3. The Self-Determination Theory. (Adapted with permission from Deci EL, Ryan, RM. *Intrinsic Motivation and Self-Determination in Human Behavior*. New York: Plenum Publishing Co: 1985.)

Self-efficacy, as previously mentioned in this chapter, is a judgment regarding your ability to perform a behavior required to achieve a certain outcome. Not surprisingly, it is critical to behavior change (8) and has been incorporated into the TTM. According to the TTM, self-efficacy is proposed to change with each stage, presumably increasing as you gain confidence, through for example, successful attempts to increase physical activity. Conversely, self-efficacy may decrease if you falter and spiral back to an earlier stage. See Figure 1.3 for a graphical display of the TTM constructs.

EVIDENCE

The TTM was first applied to physical activity in the late 1980s by Sonstroem (63) and since then its popularity has grown dramatically. Marshall and Biddle (41) conducted a meta-analysis of 91 independent samples from 71 published studies that examined at least one of the aforementioned constructs of the TTM applied to physical activity. They found the processes of change, self-efficacy, and decisional balance differed across the stages in the direction predicted by the model. They also noted that stage membership is associated with different levels of physical activity, self-efficacy, pros and cons, and processes of change. More recently, Hutchinson, Breckson, and Johnston (30) reviewed the TTM-based interventions for physical activity behavior change and found that most of the interventions failed to accurately represent all dimensions of the model. They concluded that to examine efficacy of the model, practitioners should develop physical activity interventions that accurately represent all the TTM model constructs (*i.e.*, stages of change, self-efficacy, decisional balance, and processes of change).

STEP-BY-STEP: HOW TO APPLY THE TRANSTHEORETICAL MODEL TO PHYSICAL ACTIVITY BEHAVIORS

To successfully apply the TTM to physical activity, you must first determine the person's stage of change. See From the Practical Toolbox 1.1 for a stage of change questionnaire that you can use to determine a person's stage of change. Once you know a person's stage of change you can then target the remaining TTM constructs (*i.e.*, the process of change, self-efficacy, and decisional balance; see From the Practical Toolbox 1.2 through 1.4 for questionnaires that assess these TTM constructs) in an attempt to change physical activity intentions and/or behavior, with the ultimate goal of moving a person forward along the stage of change continuum.

For *decisional balance*, you can tell if people are moving forward through the stages by looking for differences in the number of pros versus cons they list for exercise. For example, in the precontemplation stage, the cons of exercising will far outweigh the pros. Carlos DiClemente and his colleagues (25) noted that assessing the pros and cons is relevant for understanding and predicting transitions among the first three stages of change (*i.e.*, precontemplation,

From the Practical Toolbox 1.1

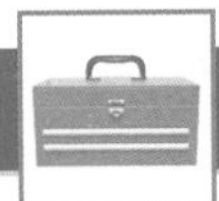

EXAMPLE OF A STAGES OF CHANGE QUESTIONNAIRE

For Exercise

The following five statements will assess how much you currently exercise in your leisure time (exercise done outside of a job). *Regular exercise* is any *planned* physical activity (*e.g.*, brisk walking, jogging, bicycling, swimming, line-dancing, tennis etc.) performed to increase physical fitness. Such activity should be performed *three or more times* per week for *20 or more minutes* per session at a level that increases your breathing rate and causes you to break a sweat (6).

Do you exercise regularly according to the definition above? **Please mark only ONE of the five statements.**

1. _____ No, and I do not intend to begin exercising regularly in the next 6 months.
2. _____ No, but I intend to begin exercising regularly in the next 6 months.
3. _____ No, but I intend to begin exercising regularly in the next 30 days.
4. _____ Yes, I have been, but for less than 6 months.
5. _____ Yes, I have been for 6 months or more.

SCORING

Item 1=Precontemplation; Item 2=Contemplation; Item 3=Preparation; Item 4=Action; Item 5=Maintenance

For Physical Activity

The following five statements will assess how much you currently engage in **regular physical activity** in your leisure time. For physical activity to be regular it must be done for *30 minutes* (or more) per day, and be done *at least* 5 days per week (67). For example, you could take three 10-minute brisk walks or ride a bicycle for 30 minutes. Physical activity includes such activities as walking briskly, biking, swimming, line dancing, and aerobics classes or any other activities where the exertion is similar to these activities. Your heart rate and/or breathing should increase, but there is no need to exhaust yourself.

Do you regularly engage in physical activity according to the definition above? **Please mark only ONE of the five statements.**

1. _____ No, and I do not intend to begin regularly engaging in physical activity in the next 6 months.
2. _____ No, but I intend to begin regularly engaging in physical activity in the next 6 months.
3. _____ No, but I intend to begin regularly engaging in physical activity in the next 30 days.
4. _____ Yes, I have been, but for less than 6 months.
5. _____ Yes, I have been for 6 months or more.

SCORING

Item 1=Precontemplation; Item 2=Contemplation; Item 3=Preparation; Item 4=Action; Item 5=Maintenance

Questionnaire for exercise: Reprinted with permission from the following source; questionnaire for physical activity: Adapted with permission from the following source:

Nigg CR and Riebe D. The Transtheoretical Model: Research review of exercise behavior and older adults. In: Burbank P and Riebe D, editors. *Promoting Exercise and Behavior Change in Older Adults: Interventions with the Transtheoretical Model.* Springer Publishing Company; 2002, p. 147–80.

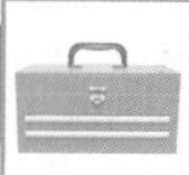

From the Practical Toolbox 1.2

PROCESSES OF CHANGE SCALE

The following experiences can affect the exercise habits of some people. Think of similar experiences you may be currently having or have had *during the past month*. Then rate how frequently the event occurs by circling the appropriate number. Please answer using the following 5-point scale:

1	2	3	4	5
Never	Seldom	Occasionally	Often	Repeatedly

1. I read articles to learn more about exercise.	1	2	3	4	5
2. I get upset when I see people who would benefit from exercise but choose not to exercise.	1	2	3	4	5
3. I realize that if I don't exercise regularly, I may get ill and be a burden to others.	1	2	3	4	5
4. I feel more confident when I exercise regularly.	1	2	3	4	5
5. I have noticed that many people know that exercise is good for them.	1	2	3	4	5
6. When I feel tired, I make myself exercise anyway because I know I will feel better afterward.	1	2	3	4	5
7. I have a friend who encourages me to exercise when I don't feel up to it.	1	2	3	4	5
8. One of the rewards of regular exercise is that it improves my mood.	1	2	3	4	5
9. I tell myself that I can keep exercising if I try hard enough.	1	2	3	4	5
10. I keep a set of exercise clothes with me so I can exercise whenever I get the time.	1	2	3	4	5
11. I look for information related to exercise.	1	2	3	4	5
12. I am afraid of the results to my health if I do not exercise.	1	2	3	4	5
13. I think that by exercising regularly I will not be a burden to the health care system.	1	2	3	4	5
14. I believe that regular exercise will make me a healthier, happier person.	1	2	3	4	5
15. I am aware of more and more people who are making exercise a part of their lives.	1	2	3	4	5
16. Instead of taking a nap after work, I exercise.	1	2	3	4	5
17. I have someone who encourages me to exercise.	1	2	3	4	5
18. I try to think of exercise as a time to clear my mind as well as a workout for my body.	1	2	3	4	5

From the Practical Toolbox 1.2 *continued*

19. I make commitments to exercise.	1	2	3	4	5
20. I use my calendar to schedule my exercise time.	1	2	3	4	5
21. I find out about new methods of exercising.	1	2	3	4	5
22. I get upset when I realize that people I love would have better health if they exercised.	1	2	3	4	5
23. I think that regular exercise plays a role in reducing health care costs.	1	2	3	4	5
24. I feel better about myself when I exercise.	1	2	3	4	5
25. I notice that famous people often say that they exercise regularly.	1	2	3	4	5
26. Instead of relaxing by watching TV or eating, I take a walk or exercise.	1	2	3	4	5
27. My friends encourage me to exercise.	1	2	3	4	5
28. If I engage in regular exercise, I find that I get the benefit of having more energy.	1	2	3	4	5
29. I believe that I can exercise regularly.	1	2	3	4	5
30. I make sure I always have a clean set of exercise clothes.	1	2	3	4	5

SCORING

Consciousness Raising – 1, 11, 21
Dramatic Relief – 2, 12, 22
Environmental Reevaluation – 3, 13, 23
Self-Reevaluation – 4, 14, 24
Social Liberation – 5, 15, 25
Counterconditioning – 6, 16, 26
Helping Relationships – 7, 17, 27
Reinforcement Management – 8, 18, 28
Self-Liberation – 9, 19, 29
Stimulus Control – 10, 20, 30

Reprinted with permission from Nigg CR and Riebe D. The Transtheoretical Model: Research review of exercise behavior and older adults. In: Burbank P and Riebe D, editors. *Promoting Exercise and Behavior Change in Older Adults: Interventions with the Transtheoretical Model.* Springer Publishing Company; 2002, p. 147–80.

contemplation, and preparation). During the action and maintenance stages, however, these decisional balance measures are much less important predictors of progress.

For *self-efficacy*, remember that your self-efficacy for exercise will increase as you progress along the stage of change continuum. Please refer to the section early on step-by-step procedures for targeting self-efficacy to give people the confidence that they can make and maintain changes in their exercise behavior.

Finally, the *process of change* enables you to understand *how* shifts in intentions and behavior occur. As previously mentioned, there are 10 processes of change that represent the behaviors, cognitions, and emotions that you engage in during the course of changing behavior. To progress through the early stages (*i.e.*, precontemplation, contemplation, and preparation), you apply cognitive, affective, and evaluative processes. As you move toward maintenance, you rely more on commitments, conditioning, contingencies, environmental controls, and support. Different strategies are most effective at different stages of change. For example, counterconditioning and stimulus control can really help you in the action and maintenance stages. But these processes are not helpful for someone who is not intending

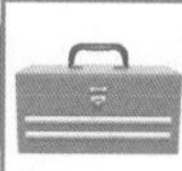

From the Practical Toolbox 1.3

SELF-EFFICACY/CONFIDENCE SCALE

This part looks at how confident you are to exercise when other things get in the way. Read the following items and fill in the circle that best expresses how each item relates to you in your leisure time. Please answer using the following 5-point scale:

1	2	3	4	5
Not at all confident	Somewhat confident	Moderately confident	Very confident	Completely confident

I am confident I can participate in regular exercise when:

1. It is raining or snowing or icy.	1	2	3	4	5
2. I am under a lot of stress.	1	2	3	4	5
3. I feel I don't have the time.	1	2	3	4	5
4. I have to exercise alone.	1	2	3	4	5
5. I don't have access to a place for exercise.	1	2	3	4	5
6. I am spending time with friends.	1	2	3	4	5

SCORING

All 6 items are a general self-efficacy scale representing the six factors. The long form (3 items per factor) may be obtained from the editor.

Reprinted with permission from Nigg CR and Riebe D. The Transtheoretical Model: Research review of exercise behavior and older adults. In: Burbank P and Riebe D, editors. *Promoting Exercise and Behavior Change in Older Adults: Interventions with the Transtheoretical Model.* Springer Publishing Company; 2002, p. 147–80.

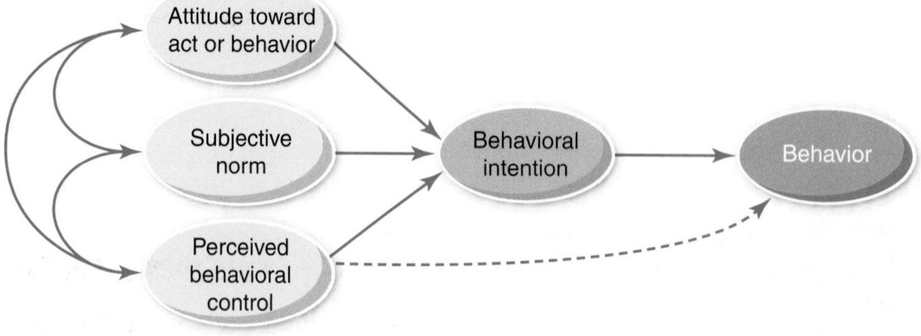

FIGURE 1.4. The Theory of Planned Behavior. (Adapted with permission from Ajzen I. The theory of planned behavior. *Organ Behav Hum Decis Process.* 1991;50:179–211.)

to take action. As another example, consciousness-raising and dramatic relief work better for someone in this stage than in the precontemplation stage.

See Figure 1.4 for a representation of how the TTM constructs work to change people's intentions and behavior.

From the Practical Toolbox 1.4

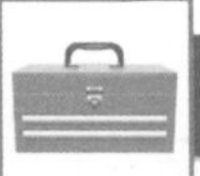

DECISIONAL BALANCE SCALE

This section looks at positive and negative aspects of exercise. Read the following items and indicate how important each statement is with respect to your decision to exercise or not to exercise in your leisure time by filling in the appropriate circle. Please answer using the following 5-point scale:

1	2	3	4	5
Not at all important	Somewhat important	Moderately important	Very important	Extremely important

1. I would have more energy for my family and friends if I exercised regularly.	1	2	3	4	5
2. I would feel embarrassed if people saw me exercising.	1	2	3	4	5
3. I would feel less stressed if I exercised regularly.	1	2	3	4	5
4. Exercise prevents me from spending time with my friends.	1	2	3	4	5
5. Exercising puts me in a better mood for the rest of the day.	1	2	3	4	5
6. I feel uncomfortable or embarrassed in exercise clothes.	1	2	3	4	5
7. I would feel more comfortable with my body if I exercised regularly.	1	2	3	4	5
8. There is too much I would have to learn to exercise.	1	2	3	4	5
9. Regular exercise would help me have a more positive outlook on life.	1	2	3	4	5
10. Exercise puts an extra burden on my significant other.	1	2	3	4	5

SCORING

PROS – 1, 3, 5, 7, 9 CONS – 2, 4, 6, 8, 10

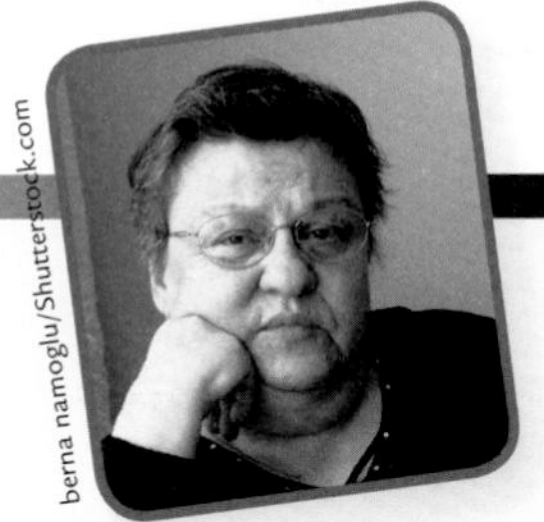

berna namoglu/Shutterstock.com

Case Scenario 1.2

Carla is a 60-year-old couch potato who is overweight. Her doctor recently diagnosed her as prediabetic and has encouraged her to start exercising. She denies having a problem and has no intention of making a change in her physical activity in the next 6 months. Carla also has a lack of motivation to become physically active and has many "excuses" for not being physically active. She does not think that physical activity is valuable in being able to help her lose her excess weight and other related health issues. She feels overwhelmed by barriers such

continued

Case Scenario 1.2 *continued*

as lack of time and lack of knowledge on how to be physically active, and she strongly feels that being physically active is impossible for her.

To help Carla, a practitioner should consider the following:

- **Stage of change:** First, determine the stage of change Carla is in. Because Carla has no intention of beginning an exercise program in the foreseeable future, she is in the precontemplation stage. Knowing her stage of change will enable a practitioner to develop a physical activity intervention that is tailored to that person's stage of change. .
- **Decisional balance:** Have Carla list her pros and cons of exercising. You want to make her more aware of the multiple benefits of changing from a sedentary to an active lifestyle. Emphasize the pros of exercising over the cons.
- **Processes of change:** Use the processes of change of dramatic relief, consciousness raising, and helping relationships to move Carla from the precontemplation to the contemplation stage. In order to do this, you can help Carla gather information about the health benefits of being physically active and how it can help her lose weight and reduce her likelihood of developing diabetes (*i.e.,* consciousness raising). You can also have Carla express her feelings about being sedentary and overweight. Finally, have Carla assess how her inactivity affects her friends and family. For example, Carla is not able to actively play with her grandchildren because she does not have the energy to do so. Also, she is not able to go for nightly walks with her husband. Educating Carla about her inactivity is critical in helping her to start thinking about becoming more active.

TAKE-HOME MESSAGES

Over the past few decades, the TTM has been increasingly applied to examine physical activity behavior. The core constructs of the TTM are the stages of change, processes of change, decisional balance, and self-efficacy.

The most frequently examined construct of the TTM in the physical activity domain has been the stages of change construct. The stages of change assesses your progression and regression through five main stages as you attempt to become physically active: precontemplation (not intending to make changes), contemplation (intending to make changes in the foreseeable future), preparation (immediate intention to change), action (actively engaging in the new behavior), and maintenance (sustaining change over time).

The processes of change are the overt and covert activities that individuals use to alter their experiences and environments to modify behavior change. Decisional balance focuses on the benefits (pros) and costs (cons) of a behavior, and is thought to be important in the decision-making process. Finally, self-efficacy is a judgment regarding one's ability to perform a behavior required to achieve a certain outcome. It is important to apply all the applicable TTM constructs (*i.e.,* processes of change, self-efficacy, decisional balance) when attempting to change people's physical activity motivation and behavior.

SELF-DETERMINATION THEORY

Note: This theory is presented here for chapter completeness. A more comprehensive approach for using this theory is presented in Chapter 5.

CONCEPT OVERVIEW

WHAT IT IS AND WHY IT WORKS

Self-Determination Theory (SDT) (24) is a practical theory that was developed to explain affective, cognitive, and behavioral responses in an achievement domain (*i.e.,* an area that you can set goals to strive for, particularly in terms of competence relevant activities such as academics) and it can be applied to physical activity to understand your motives. SDT is based on the concept that you have three primary psychological needs:

- The need for *competence* (*i.e.,* ability to effectively perform a behavior)
- The need for *relatedness* (*i.e.,* social connections with others)
- The need for *autonomy* (*i.e.,* independence to make own decisions)

As a result, you seek challenges to satisfy at least one of these three basic needs.
SDT also suggests that three types of motivation drive your behaviors (see Figure 1.3):

- **Amotivation:** On one end of the continuum, *amotivation* is the absence of motivation. In terms of exercise behavior, you may show amotivation toward being physically active for a number of reasons, such as a lack of self-discipline to fit exercise into your daily routine or the belief that exercise is not necessary and will not result in a desired outcome (*i.e.,* weight loss).
- **Extrinsic motivation:** Next on the continuum is *extrinsic motivation*, which is often viewed negatively and is not an ideal means of motivating you to perform specific behaviors. However, in terms of exercise behavior, it is important to note that being extrinsically motivated to be physically active is not necessarily a bad thing since exercising to lose weight and improve your health are technically considered to be extrinsic motives, but they are great reasons for you to be physically active. Deci and Ryan (24) described four types of extrinsic motivation:
  - **External regulation:** The least self-determined of these four, this is the process of performing a behavior because of an external reward (*i.e.,* exercising to receive praise from others or monetary compensation) or to avoid punishment (*i.e.,* exercising to avoid being scolded by a significant other).
  - **Introjected regulation:** Describes behavior that is contingent on self-imposed pressures such as exercising to avoid feelings of guilt.
  - **Identified regulation:** Is a more autonomous form of extrinsic motivation driven by your personal goals (*i.e.,* exercising to lose weight or running to train for a 5k).
  - **Integrated regulation:** Is the most self-determined type of extrinsic motivation that includes engaging in a behavior to confirm your sense of self (*i.e.,* I am a cyclist or a runner and this is what I do). However, integrated regulation is still considered extrinsic because the goals you are trying to achieve are for reasons extrinsic to yourself, rather than the inherent enjoyment or interest in the task.

continued

- **Intrinsic motivation:** Is engaging in a behavior for reasons of pleasure, enjoyment, and fun.

SDT examines predictors of physical activity including factors in the environment (*i.e.*, rewards, positive feedback), within the person (*i.e.*, basic psychological needs), and allows for the examination of important psychological outcomes as a result of the physical activity (*i.e.*, perceived competence) (28). SDT provides useful guidelines for practitioners to use for targeting how to motivate people for physical activity.

EVIDENCE

Much of the initial research using SDT within the physical activity domain has been correlational in nature (18). Correlational designs are important for identifying the antecedents of physical activity behavior and the underlying mechanisms that are associated with these antecedents, but such designs are limiting. Therefore, experimental designs are needed to establish causality.

There are limited experimental and interventional studies applying SDT within a physical activity context. Most of the early work was focused on the sports domain (20,21,69); but recently researchers have focused on experimental methods that examine specific constructs of SDT and their effects on exercise behavior. Researchers have demonstrated that manipulations designed at changing self-determined motivation resulted in changes in exercise intentions that furthermore resulted in changes in exercise behavior (19). There have also been recent advances in the development of interventions in applied settings using SDT to increase motivation for physical activity in students (26,70), promote leisure physical activity in sedentary young adults (48), understand physical activity motives in cancer survivors (49) and increase physical activity in overweight women (59–61).

Despite these recent successes, there is still a need for further research examining the role of autonomy-supportive techniques to change self-determined motivation and physical activity behavior (*e.g.*, providing participants with options about intensity, frequency, and type of exercise-related activities; praising participants for improvements in techniques and fitness). Researchers and practitioners should teach these strategies to individuals so they have the tools to engage in physical activity behavior on their own after the intervention has ended. Future research is also needed to better understand the underlying mechanisms that are not only important for initial behavior change, but for long-term adherence to physical activity behavior.

STEP-BY-STEP: HOW TO APPLY SELF-DETERMINATION THEORY TO PHYSICAL ACTIVITY BEHAVIORS

To effectively use SDT to promote physical activity behavior and adherence, Kilpatrick and colleagues (36) developed the following set of guidelines for practitioners:

Step 1: Provide Choice of Activities to Promote Autonomy

Make a conscious effort to involve people in the decision-making process to promote both autonomy and self-determination. For example, giving a person the ability to choose the type of physical activity they enjoy most will promote autonomy while also increasing enjoyment. These are essential steps in "hooking" a person on engaging in physical activity. Also, providing multiple activities to choose from is more likely to lead to increased independence rather than forcing people to do one activity without any other options.

Step 2: Provide a Rationale for Activities

Explain why a person is engaging in physical activity, how the activity has health benefits, and which aspects of fitness will improve as a result of the physical activity. Giving someone a rationale and purpose not only creates a sense of autonomy, but it is also likely to lead to positive perceptions of the activity, which is more likely to foster the development of intrinsic motivation.

Step 3: Provide Positive Feedback so Individuals Gain a Sense of Competence

Positive feedback includes praise as well as constructive criticism for improving a behavior. The type of feedback will vary depending on their skill level. For instance, a highly skilled and experienced exerciser may perceive corrective or instructional feedback as more helpful than positive reinforcement, while a novice exerciser may respond favorably to praise and encouragement. Positive feedback has been shown to foster confidence and competence, which in turn will lead to greater enjoyment of the activity and stronger intrinsic motivation.

Step 4: Promote Process Goals That Are Moderately Difficult

Process goals focus on the tasks necessary to achieve goals—that is, the specific steps for successfully performing a behavior. Practitioners should create an environment based on competence rather than competition against others and encourage individuals to measure their success relative to their own performances rather than comparing to others. Also, setting moderately difficult goals are likely to result in short-term success that can foster competence. If the goals are too difficult, failure may be more likely to occur, which will lead to decreased confidence and motivation for that behavior.

Step 5: Promote the development of social relationships

Adherence is more likely to occur when people build social connections, which in turn leads to greater satisfaction and increases the likelihood of long-term physical activity maintenance.

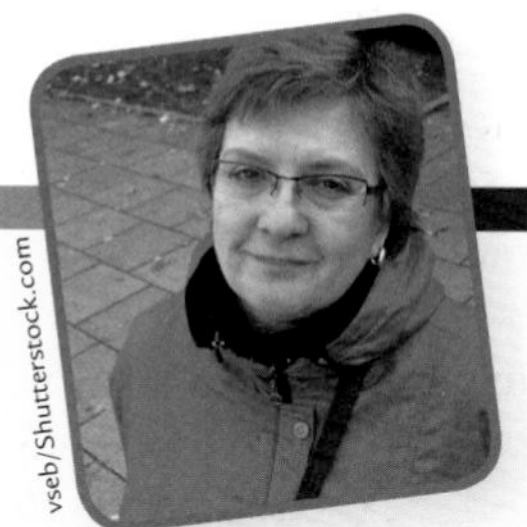
vseb/Shutterstock.com

Case Scenario 1.3

INTROJECTED REGULATION

Susie is in her mid 40s. She has been exercising irregularly for the past year (*i.e.*, goes to the gym 4 or 5 days a week for a month and then not again for another 3 months). Her main motivation for going to the gym or going out for a run is to improve her appearance for different events such as a friend's wedding or a party with friends. She is exhibiting extrinsic motives for being physically active driven by a need to look aesthetically better when she has to see friends or family. As a result, Susie is not adhering to a regular exercise regimen or exercising for inherent pleasure or to improve her overall health.

Susie would benefit from a program that requires her to set moderately difficult goals such as exercising every week, 3 to 5 days a week and not quitting once she sees results that she wants. Susie should pick the activities that she wants to do to promote autonomy and to make sure the activities she is engaging in are enjoyable for her. Also, Susie should set personal goals to achieve (*i.e.*, run a 5k) so that she can experience mastery of these tasks as well as feelings of pride and satisfaction (see From the Practical Toolbox 1.5 for an example goal setting sheet). Finally, Susie should be encouraged to take group fitness classes to promote relatedness and satisfy her need for social interactions.

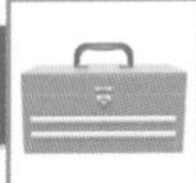

From the Practical Toolbox 1.5

GOAL SETTING AND SELF-DETERMINATION THEORY EXAMPLE

Short-term goal #1	Short-term goal #2	Long-term goal #1	Long-term goal #2
Goal:	**Goal:**	**Goal:**	**Goal:**
When do I want to accomplish this goal by?	When do I want to accomplish this goal by?	When do I want to accomplish this goal by?	When do I want to accomplish this goal by?
How will I work on this?	How will I work on this?	How will I work on this?	How will I work on this?
Where will I work on this?	Where will I work on this?	Where will I work on this?	Where will I work on this?
How realistic is it that I will accomplish this goal?	How realistic is it that I will accomplish this goal?	How realistic is it that I will accomplish this goal?	How realistic is it that I will accomplish this goal?
How difficult is this goal for me to achieve?	How difficult is this goal for me to achieve?	How difficult is this goal for me to achieve?	How difficult is this goal for me to achieve?

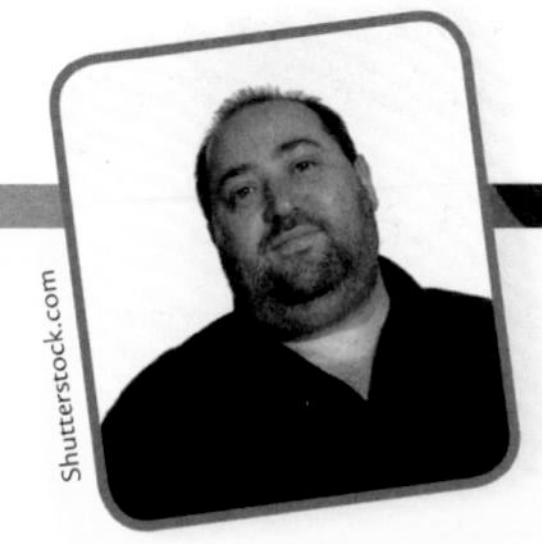
Shutterstock.com

Case Scenario 1.4

AMOTIVATION

Justin was a high school football player who was previously in good physical shape due to team workouts and weightlifting. However, once he entered college, his regular exercise routine stopped and he continued this "no exercise" routine through his 20s. Justin does not see any reason to be physically active now that he is no longer playing football. He lacks any form of discipline or motivation to go to the gym on a regular basis. He knows that he is a few pounds overweight, but does not see any problem with the extra pounds he has gained since high school. He believes he is perfectly healthy and has no need to exercise.

To help Justin, there are several important things a practitioner or interventionist needs to consider. They need to explain to Justin the importance of physical activity for his health. Since Justin is slightly overweight, they should explain the consequences that are likely to occur if he continues to lead a sedentary lifestyle (*i.e.,* development of obesity, metabolic syndrome, heart disease). Justin has no motivation to be physically active; therefore, the goal would be for him to eventually achieve intrinsic motivation toward being active.

A program designed to encourage Justin to develop intrinsic motivation should be aimed at enhancing his sense of competence and autonomy within a positive, supportive environment where social interactions can take place. Justin should be able to choose the types of activities he wishes to engage in so that he has a sense of ownership and control over his workout routine to enhance his sense of autonomy toward exercise. Having choice in the type of activity he does will also make the activity more enjoyable for Justin and increase the likelihood that he continues to be physically active. Also, developing a program that allows Justin to feel successful in mastering his choice of activity will help to develop his feelings of competence. Finally, group exercise may be beneficial in addition to exercising on his own because it fulfills his sense of relatedness and will develop social support toward being active.

As a novice exerciser, Justin would start with simple, low-intensity activities that he can master and thus develop feelings of satisfaction toward being active. It is likely that Justin will first experience extrinsic rewards from being active (*i.e.,* weight loss, improved mood) and hopefully continued exercise behavior will be enjoyable and satisfying, such that Justin develops intrinsic motives for being active. Also, over time, the duration and intensity of his exercise can be increased so that he continues to be challenged and does not get bored with his exercise routine.

Therefore, incorporating all three basic needs (autonomy, competence, and relatedness) are important so that Justin can move from being amotivated to being intrinsically motivated toward exercising. However, it is important to note that it may not be necessary to target all three basic needs when intervening with individuals as it may be too overwhelming for certain individuals. It is important to tailor the intervention design to the individual and target the needs of that individual that will be the most influential in helping them become more intrinsically motivated to be physically active.

TAKE-HOME MESSAGES

SDT specifies that individuals seek behaviors that satisfy three basic needs: competence, autonomy, and relatedness. The theory furthermore indentifies three forms of motivation (amotivation, extrinsic motivation, and intrinsic motivation) that drive individuals' achievement behaviors. Following the recommendations provided in this chapter to target individuals' sense of autonomy and competence, self-determination theory can be easily incorporated into practice to promote and encourage physical activity.

Theory of Planned Behavior

CONCEPT OVERVIEW

WHAT IT IS AND WHY IT WORKS

The Theory of Planned Behavior (TPB) is a theory about the link between your attitudes and behaviors. Ajzen (3) defined behavior in terms of a single action (taking an aerobics class), directed at a specified target (fitness center) in a given context (YMCA community center), and at a specified time (Tuesday nights at 5pm) (27). Ajzen proposed the TPB as an extension of the Theory of Reasoned Action (5). The TPB is one of the most predictive persuasion theories, and it has guided a large majority of the physical activity theory-based research (3). This theory specifies that some or all of the following four main psychological variables influence your behavior (see Figure 1.4):

- **Intention: Intending** to perform a behavior is the main determinant of whether or not you engage in that behavior. Intention is reflected in your willingness and how much effort you are planning to exert to perform the behavior. The stronger your intention to perform a behavior, the more likely you will engage in that behavior. Thus, if you have a strong intent to go biking this afternoon, you are more likely to do it. As might be expected, your intention can weaken over time. The longer the time between intention and behavior, the greater the likelihood that unforeseen events will produce changes in your intention. For example, you may intend to go for a long bike ride on the weekend. However, bad weather may make it difficult to safely take a long ride, and thus, even though you have a strong intent, you will not be able to go for a bike ride. Your intention, or level of motivation, is influenced by your attitude about the behavior, the perceived social pressures to do the behavior (*i.e.,* subjective norm), and the amount of perceived control over performing the behavior (*i.e.,* perceived behavioral control). These are described in more detail in the following.
- **Attitude:** Is your positive or negative evaluation of performing a behavior. For example, an older adult may have a negative attitude toward engaging in a vigorous physical activity such as running, but have a positive attitude toward

walking in the neighborhood. Your attitude toward a specific behavior (whether it be walking or running for example) is a function of your *behavioral beliefs*, which refer to the perceived consequences of carrying out a specific action and your evaluation of each of these consequences. For example, your beliefs about playing doubles tennis could be represented by both positive expectations (*e.g.*, it will improve my social life because I will meet lots of people) and negative expectations (*e.g.*, it will reduce my time with family). In shaping a physical activity behavior, you evaluate the consequences attached to each of these beliefs. Common behavioral beliefs for physical activity are that it improves fitness/health, improves physical appearance, is fun/enjoyable, increases social interactions, and improves psychological health (65).

- **Subjective norm:** Is your perceived social pressure to perform or not perform a particular behavior. Subjective norm is from your *normative beliefs*, which are determined by the perceived expectations of important significant others (*e.g.*, family, friends, physician, priest) or groups (*e.g.*, classmates, teammates, church members) and by your motivation to comply with the expectations of these important significant others. For example, a mother may feel that her pregnant daughter should not exercise during her pregnancy. The daughter, however, may not be motivated to comply with her mother's expectations, and thus she walks regularly throughout her pregnancy.
- **Perceived behavioral control:** Represents your perceived ease or difficulty of performing a behavior. You may hold positive attitudes toward a behavior and believe that important others would approve of your behavior. However, you are not likely to form a strong intention to perform that behavior if you believe you do not have the resources or opportunities to do so (27). For example, you may have a positive attitude and enjoy swimming; however, if you do not have access to a pool, you will not be able to perform this behavior. Perceived behavioral control is a function of *control beliefs,* which represent the perceived presence or absence of required resources and opportunities (*e.g.*, "there is a road race this weekend"), the anticipated obstacles or impediments to behavior (*e.g.*, "the probability of rain on the weekend is 95%"), and the perceived power of a control factor to facilitate or inhibit performance of the behavior (*e.g.*, "even if it rains this weekend, I can still participate in the road race") (4). The most common control beliefs for physical activity are lack of time, lack of energy, and lack of motivation (65).

EVIDENCE

Several statistical reviews have supported the TPB for explaining and predicting a wide variety of physical activities across many populations, such as ethnic minorities, youth, pregnant women, cancer patients, cancer survivors, and older adults, just to name a few (5,12,29,33,34,66). In general, the research has found that intention is the strongest

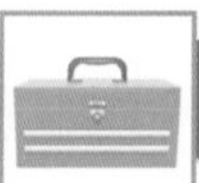

From the Practical Toolbox 1.6

THEORY OF PLANNED BEHAVIOR BELIEF ITEMS

Instructions. The following questions relate to your walking behavior during cancer treatment. List as many that apply to you in the space provided below.

List the main advantages of walking during your cancer treatment ***[behavioral beliefs]***

List the main disadvantages of walking during your cancer treatment ***[behavioral beliefs]***

List the main factors that prevented you from walking during your cancer treatment ***[control beliefs]***

List the main factors that helped you in walking during your cancer treatment ***[control beliefs]***

From the Practical Toolbox 1.6 *continued*

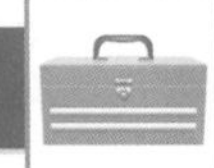

List the individuals or groups who were/are most important to you when you thought/think about walking during your cancer treatment ***[normative beliefs]***

____

____

____

____

____

____

Source: http://people.umass.edu/aizen/tpb.html

determinant of your behavior, followed closely by perceived behavioral control. And your intention to perform a behavior is largely influenced by your attitude and perceived behavioral control, followed by the subjective norm. It is important to note though that the influence of each of the TPB constructs can vary from population and context.

STEP-BY-STEP: HOW TO APPLY THE TPB TO PHYSICAL ACTIVITY

A strength of the TPB is that an *elicitation study* forms the basis for developing questions to assess the TPB constructs in a specific population. The elicitation study enables you to determine the specific beliefs for a specific population. This is very important because beliefs vary by population and even by activity. For example, the main behavioral beliefs for breast cancer survivors are that physical activity "gets my mind off cancer and treatment, makes me feel better and improves my well-being, and helps me maintain a normal lifestyle." In comparison, the main behavior beliefs for pregnant women are that exercise "improves my mood and reduces physical limitations common to pregnancy, such as nausea." Because beliefs vary by population, researchers and practitioners are strongly encouraged to refer to research that has already determined the physical activity beliefs of your specific intervention population (*e.g.,* postpartum women, cancer survivors, high school students). If physical activity beliefs for a practitioner's population of interest have not been determined, then it is recommended that you conduct a pilot study (*i.e.,* known as an elicitation study) to determine the pertinent beliefs concerning a behavior for your specific population. Protocol suggested by Ajzen and Fishbein (65) for conducting elicitation studies include:

- Using open-ended questions to determine the important behavioral, normative, and control beliefs in a small sample of the targeted population (see From the Practical Toolbox 1.6);
- Carrying out a content analysis (*i.e.,* a simple frequency count) to determine which beliefs are most salient; and
- Developing structured items from the content analysis (see From the Practical Toolbox 1.7).

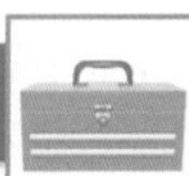

From the Practical Toolbox 1.7

EXAMPLES OF THEORY OF PLANNED BEHAVIOR ITEMS

Note. These items are for pregnant women in their first trimester. Reword to reflect the population you are studying.

Regular exercise behavior is participating in 30 minutes of accumulated moderate exercise on most, if not all, days of the week. This exercise can be done at one time (*e.g.*, 30 minutes of continuous walking or jogging) or accumulated in the day (*e.g.*, walking 10 minutes in the morning and 20 minutes in the evening). Examples of activities often done during pregnancy include walking, aqua-aerobics, and low impact fitness classes.

In this survey, we are interested in your personal opinions regarding regular exercise during the first three months of pregnancy (*i.e.*, your first trimester). Although some of the questions may appear very similar, each addresses a somewhat different issue. Please read each question carefully and reply by circling the number that best reflects your opinion.

1. For me to exercise regularly during my first trimester will be:

Useless						Useful
1	2	3	4	5	6	7

2. For me to exercise regularly during my first trimester will be:

Unenjoyable						Enjoyable
1	2	3	4	5	6	7

3. For me to exercise regularly during my first trimester will be:

Unpleasant						Pleasant
1	2	3	4	5	6	7

4. For me to exercise regularly during my first trimester will be:

Foolish						Wise
1	2	3	4	5	6	7

5. For me to exercise regularly during my first trimester will be:

Boring						Interesting
1	2	3	4	5	6	7

6. For me to exercise regularly during my first trimester will be:

Harmful						Beneficial
1	2	3	4	5	6	7

From the Practical Toolbox 1.7 *continued*

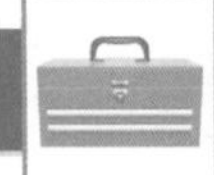

7. For me to exercise regularly during my first trimester will be:

Bad						Good
1	2	3	4	5	6	7

8. Most people who are important to me want me to exercise regularly during my first trimester.

Extremely Likely						Extremely Unlikely
1	2	3	4	5	6	7

9. Most women who are important to me have themselves exercised regularly during their first trimester.

Extremely Likely						Extremely Unlikely
1	2	3	4	5	6	7

10. Most pregnant women will themselves exercise regularly during their first trimester.

Extremely Likely						Extremely Unlikely
1	2	3	4	5	6	7

11. Most people whose opinion I value think that I should exercise regularly during my first trimester.

Extremely Likely						Extremely Unlikely
1	2	3	4	5	6	7

12. Most people I care about would approve of my exercising regularly during my first trimester.

Extremely Likely						Extremely Unlikely
1	2	3	4	5	6	7

13. My doctor or health care provider thinks that I should participate in regular exercise during my first trimester.

Disagree						Agree
1	2	3	4	5	6	7

14. I will exercise regularly during my first trimester.

Definitely Not						Definitely
1	2	3	4	5	6	7

continued

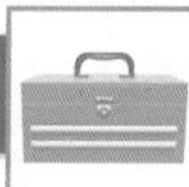

From the Practical Toolbox 1.7 *continued*

15. Whether I exercise regularly during my first trimester is completely up to me.

Disagree						Agree
1	2	3	4	5	6	7

16. Exercising regularly during my first trimester is under my control.

Not at All						Completely
1	2	3	4	5	6	7

17. If I want to, I can easily exercise regularly during my first trimester.

Extremely Likely						Extremely Unlikely
1	2	3	4	5	6	7

18. I intend to exercise regularly during my first trimester.

Definitely False						Definitely True
1	2	3	4	5	6	7

19. I plan to exercise regularly during my first trimester.

Definitely False						Definitely True
1	2	3	4	5	6	7

20. My goal is to exercise regularly during my first trimester.

Definitely False						Definitely True
1	2	3	4	5	6	7

21. I exercised regularly during my first trimester.

Definitely False						Definitely True
1	2	3	4	5	6	7

22. I had the ability to exercising regularly during my first trimester.

Definitely False						Definitely True
1	2	3	4	5	6	7

From the Practical Toolbox 1.7 *continued*

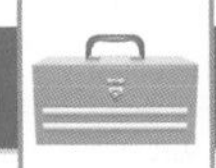

23. For me to exercise regularly during my first trimester is:

Impossible						Possible
1	2	3	4	5	6	7

24. I am determined to exercise regularly during my first trimester.

Definitely Not						Definitely
1	2	3	4	5	6	7

Theory of Planned Behavior Global Items Information

Attitude: Items 1, 2, 3, 4, 5, 6, and 7
Subjective Norm: Items 8, 9, 10, 11, 12, and 13
Perceived Behavioral Control: Items 15, 16, 17, 22, and 23
Intention = Items 14, 18, 19, 20, 24
Behavior = Item 21

Source: http://people.umass.edu/aizen/tpb.html

Ajzen and Fishbein (65) proposed that structured items that arise from the elicitation study should be specific to the target at which the behavior is directed, the action or specificity of the behavior under study, and the context and time in which the behavior is being performed. This means, for example, that when trying to develop a walking intervention for older adults, you should ask a sample of older adults to: "list the main advantages of walking briskly 3 times a week for 30 minutes outside during the summer." This information will help you develop an intervention based on the salient behavioral beliefs of these older adults that is specific to the behavior. According to the TPB, once beliefs are modified, intention will be altered and the desired behavior change will occur (4,66).

The relative contribution of the TPB constructs may fluctuate from context to context. Thus, before interventions using this framework are implemented, the predictive ability of these constructs with the specific population and specific context should first be tested.

The TPB is useful in identifying psychosocial determinants of physical activity, and thus it is useful for developing community and individual exercise programs. For example, exercise programs that offer a positive experience would obviously increase the intention to exercise, which in turn influences exercise behavior. Positive behavioral beliefs and their evaluation may be enhanced if you are given experiences with enjoyable types of physical activities and then are gradually encouraged to increase the intensity, duration, and frequency of those activities. Perceived behavioral control is an important factor in the intention to be physically active (13,51). When you perceive physical activity as difficult to do, intention is low. Overcoming barriers such as lack of time, competing demands and other obligations, and feelings of inability should enhance perceptions of control about carrying out physical activity. The next step in research using the TPB is to determine whether belief-based programs will lead to increased levels of physical activity and to determine whether beliefs about physical activity behavior change as one initiates and continues to engage in physical activity behaviors (52).

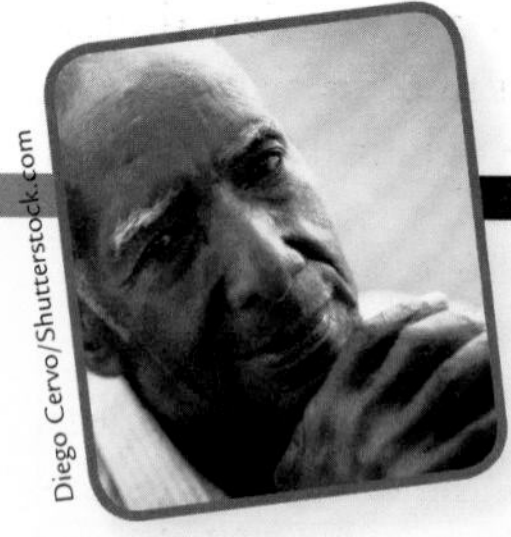
Diego Cervo/Shutterstock.com

Case Scenario 1.5

Bill is a 75-year-old retired school teacher who lives alone and likes to garden and do yard work in the summer months. This keeps him very active because he typically spends about two hours a day outside doing various yard activities from mowing the grass to raking to picking weeds. However, during the colder winter months, Bill tends to become sedentary and retreats to watching television to fill the time that he normally spends doing yard work in the summer. Because of Bill's advancing age and the fact that he lives alone, his doctor is concerned that he is not active enough during the entire year. His doctor wants Bill to maintain a more constant level of physical activity during all months of the year so that he has a high level of functional physical activity to ensure that he can perform day-to-day activities such as getting himself dressed, avoiding falling, and doing household chores.

To help Bill, a practitioner should consider the following:

- **Behavioral beliefs:** Have Bill make a list of activities that he may enjoy doing in the winter as well as the summer.
- **Normative beliefs:** Have Bill establish some winter activities that he can do with friends, such as mall walking. Have him identify friends and family that will support the types of activities he will be doing and make sure they are aware of his goals so they can provide the perceived support he needs.
- **Control beliefs:** Provide Bill with a list of issues that may arise (such as bad weather) that may make it difficult to be active in the winter, and then provide Bill with the skills to overcome these issues. For example, if the weather is too cold or stormy to do activities outside, provide him with activities that he can do inside (*e.g.,* exercise videos, home exercise equipment).
- **Intention:** Provide him with a motivational plan for year-round activities.

TAKE-HOME MESSAGES

Changing your behavior is very difficult to do, especially when you are dealing with a complex health behavior such as physical activity. To increase the success of predicting, understanding, explaining, and changing physical activity behavior, researchers and practitioners should use a theoretical framework such as the TPB as a guide (68). Researchers have found support for the utility of attitude, perceived behavioral control, and to a lesser extent, subjective norm in explaining people's intention to becoming physically active. Also, research has found a strong relationship between your intention to be active and whether you do the behavior. Furthermore, your perception of control over engaging in physical activity can also directly predict behavior. In short, because of the success of the TPB for explaining and predicting physical activity behavior, it offers you a useful framework to guide physical activity interventions.

OTHER THEORIES TO CONSIDER

While a detailed overview of several, frequently used theories and models applied to physical activity behaviors has been provided in this chapter, there are nonetheless other conceptual frameworks that have been used in the exercise domain. While they have been used less frequently than other frameworks, these are important to consider because to date there is no single "exercise theory" that consistently and effectively explains and predicts exercise behavior. In the following, you will find a brief explanation of the Health Belief Model, Relapse Prevention, and the Social Ecological Model.

THE HEALTH BELIEF MODEL

The Health Belief Model (HBM) (32) is one of the most widely recognized conceptual frameworks for health behavior. The main hypothesis is that behavior depends on two conditions: (a) value placed by you on a particular goal and (b) your estimate of the likelihood that a given action will achieve the goal (32). When these two conditions are viewed within the context of health-related behaviors, the focus is either on the desire to avoid illness (or if already ill, to get healthy) or the belief that a specific action will prevent or improve illness. Thus, HBM is most useful as a framework when a chronic disease (*e.g.*, cancer, diabetes, cardiovascular disease) is imminent.

The first component of HBM is *perceived susceptibility*, or your belief that you are personally susceptible to a particular illness (*e.g.*, my chances of developing prostate cancer are high because it runs in the family). *Perceived severity* is your opinion of the seriousness of a condition and its consequences (*e.g.*, cancer is a serious disease that can reduce my quality of life and if not effectively treated, can take my life).

The first four constructs of HBM represent your readiness to take action:

- **Perceived benefits:** Represents your opinion of the efficacy of the advised action to reduce risk or seriousness of impact. For example, whether you believe that engaging in regular physical activity (*e.g.*, 30 minutes of moderate-intensity physical activity a day) can reduce your cancer risk.
- **Perceived barriers:** Are your perceptions of the physical and psychological costs of the advised action. For example, you may believe that physical activity can reduce your cancer risk, but barriers such as inexperience with physical activity, low motivation, lack of time, and physical discomfort (*e.g.*, radiation treatment causes soreness) may reduce or altogether prevent the likelihood that action takes place.
- **Cues to action:** These trigger your readiness to take action and stimulates the actual behavior. Examples of Cues to Action include those that are personal (*e.g.*, breathlessness when walking up stairs or a family member or friend who becomes sick) as well as strategies that provide "how-to" information or instructions on the behavior, promoting awareness about disease risks, and providing reminders or prompts (*e.g.*, phone calls, texts, notes) to initiate the behavior.
- **Self-Efficacy:** This recent addition to the model (for a full description of this construct, see the "Self-Efficacy Theory" section earlier in this chapter), which represents your confidence in your ability to take action. Strategies to increase self-efficacy include training/guided instruction, multiple opportunities for success with the desired behavior, and verbal praise for positive reinforcement.

RELAPSE PREVENTION

Relapse prevention (40) is a cognitive-behavioral approach with the goal of identifying or preventing high-risk situations. This model is most useful as a framework when setbacks (or relapses) are common, particularly with high-risk behaviors such as substance or alcohol abuse, obsessive-compulsive behavior, and depression. Typically these behaviors are high in frequency and undesired—thus, it may seem less applicable to apply this framework to physical activity, which is a desired behavior, yet often of low frequency. Nevertheless, this model can provide some insight regarding the antecedents of exercise cessation—when you reduce or stop exercising altogether.

Marlatt and Gordon (40) identified three primary triggers of relapse (in the case of exercise, exercise cessation):

- Personal conflict
- Negative emotional states
- Social pressures

In particular, negative emotional states (*e.g.*, depression, anger, stress) and social pressures (*e.g.*, increased pressure from school or work colleagues to engage in activities other than exercise) are common predictors of inactivity.

A key to preventing relapse is having effective coping strategies. When coping strategies are strong (*e.g.*, self-awareness, optimistic outlook, supportive family/friends), self-efficacy is higher and you have a reduced chance of relapse (exercise cessation). However, when coping strategies are poor or absent, self-efficacy is low and attributions are negative (*e.g.*, feelings of helplessness, lack of control), and in turn, relapse (or exercise cessation) is likely. Therefore, understanding and identifying effective coping strategies is an effective way to prevent exercise cessation.

THE SOCIAL ECOLOGICAL MODEL

The Social Ecological Model is a framework for understanding multiple levels of influence on behavior. It emphasizes that the individual is responsible for engaging in healthy behaviors, but it also considers that surrounding social and environmental pressures and manipulations are key determinants of taking action.

This approach has several adaptations. The most commonly used in the exercise domain is based on Bronfenbrenner's (15,16) Ecological Systems Theory which divides environmental factors into four main influences. These factors can be illustrated as an "onion" (see Figure 1.5):

- The *individual* is at the center of this system.
- The next layer is the *microsystem*, or the immediate systems in which you interact (*e.g.*, family, school, work environments, parks, gyms, etc.).

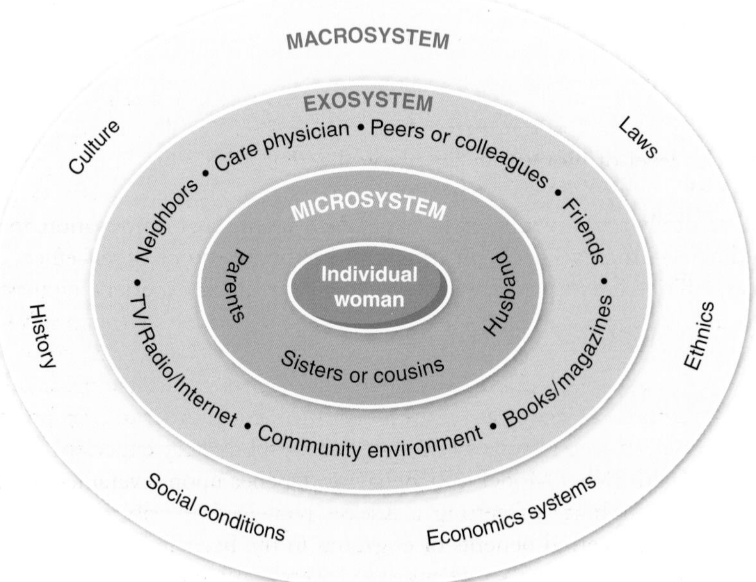

FIGURE 1.5. The Social Ecological Model. (Adapted with permission from Bronfenbrenner U. Toward an experimental ecology of human development. *Am Psychol*. 1977;32:513–31.)

- The *mesosystem*, which is the next level of influence, represents the interaction of multiple individual systems. For example, the influences of parents (home microsystem) and teachers (school microsystem).
- The final two systems represent the most global or broader environmental influences. The *exosystem* represents external systems such as school or community boards, and the *macrosystem* encompasses all other systems (*e.g.*, government, economic, social, etc.).

The closer the system is to the individual, the stronger the direct influence it has on that person's behavior.

The Social Ecological Model is a useful framework for guiding physical activity behavior when the role of the environment plays a key factor in the behavior change. For example, in order for a community to be able to engage in active commuting such as biking or walking to work, there must be good access to bike/walking paths, basic infrastructure to support it (*e.g.*, sufficient sidewalk space, good flow of sidewalks and paths to main locations, bike racks, etc.), and connectivity of rural and urban areas (*e.g.*, rails to trails for longer commutes vs. only highway access to main areas). Social ecological models have become more popular in recent years as interest has increased in how the built environment may facilitate exercise initiation and maintenance.

INCORPORATING THEORY-BASED TECHNIQUES AND PRINCIPLES INTO PRACTICE

Now that the importance of theories and models has been established, and the theories have been explained, the next step is to understand how to incorporate theory-based strategies and principles into practice. Theories provide a logic model or roadmap for where to focus your efforts. They help to identify where to start and how to navigate the journey.

The foundation of a logic model is identifying the *behavioral antecedents*—or factors that precede the behavior—and then understanding how these antecedents influence the likelihood of a future behavior (37). By identifying these important antecedents, you can determine key targets for intervention, and in turn develop and implement more effective programs.

For example, in the Theory of Planned Behavior (1,4), one's intention (level of motivation) is identified as a primary determinant (behavioral antecedent) of behavior. The greater the level of motivation for physical activity, the more likely a person will engage in physical activity behaviors. Thus, according to this theory, in order to get people to be more physically active, you need to target their intention, or motivation, for the behavior.

In the Self-Efficacy Theory (9), the most important source of self-efficacy, or your belief in your abilities, is past performance accomplishments or experiencing mastery. When you successfully carry out a task, you will believe that you have the capabilities necessary to engage in the behavior in the future. For example, if you walk in a 5k event and successfully complete the race, you will have a greater belief that you can accomplish another event like this in the future. Therefore, according to this theory, in order to help promote behavioral change, you need to find ways of creating successful mastery experiences.

In the Health Belief Model (32), behavior depends upon several factors, including your perceived susceptibility of getting a disease, perceived severity of the condition and its consequences, perceived benefits of engaging in the behavior for reducing risk, perceived barriers or costs of doing the behavior, and your confidence in your ability to take action and start the behavior. For example, if you are a sedentary person, you may believe that you could have a heart attack (perceived susceptibility is likely), that inactivity can lead to a heart attack (perceived severity is great), and that starting to engage in physical activity will reduce this risk (perceived benefits) without causing negative side effects of excessive difficulty (low perceived barriers).

The point is that theories provide you with the basic starting foundation. It is important to note that no single theory or model explains the broad scope of all health behaviors; or more specifically, explains 100% of physical activity behavior. You need to take into consideration the target individual or audience, environmental factors that may influence behavior, as well as other factors. In addition, a combination of theories may provide the best explanation for variations in behavior (37).

TAKE-HOME MESSAGE

This chapter reviewed the basic principles of behavior change as well as provided an overview of several theories and models that can provide you with a useful foundation to promote physical activity. While there is not a single theory of physical activity behavior change, the most important aspect is choosing a conceptual framework that provides a good understanding of the key factors that influence physical activity behavior in the target population. After all, these antecedents (thoughts, beliefs, barriers, etc.) are what provide us with clues about "the how and why" a behavior occurs (or doesn't occur) in order to initiate physical activity behavior change and sustain long-term maintenance.

REFERENCES

1. Ajzen I. *Attitudes, Personality, and Behavior.* Chicago (IL): Dorsey Press: 1988.
2. Ajzen I. *Construction of a standard questionnaire for the theory of planned behavior;* [cited 2012 May 11]. Available from: http://people.umass.edu/aizen/pdf/tpb.measurement.pdf
3. Ajzen I. The theory of planned behavior. *Organ Behav Hum Decis Process.* 1991;50:179–211.
4. Ajzen I, Driver B. Prediction of leisure participation from behavioral, normative, and control beliefs: An application of the theory of planned behavior. *Leisure Sci.* 1991;13:185–204.
5. Ajzen I, Fishbein M. *Understanding Attitudes and Predicting Social Behavior.* Englewood Cliffs (NJ): Prentice Hall: 1980.
6. American College of Sports Medicine. *ACSM's guidelines for exercise testing and prescription.* 6th ed. Philadelphia (PA): Lippincott, Williams & Wilkins: 2000.
7. Bandura A. Self-efficacy. In: Ramachaudran VS, editor. *Encyclopedia of Human Behavior Volume 4.* New York: Academic Press; 1994. p. 71–81.
8. Bandura A. *Self-efficacy: The Exercise of Control.* New York (NY): W. H. Freeman: 1997.
9. Bandura A. *Social Foundations of Thought and Action.* Englewood Cliffs (NJ): Prentice Hall: 1986.
10. Bao W, Ma A, Mao L, et al. Diet and lifestyle interventions in postpartum women in China: Study design and rationale of a multicenter randomized controlled trial. *BMC Public Health.* 2010;10:103–10.
11. Bazzano AT, Zeldin AS, Diab, IR, Garro NM, Allevato NA, Lehrer D. The Healthy Lifestyle Change Program: A pilot of a community-based health promotion intervention for adults with developmental disabilities. *Am J Prev Med.* 2009; 37(6):S201–8.
12. Blanchard C, Fisher J, Sparling P, Nehl E, Rhodes R, Courneya K, Baker F. Understanding physical activity behavior in African American and Caucasian college students: An application of the theory of planned behavior. *J Am Coll Health.* 2008;56(4): 341–6.
13. Blue CL. The predictive capacity of the theory of reasoned action and the theory of planned behavior in exercise behavior: An integrated literature review. *Res Nurs Health.* 1995;18(2):105–21.
14. Bouchard C, Shephard RJ, Stephen T. *Physical Activity, Fitness, and Health.* Champaign (IL): Human Kinetics: 1994.
15. Bronfenbrenner U. *The Ecology of Human Development.* Cambridge (MA): Harvard University Press: 1979.
16. Bronfenbrenner U. Toward an experimental ecology of human development. *Am Psychol.* 1977; 32:513–31.
17. Catania AC. *Learning.* 3rd ed. Englewood Cliffs (NJ): Prentice-Hall: 1992.
18. Chatzisarantis NL, Hagger MS, Biddle SJ, Smith B, Wang JC. A meta-analysis of perceived locus of causality in exercise, sport, and physical education contexts. *J Sport Exerc Psychol.* 2003;25:284–306.
19. Chatzisarantis NL, Hagger MS. Effects of an intervention based on self-determination theory

on self-reported leisure-time physical activity participation. *Psychol Health.* 2009;24(1):29–48.

20. Cury F, Da Fonsesca D, Rufo M, Peres C, Sarrazin P. The trichotomous model and investment in learning to prepare for a sport test: A mediational analysis. *Br J Educ Psychol.* 2003;73:529–43.
21. Cury F, Da Fonseca D, Rufo M, Sarrazin P. Perceptions of competence, implicit theory of ability, perception of motivational climate, and achievement goals: A test of trichotomous conceptualization of endorsement of achievement motivational in the physical education setting. *Percept Mot Skill.* 2002;95(1):233–44.
22. Contento IR, Koch PA, Lee H, Calabrese-Barton A. Adolescents demonstrate improvement in obesity risk behaviors after completion of choice, control and change, a curriculum addressing personal agency and autonomous motivation. *J Am Diet Assoc.* 2010;110(12):1830–9.
23. Cramp AG, Brawley LR. Sustaining self-regulatory efficacy and psychological outcome expectations for postnatal exercise: Effects of a group-mediated cognitive behavioural intervention. *Br J Health Psychol.* 2009;14(Pt3):595–611.
24. Deci EL, Ryan, RM. *Intrinsic Motivation and Self-Determination in Human Behavior.* New York (NY): Plenum Publishing Co: 1985.
25. DiClemente CC, Prochaska JO, Velicer WF, Fairhurst S, Rossi JS, Velasquez WE. The process of smoking cessation: An analysis of precontemplation, contemplation, and preparation stages of change. *J Consult Clin Psychol.* 1991;59(2):295–304.
26. Edmunds JK, Ntoumanis N, Duda JLD. Testing a self-determination theory based teaching style in the exercise domain. *Eur J Soc Psychol.* 2008; 38:375–88.
27. Fishbein M, Ajzen I. *Predicting and Changing Behavior: The Reasoned Action Approach.* New York: Taylor & Francis Group; 2010.
28. Hagger M, Chatzisarantis N. Self-determination theory and the psychology of exercise. *Int Rev Sport Exerc Psychol.* 2008;1(1):79–103.
29. Hausenblas HA, Symons Downs D. Prospective examination of the theory of planned behavior applied to exercise behavior during women's first trimester of pregnancy. *J Reproduct Infant Psychol.* 2004;22:199–210.
30. Hutchinson AJ, Breckson JD, Johnston LH. Physical activity behavior change interventions on the transtheoretical model: A systematic review. *Health Educ Behav.* 2009;36(5):829–45.
31. Janis IL, Mann L. *Decision-making: A Psychological Analysis of Conflict, Choice, and Commitment.* New York (NY): Free Press: 1977.
32. Janz N, Becker M. The health belief model: A decade later. *Health Educ Q.* 1984;11(1):47.
33. Jones LW, Guill B, Keir ST, et al. Using the theory of planned behavior to understand the determinants of exercise intention in patients diagnosed with primary brain cancer. *Psychooncology.* 2007;16(3):232–40.
34. Karvinen KH, Courneya KS, Campbell KL, et al. Correlates of exercise motivation and behavior in a population-based sample of endometrial cancer survivors: An application of the theory of planned behavior. *Int J Behav Nutr Phys Act.* 2007;4:20–30.
35. Keller C, Fleury J, Gregor-Holt N, Thompson T. Predictive ability of social cognitive theory in exercise research: An integrated literature review. *Online J Knowl Synth Nurs.* 1999;6:2.
36. Kilpatrick M, Hebert E, Jacobsen D. Physical activity motivation: A practitioner's guide to self-determination theory. *J Phys Educ Recreat Dance.* 2002;73:36–41.
37. Langlois MA, Hallam JS. Integrating multiple health behavior theories into program planning: The PER worksheet. *Health Promot Pract.* 2010;11(2):282–8.
38. Lox CL, Martin Ginis KA, Petruzzello SJ. *The psychology of exercise: Integrating theory and practice.* 3rd ed. Scottsdale (AZ): Holcomb Hathaway Publishers: 2010.
39. Marcus BH, Dubbert PM, Forsyth LH, et al. Physical activity behavior change: Issues in adoption and maintenance. *Health Psychol.* 2000; 19: 32–41.
40. Marlatt GA, Gordon JR. *Relapse Prevention: Maintenance Strategies in the Treatment of Addictive Behaviors.* New York: Guilford: 1985.
41. Marshall SJ, Biddle SJ. The transtheoretical model of behavior change: A meta-analysis of applications to physical activity and exercise. *Ann Behav Med.* 2001;23(4):229–46.
42. Martin G L, Pear JJ. *Behavior Modification: What It Is and How to Do It.* 7th ed. Englewood Cliffs (NJ): Prentice-Hall: 2003.
43. McAuley E. Enhancing psychological health through physical activity. In: Quinney HA, Gauvin L, Wall AET, editors. *Toward Active Living: Proceedings of the International Conference on Physical Activity, Fitness, and Health.* Champaign (IL): Human Kinetics; 1994. p. 83–90.
44. McAuley E, Bane SM, Mihalko SL. Exercise in middle-age adults: Self-efficacy and self-presentation outcomes. *Prev Med.* 1995;24(4):319–28.
45. McAuley E, Mihalko SL. Measuring exercise-related self-efficacy. In Duda, JL, editor. *Advances in Sport and Exercise Psychology Measurement*: Morgantown: Fitness Information Technology; 1998. p. 371–90.
46. Miller NE, Dollard J. *Social Learning and Imitation.* New Haven (CT): Yale University Press: 1941.
47. Mosher CE, Fuemmeler BF, Sloane R, et al. Change in self-efficacy partially mediates the effects of the FRESH START intervention on cancer survivors' dietary outcomes. *Psychooncology.* 2008; 17(10): 1014–23.
48. Patrick H, Canevello A. Methodological overview of a self-determination theory based computerized intervention to promote leisure-time physical activity. *Psychol Sport Exerc.* 2011;12(1):13–19.
49. Peddle CJ, Plotnikoff RC, Wild TC, Au H, Courneya KS. Medical, demographic, and psychological correlates of exercise in colorectal cancer survivors: an application of self-determination theory. *Support Care Cancer.* 2008;16(1):9–17.
50. Peterson GB. A day of great illumination: B. F. Skinner's *discovery* of shaping. *J Exp Anal Behav.* 2004;82(3):317–28.

51. Plotnikoff R, Lippke S, Courneya K, Birkett N, Sigal, R. Physical activity and diabetes: An application of the theory of planned behavior to explain physical activity for Type 1 and Type 2 diabetes in an adult population sample. *Psychol Health.* 2010; 25:7–23.
52. Plotnikoff RC, Lubans DR, Costigan SA, et al. A test of the theory of planned behavior to explain physical activity in a large population sample of adolescents from Alberta, Canada. *J Adolesc Health.* 2011;49(5):547–59.
53. Prochaska JO, DiClemente CC. *The Transtheoretical Approach: Crossing Traditional Boundaries of Change.* Homewood (IL): Dorsey: 1984.
54. Prochaska JO, DiClemete CC. Toward a comprehensive model of change. In Miller WR, Heather N, editors. *Treating Addictive Behaviors: Processes of Change.* New York: Plenum; 1986. p. 3–27.
55. Prochaska JO, Marcus BH. The Transtheoretical Model: Applications to exercise. In: Dishman RK, editor. *Advances in Exercise Adherence.* Champaign (IL): Human Kinetics; 1994. p. 161–80.
56. Prochaska JO, Velicer WF. The transtheoretical model of health behavior change. *Am J Health Promot.* 1997;12:38–48.
57. Reed GR, Velicer WF, Prochaska JO, Rossi JS, Marcus BH. What makes a good algorithm: Examples from regular exercise. *Am J Health Promot.* 1997;12(1):57–66.
58. Schmidt RA, Wrisberg C. *Motor Learning and Performance.* 4th ed. Champaign (IL): Human Kinetics: 2004.
59. Silva MN, Markland DA, Minderico CS, et al. A randomized controlled trial to evaluate self-determination theory for exercise adherence and weight control: Rationale and intervention description. *BMC Public Health.* 2008;8:234–47.
60. Silva MN, Markland DA, Vieira PN, et al. Helping overweight women become more active: Need support and motivational regulations for different forms of physical activity. *Psychol Sport Exerc.* 2010;11:591–601.
61. Silva MN, Vieira PN, Coutinho SR, et al. Using self-determination theory to promote physical activity and weight control: A randomized controlled trial in women. *J Behav Med.* 2010;33(2):110–22.
62. Skinner BF. *The Technology of Teaching.* New York: Appleton-Centry-Crofts: 1968.
63. Sonstroem RJ. Stage model of exercise adoption. In: *Proceedings of the 85th Annual Meeting of the American Psychological Association*; 1987 Aug 26–30: San Francisco.
64. Sweet SN, Tulloch H, Fortier MS, Pipe AL, Reid RD. Patterns of motivation and ongoing exercise activity in cardiac rehabilitation settings: A 24-month exploration from the TEACH Study. *Ann Behav Med.* 2011;42(1):55–63.
65. Symons Downs D, Hausenblas HA. Elicitation studies and the theory of planned behavior: A systematic review of exercise beliefs. *Psychol Sport Exer.* 2005a;6:1–31.
66. Symons Downs D, Hausenblas HA. Exercise behavior and the theories of reasoned action and planned behavior: A meta-analytic update. *J Phys Act Health.* 2005b;2:76–97.
67. United States Department of Health and Human Services. *2008 Physical Activity Guidelines for Americans.* Washington, D.C.: U.S. Department of Health and Human Services, Secretary of Health and Human Services; 2008. Available from: http://www.health.gov/PAGuidelines/guidelines/default.aspx.
68. Vallance JK, Courneya KS, Plotnikoff RC, Mackey JR. Analyzing theoretical mechanisms of physical activity behavior change in breast cancer survivors: Results from the activity promotion (ACTION) trial. *Ann Behav Med.* 2008;35(2):150–8.
69. Vallerand RJ, Reid G. On the causal effects of perceived competence on intrinsic motivation: A test of Cognitive Evaluation Theory. *J Sport Psychol.* 1984;6:94–102.
70. Weinberg RS, Gould D. *Foundations of Sport and Exercise Psychology.* 5th ed. Champaign (IL): Human Kinetics: 2011.

FURTHER WEB RESOURCES

The following Web site provides useful information on how to develop theory of planned behavior questionnaires and intervention:
http://people.umass.edu/aizen/tpb.html

The following Web site includes an extensive list of questionnaires used to assess constructs of Self-Determination Theory, with some specifically in an exercise context (*i.e.,* motives for physical activity):
http://www.psych.rochester.edu/SDT/questionnaires.php

CHAPTER 2

Assessing Your Client's Physical Activity Behavior, Motivation, and Individual Resources

Sonia Lippke, Claudia Voelcker-Rehage, and Ute Bültmann

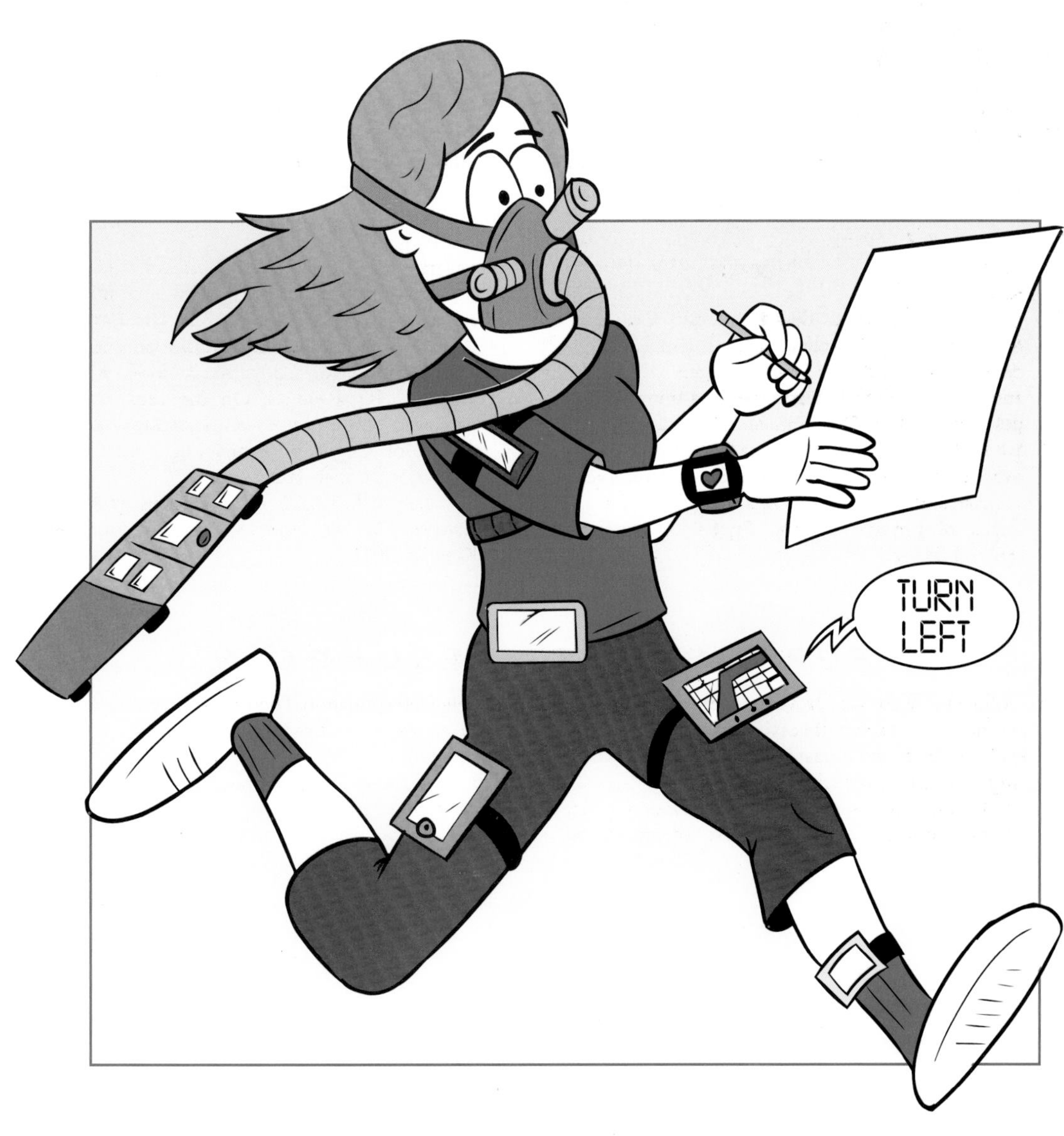

INTRODUCTION: ASSESSING INDIVIDUALS' PHYSICAL ACTIVITY AND MOTIVATION

Most organizations, like the American College of Sports Medicine (ACSM), provide *guidelines* to perform physical activity regularly (8). Specifically, the ACSM recommends to engage in. . .

- *moderate*-intensity cardiorespiratory exercise training for 30 minutes or more per day on 5 or more days per week, or
- *vigorous*-intensity cardiorespiratory exercise training for 20 minutes or more per day on 3 or more days per week, or
- a *combination* of moderate- and vigorous-intensity exercise to accumulate a total energy expenditure of 500–1000 or more MET minutes per week; and additionally
- *resistance* exercises for each of the major muscle groups a minimum of 2 days per week and
- *neuromotor exercise* (functional fitness training) involving balance, agility, and coordination for each of the major muscle-tendon groups (a total of 60 seconds per exercise) a minimum of 2 days per week.

The activity can be performed in bouts of 10 minutes as part of daily living, or as part of a fitness program. Although these guidelines are helpful, they also raise many practical questions (see Figure 2.1).

To best answer the questions found in Figure 2.1, we require an understanding of motivation and behavior, as well as other individual variables such as needs, wishes, fears, and barriers to physical activity. Such information can be acquired from those individuals whom we want to help. Different aspects or variables are important to assess within a person. Besides these, it is inevitable that environmental characteristics, such as the availability of proper facilities, also influence exercise behavior. *Ecological frameworks,* like the model by Bronfenbrenner (6), describe different levels: individual, social, physical environment, and policy (Figure 2.2).

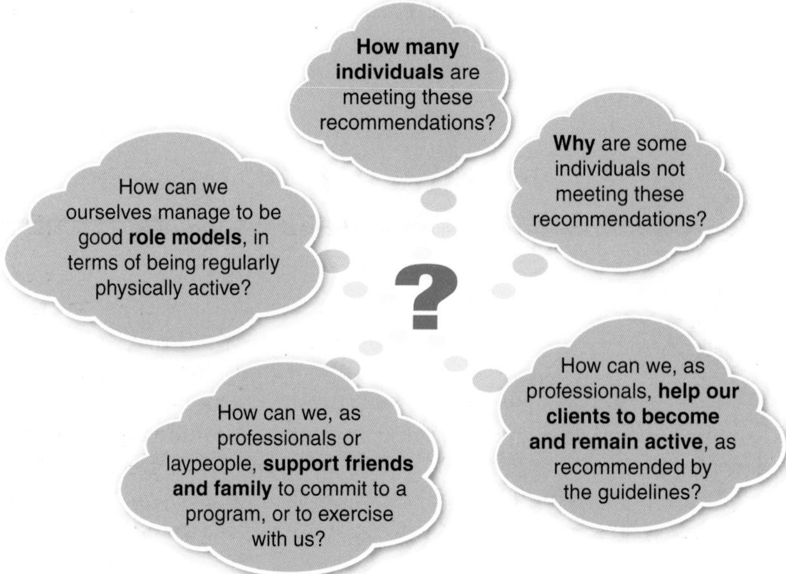

FIGURE 2.1. Practical questions arising from recommended physical activity guidelines.

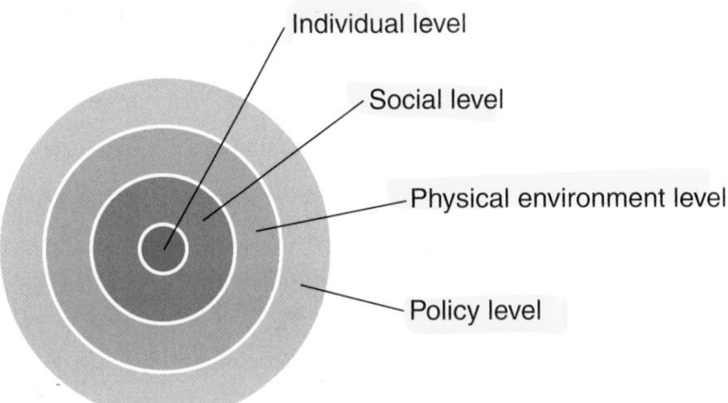

FIGURE 2.2. Ecological model of physical activity.

This chapter will focus only on the two inner levels shown in Figure 2.2 (individual and social levels), as we can directly assess how individuals perceive their environment, and what their expectations and (perceived) barriers are. The two outer levels are important as well, and are presented in Chapter 7.

Step-by-Step

As professionals working with clients, we need information about our clients' thoughts, expectations, perceptions, and competencies regarding health behaviors to help them adequately. For doing so, a good way is to determine:

1. The target population
2. The physical activity behavior of interest
3. Related behaviors of interest
4. Psychological and social (mediator/predictor) variables of interest
5. The measurement strategy

On the basis of this information, a measurement and assessment plan can be set up.

Case Scenario 2.1 demonstrates the practical application of the preceding steps when faced with the task of helping people become and remain physically active. Such a scenario might occur in any environment in which people work, learn, meet, or simply spend time.

Case Scenario 2.1

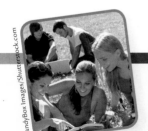

CandyBox Images/Shutterstock.com

Consider a university with a relatively small and young campus, with 1,500 students and 450 faculty and staff members (=target population). Currently, *physical exercise programs* exist for students and employees. A *recreation center* hosts a rowing tank, gyms, and a well-equipped fitness facility. The wide variety of fitness equipment includes cardiovascular equipment, free weights, and resistance training machines. Additionally, a *gymnasium* provides athletic grounds and sports equipment, such as balls, nets, and rowing equipment. The question is how many people are performing physical activities within the *physical exercise programs*, in the *recreation center* and the *gymnasium* (=physical activity behavior of interest).

continued

Case Scenario 2.1 *continued*

In addition to changing rooms and bathroom facilities in the center, different buildings on campus provide *showers* for those students and employees who cycle to the campus (=related behaviors of interest).

A small interviewing (=measurement strategy) shows that (a) 30% of the university's students and employees engage in at least one physical exercise program once a week. It also reveals that (b) an additional 25% of students and employees would be interested in using it (=psychological and social variables). Finally, (c) the university board is not satisfied with the user numbers in the recreation center, and seeks better utilization (=psychological and social variables).

For this scenario, we can apply questions exploring how to help individuals engage in and maintain the recommended activity levels. How can we answer the question how to help individuals? There are different approaches:

1. We can generate some solutions ourselves.
2. We can ask students, faculty, staff, alumni, and the public, or a representative sample of those parties, what they desire, like and dislike.
3. We can look into the literature and previous good examples to search for theories and evidence to base our own developments on.

A combination of all these approaches would certainly be the most favorable. However, to meet the needs of the people, we must begin with understanding and assessing them.

CONCEPT OVERVIEW

If our aim is to understand individual and social factors, and design strategies that help to improve the behavior of individuals, we require additional information. Only if we understand what people do (*e.g.*, physical activity level), feel (*e.g.*, perceived barriers to activity), and think (*e.g.*, motivation), can we adequately tailor our intervention to each individual. Moreover, assessment is equally important in order to evaluate if our intervention was satisfactory and achieved desired outcomes.

In particular, describing how to measure aspects of an individual that affect health behavior is imperative for the following chapters of this book, because it allows us to understand individuals and their feelings, thoughts, and aims better. The goal of such measurements is to accurately assess the behavior, needs and preconditions of the client, such as intention or self-efficacy. When this is achieved, results of the assessment and measurement can be used for optimally designing and modifying health interventions to each individual. Further, when we establish which aspects should be changed throughout an intervention (such as intention), or what the outcome of an intervention should look like (*e.g.*, behavior change or behavior maintenance), interventions can be tailored adequately and evaluated accordingly. In this chapter, we provide example assessment scenarios to display practical implications of the information at the individual and social level. We also demonstrate possible tools or items that are useful for assessment. These tools generally originate from validated questionnaires published in research papers, and references to these studies are provided throughout the chapter. Furthermore, we refer to useful Web-sources in which these assessment tools can also be found.

TAKE-HOME MESSAGE

Assessment opens avenues for understanding and addressing individuals' behaviors, motivations, and determinants of behavior. With the results from assessments, we are able to design appropriate interventions and evaluate their effectiveness.

Assessment Modes

A *health behavior* is any behavior that improves health and well-being, which in turn helps to prevent the onset or progression of morbidity, as well as premature mortality. Thus, physical activity can be a health behavior if it is performed with appropriate intensity and frequency. Health behaviors also include risk reduction behaviors, such as limiting sedentary activities like television watching. Although many people are well aware that they should perform health behaviors on a regular basis, reports show that alarming numbers of people are not meeting the physical activity recommendations (8). This is especially the case for those who have disabilities and chronic illnesses.

To better cover different aspects of physical activity behavior, assessment of physical activity could cover the different aspects displayed in Table 2.1.

As you can see, there is more than just the pure behavior in terms of movements an observer would see if he or she monitors the individuals from the outside; psychological aspects such as easiness of execution are important as well. That is, some components of a behavior can be obtained through observation and other objective measures. However, not all facets can be observed or measured by means of physiological indicators, so self-report measures are also used (18). The advantages and disadvantage of various assessment modes are shown in Table 2.2.

Tools for Assessing Self-Reported Information

Self-reported information (questionnaires/interviews) is often used to measure physical activity and its determinants. While physical activity can also be assessed by objective methods, such as observation or physiological measures, influences like motivation are typically measured by self-reports. Although the validity (degree to which measurement actually measures what it should measure) of self-reports of behavior is not always assured, they are rather easy to obtain in comparison to objective measures.

The type of interview used can vary in usefulness, depending on the specific approach. Narrative and unstructured interviews utilize methods in which little or no predefined questions are asked, and questions are instead open ended (*i.e.*, the interviewee can respond

TABLE 2.1 Different Aspects of Behavior Assessment

Aspect	Example
Energy expenditure	kcal, MET (metabolic equivalent)
Length of behavior time	Time (minutes per week)
Frequency of behavior	Number of times per week
Easiness of executing (intensity)	How demanding it is to perform the intended activity

Note: For measuring and calculating MET (1, 7).

TABLE 2.2 Different Assessment Modes: Advantages and Disadvantages

	Subjective Assessment	*Objective Measures*
Content	**Perceived Value**	**Outside Measures**
Method	Person is directly asked about his or her behavior • Interviews, • Questionnaires, or • Diary logs and self-monitoring strategies.	Behavior is monitored with a device, like pedometer or accelerometer (tracking steps or movements), or by direct observation (attendance rates; observing which products are bought or used for exercising, etc.).
Advantage	Individual resources and impediments such as intention, inner temptations, perceived self-efficacy and perceived social support, can only be measured subjectively.	Less likely to be biased by social desirability (tendency to present oneself in a more favorable manner than is actually true) and answering tendencies (*e.g.*, to agree to questions)
Disadvantage	Social desirability (to present oneself in a more positive view) affects validity and reliability of measures.	Most are more challenging (time consuming, expensive) to gather.

in a narrative text form, instead of in the form of "yes-no" or multiple choice answers). These interviews often result in very different outcomes. This can complicate the comparison of information from multiple interviews (*e.g.*, of one person interviewed several times). Alternatively, interviews can also be organized like questionnaires, providing well-defined question-and-answer options. This restricts gathered information to a range of selected answers, making it easier to compare. While the main difference between interviews and questionnaires is how the clients disclose themselves, they each have distinct advantages, as well as some similar traits. An interviewer requires the client to reveal all answers to the interviewer. In a questionnaire, however, the answering procedure is anonymous, which may reduce *social desirability bias*. For example, social desirability bias may cause the client to report more health behavior than they actually performed. Alternatively, interviews allow the interviewer to clarify questions for the client; an advantage not as likely with questionnaires. The anxiety of sharing personal information can occur in both questionnaires and interviews.

Diary log techniques and self-monitoring strategies can be very similar to questionnaires. With these techniques, clients are asked to monitor, say, the amount of their daily steps by carrying a pedometer and entering the daily number it reads into a log. Such a log can be a hard-copy book or an electronic book version. The latter provides the option to receive immediate feedback relating to the performed steps. For example, *individual/ipsative*: "Today, you performed 7000 steps. That is two times more than yesterday." Or *normative*: "Today, you performed 7000 steps. That is less than the recommended 10,000 steps/day."

TIME CONSIDERATIONS

When designing self-report surveys to assess information, several aspects are important to consider. First, the nature of the behavior should be considered: Whether the behavior in question may consist of an action performed on a *single occasion*, or a *repeatedly performed action*. For example, we might be interested in learning whether a person participates in regular physical activity (which can be measured by means of the PAR-Q—see the description later in this chapter and 22,23), or in a sports event (single occasion). The answer to either of these can then only be dichotomous, providing a "yes" or "no" response. Physical exercise, however, has to be performed repeatedly in order to be health promoting. Thus, we are now interested in a repeatedly performed behavior.

- Second, physical activity can be assessed over the course of a defined time span (*e.g.*, "How often did you exercise during the last month?"), or measured by questioning the typical quantity and frequency of the behavior (*e.g.*, "How often do you exercise during a typical week?"). Additionally, in the case of an accident or some other health conditions preventing one from performing his or her typical activities, individuals should receive a concrete instruction, such as thinking about the month prior to that incident. Any health incident should be considered and taken into account when evaluating the information.
- Third, the optimal period for measurement should be considered. The course of a defined time span should be assessed if there are clear reasons for doing so. Defining a time span is recommended for the following situations:

1. If behavior change process is expected to occur—for example, after an intervention,
2. If a special interval was predicted by social-cognitive variables at an earlier point in time, such as predicting participation in a marathon half a year after measuring the intention to do so, or
3. If the individual has been in an unusual condition—for example, after a surgery or vacation.

Alternatively, having no time frame is sometimes advantageous, as specific time frames might be arbitrary: Why should a person who intends to adopt a physical activity in 6 months and 1 day be different from a person intending to start a physical activity in 5 months and 20 days or from a person intending to change within 6 months? There is no empirical evidence for this specific cutoff of 5 months and 20 days or 6 months. Contemporary assessments measure stages of change (see examples in Table 2.3) without using a specific time frame (10, 11).

PRECISION OF MEASUREMENT

- The precision of measurement must also be considered. The level of comprehensiveness of behavior can be very broad (*e.g.*, "I follow an active lifestyle"), or more precisely defined in terms of duration (*e.g.*, "I bicycle to work every day, which takes about 30 minutes"). In order to have precise measurements, questions are asked about frequency and duration of exercising (*e.g.*, "How many days per week did you perform sports activities? How many hours and minutes did one session last?"). Alternatively, the answers can be given on rating scales with verbal anchors (*e.g.*, *less than 1 time a month or never* (1), *1–3 times a month* (2),

TABLE 2.3 Stages of Change Assessment

Instruction: Please think about your typical week. Did you engage in physical activity at least 5 days per week, for 30 minutes or more at a time (or a total of 2.5 hours during the week), in such a way that you were moderately exhausted? From the following statements, please choose the one that describes you most accurately by checking the number.

No, and I do not intend to start	*1*
No, but I am considering it	*2*
No, but I seriously intend to start	*3*
Yes, but it is rather difficult for me	*4*
Yes, and it is rather easy for me	*5*

Adapted with permission from Lippke S, Ziegelmann JP, Schwarzer R, and Velicer WF (2009). Validity of stage assessment in the adoption and maintenance of physical activity and fruit and vegetable consumption. *Health Psychology*, 28(2), 183–193.

approximately once a week (3), *between 2 and 3 times a week* (4), *4–5 times a week* (5), and *(almost) every day* (6)). In order to rate statements broadly, answers can be given on a rating scale that ranges from *not at all* (1) to *exactly* (6).

Objective Measures: Rationale, Tools, and Advantages

Some objective measures (such as steps performed during a week measured with a pedometer, and others as shown in Table 2.4) typically have higher accuracy than subjective ones (measured by means of an interview). This is because individuals do not have to respond to questions themselves. Instead, physical activity level is collected with tools such as physical activity motion detector monitoring (such as a pedometer, or accelerometers).

Modern technologies (*e.g.,* mobile phones, GPS technology), which track movements of the individual, could also be a solution. This must be assessed carefully, however, as accurate instruction and compliance of the individual is required as the main basis for gaining reliable information. Only if the person actually uses the pedometer appropriately, can it monitor physical activity correctly. The devices mentioned are normally small and not cumbersome for the client. They are affordable and come in a variety of brands, most of which should be reliable and valid.

Attendance rates within a recreation center can also be used as an objective observational measure. If members of a recreation center have to check in for their training, these measurements are relatively objective. However, if people forget to check in for a training or someone else checks in for the client, data might be inaccurate. Errors may be occurring if one is not only interested in attendance rates but also general physical activity during the day—*e.g.,* people may also train in other environments (such as a park).

Typical physiological objective measures (Table 2.4) capture the physical activity level, or fitness and functionality of the individual. Physical activity and fitness are related but not the same. Behavior can lead to an improvement in fitness and functionality, and lack of fitness and functionality may obstruct behavior.

TABLE 2.4 Examples of Objective Measures to Assess Physical Activity Level and Physical Fitness

Measure of . . .	Test and Material Needed (Example)
. . . *Physical activity*	
Number of steps	Pedometer
Acceleration forces	Accelerometer, GPS, mobile phones
. . . *Physical fitness*	
Cardiovascular fitness	VO_2Max test (spiroergometry) on the treadmill, stationary bike, rowing machine etc. Rockport 1-mile walk test
Heart rate / heart rate variability	Heart rate measurement device
Grip strength	Hand grip dynamometer
Flexibility	Measure tape/stick
Postural stability	Force platform, one leg stance

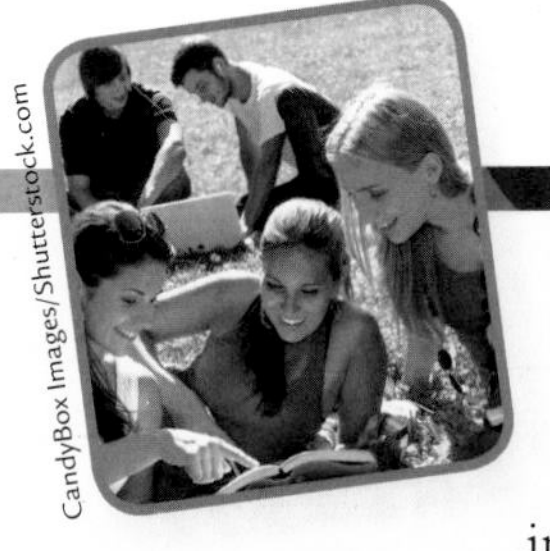
CandyBox Images/Shutterstock.com

Case Scenario 2.2

Let's think again about the physical activity of individuals connected to the university. A task force of researchers decides to speak with students, faculty, staff, and alumni, as well as family of staff, and people living in the neighborhood of the campus, to obtain information about these individuals' physical activity levels. The goal is to learn more about their past behavior and experiences at the university, what they like and dislike about the fitness options at the campus, and whether they want support in committing to a weekly routine of physical activity. The process is as follows: First, the task force selects a group of participants representative of the population. To do this, three to five individuals from each group are selected, recruited, and *interviewed*.

Possible questions include:

- "Are you performing 30 minutes of moderate-intensity physical activity daily?"
- If *no*: "What challenges prevent you from doing so?"; "What could be changed to assist you in becoming more active?"
- If *yes*: "What do you think would motivate inactive people to be as active as you are?"

Next, *closed-end questions* are developed on the basis of those answers. The generated questions are sent out by e-mail to all students, faculty, staff, and alumni. Family of staff are to be approached personally. All people of interest then receive questions like:

- "If you think about the following potential changes on campus, would they help you perform 30 minutes of moderate-intensity physical activity daily?" Please indicate your answer on the following scale from "*not at all*" (1) to "*very much*" (6).
    (a) If you get tips on how to schedule your training into your working day. 1–2–3–4–5–6
    (b) If you get (more) personal assistance during your workout. 1–2–3–4–5–6
    (c) If your friends and/or family could work out with you. 1–2–3–4–5–6

This allows people to indicate their past behavior and beliefs.

We now know something about the individuals who answered the questions. With that, we can tailor our interventions to the needs of the individuals.

TAKE-HOME MESSAGE

When assessing behavior, both objective and subject measures can be collected. Motivation and other psychological variables (see the following sections) are typically measured by perceived or subjective means. The variety of objective and subjective assessment options provides a number of different advantages, but also several restrictions. One should be aware of these when choosing a measurement tool or designing a project.

OBTAIN HEALTH INFORMATION/HISTORY TO ENSURE SAFE PARTICIPATION IN PHYSICAL ACTIVITY AND EXERCISE

CONCEPT OVERVIEW

Knowing about the health of oneself or of a client is important in order to exercise appropriately. The health status determines whether a specialist should be consulted to evaluate the safety of exercising. The recommended preparticipation questionnaires according to *ACSM's Guidelines for Exercise Testing and Prescription* (3) are the Physical Activity Readiness Questionnaire (PAR-Q, 22, 23) and the AHA/ACSM Health/Fitness Facility Preparticipation Screening Questionnaire. For a more specific, in-depth, and detailed preactivity screening process, the PAR-Q and AHA/ACSM Health/Fitness Facility Pre-participation Screening Questionnaire may be combined with tools like the Health Risk Appraisal (HRA) or Health History Questionnaire (HHQ) (24).

These four assessment tools—the PAR-Q, the AHA/ACSM Health/Fitness Facility Preparticipation Screening Questionnaire, the HRA, and the HHQ—are all standardized questionnaires used to identify health risk factors of exercising for an individual. Their purpose is to obtain medical clearance for a person, refer a person to his or her doctor, use the information to modify their program, etc. Thus, it is important for both the individual who intends to start exercising, and the professionals who provide the environment, to know about any risk factors and contraindications. Moreover, such assessments provide the opportunity to follow up with clients over time and track improvements and obstacles, and should therefore be repeated on a regular basis, perhaps weekly or annually. More detailed variations of the PAR-Q exist: The PAR-MEDX and the PAR-MEDX for Pregnancy are longer questionnaires. If individuals respond to these more detailed versions properly, exercise prescription can be done more accurately. (See From the Practical Toolbox 2.1 for more information about the PAR-Q, the PARmed-X, and the PARmed-X for Pregnancy.)

The four assessments can be found on the Internet as follows:

- PAR-Q at http://www.csep.ca/english/view.asp?x=698
- AHA/ACSM Health/Fitness Facility Preparticipation Screening Questionnaire at http://circ.ahajournals.org/content/97/22/2283.full.pdf
- HRA at http://www.cdc.gov/nccdphp/dnpao/hwi/downloads/HRA_checklist.pdf
- HHQ at http://www.hr.emory.edu/blomeyer/docs/HealthHistory Questionnaire2007.pdf

Two of these assessments will be described briefly in the following subsections.

From the Practical Toolbox 2.1

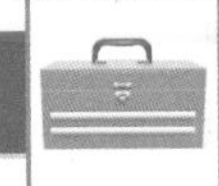

SCREENING FOR EXERCISE PREPAREDNESS

Lauren Capozzi and S. Nicole Culos-Reed

When screening someone for exercise, it is important to recognize certain population characteristics that may be contraindicated. Using the appropriate screening tool is the first step to ensuring someone's safety.

PAR-Q and YOU

This questionnaire is for people aged 15–69. This one-page form helps people to know if they need to check with their physician before engaging in physical activity. See Figure 2.3; this form is also available at http://www.csep.ca/english/view.asp?x=698.

PARmed-X

This is a physical activity–specific checklist used by physicians with patients who have responded "yes" to one or more questions on the PAR-Q. This form is available at http://www.csep.ca/english/view.asp?x=698.

PARmed-X for Pregnancy

This is a physical activity–specific checklist used by physicians with patients who are pregnant prior to attending prenatal fitness class or performing other exercise. This form is available at http://www.csep.ca/english/view.asp?x=698.

AHA/ACSM Health Fitness Facility Preparticipation Screening

This form (see Figure 2.4) provides an in-depth analysis of specific cardiovascular and other risk factors that could be affected by physical activity participation. It also recommends whether or not someone needs to contact his or her health care provider prior to exercise.

Informed Consent

This form (see Figure 2.5) ensures that individuals are aware of exercise testing and training procedures and that both parties (the individual and the exercise professional) understand the implications related to all possible outcomes.

continued

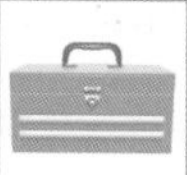

From the Practical Toolbox 2.1 *continued*

Physical Activity Readiness
Questionnaire - PAR-Q
(revised 2002)

PAR-Q & YOU

(A Questionnaire for People Aged 15 to 69)

Regular physical activity is fun and healthy, and increasingly more people are starting to become more active every day. Being more active is very safe for most people. However, some people should check with their doctor before they start becoming much more physically active.

If you are planning to become much more physically active than you are now, start by answering the seven questions in the box below. If you are between the ages of 15 and 69, the PAR-Q will tell you if you should check with your doctor before you start. If you are over 69 years of age, and you are not used to being very active, check with your doctor.

Common sense is your best guide when you answer these questions. Please read the questions carefully and answer each one honestly: check YES or NO.

YES	NO	
☐	☐	**1. Has your doctor ever said that you have a heart condition and that you should only do physical activity recommended by a doctor?**
☐	☐	**2. Do you feel pain in your chest when you do physical activity?**
☐	☐	**3. In the past month, have you had chest pain when you were not doing physical activity?**
☐	☐	**4. Do you lose your balance because of dizziness or do you ever lose consciousness?**
☐	☐	**5. Do you have a bone or joint problem (for example, back, knee or hip) that could be made worse by a change in your physical activity?**
☐	☐	**6. Is your doctor currently prescribing drugs (for example, water pills) for your blood pressure or heart condition?**
☐	☐	**7. Do you know of any other reason why you should not do physical activity?**

If you answered

YES to one or more questions

Talk with your doctor by phone or in person BEFORE you start becoming much more physically active or BEFORE you have a fitness appraisal. Tell your doctor about the PAR-Q and which questions you answered YES.

- You may be able to do any activity you want — as long as you start slowly and build up gradually. Or, you may need to restrict your activities to those which are safe for you. Talk with your doctor about the kinds of activities you wish to participate in and follow his/her advice.
- Find out which community programs are safe and helpful for you.

NO to all questions

If you answered NO honestly to all PAR-Q questions, you can be reasonably sure that you can:

- start becoming much more physically active – begin slowly and build up gradually. This is the safest and easiest way to go.
- take part in a fitness appraisal – this is an excellent way to determine your basic fitness so that you can plan the best way for you to live actively. It is also highly recommended that you have your blood pressure evaluated. If your reading is over 144/94, talk with your doctor before you start becoming much more physically active.

DELAY BECOMING MUCH MORE ACTIVE:

- if you are not feeling well because of a temporary illness such as a cold or a fever – wait until you feel better; or
- if you are or may be pregnant – talk to your doctor before you start becoming more active.

PLEASE NOTE: If your health changes so that you then answer YES to any of the above questions, tell your fitness or health professional. Ask whether you should change your physical activity plan.

Informed Use of the PAR-Q: The Canadian Society for Exercise Physiology, Health Canada, and their agents assume no liability for persons who undertake physical activity, and if in doubt after completing this questionnaire, consult your doctor prior to physical activity.

No changes permitted. You are encouraged to photocopy the PAR-Q but only if you use the entire form.

NOTE: If the PAR-Q is being given to a person before he or she participates in a physical activity program or a fitness appraisal, this section may be used for legal or administrative purposes.

"I have read, understood and completed this questionnaire. Any questions I had were answered to my full satisfaction."

NAME ____________________

SIGNATURE ____________________ DATE ____________________

SIGNATURE OF PARENT ____________________ WITNESS ____________________
or GUARDIAN (for participants under the age of majority)

Note: This physical activity clearance is valid for a maximum of 12 months from the date it is completed and becomes invalid if your condition changes so that you would answer YES to any of the seven questions.

continued on other side...

FIGURE 2.3. Par-Q & You, Physical Activity Readiness Questionnaire (PAR-Q) form. Reprinted from *Canada's Physical Activity Guide to Healthy Active Living* [Internet]. Ontario (Canada): Public Health Agency of Canada; [cited 2007 Jun 15]. Permission from the Canadian Society for Exercise Physiology, http://www.csep.ca. © 2002.

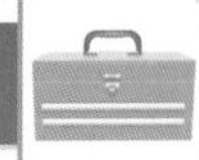

Assess your health status by marking all *true* statements

History

You have had:

___ a heart attack
___ heart surgery
___ cardiac catheterization
___ coronary angioplasty (PTCA)
___ pacemaker/implantable cardiac defibrillator/rhythm disturbance
___ heart valve disease
___ heart failure
___ heart transplantation
___ congenital heart disease

Symptoms

___ You experience chest discomfort with exertion
___ You experience unreasonable breathlessness
___ You experience dizziness, fainting, or blackouts
___ You experience ankle swelling
___ You experience unpleasant awareness of a forceful or rapid heart rate
___ You take heart medications

Other health issues

___ You have diabetes
___ You have asthma or other lung disease
___ You have burning or cramping sensation in your lower legs when walking short distance
___ You have musculoskeletal problems that limit your physical activity
___ You have concerns about the safety of exercise
___ You take prescription medications
___ You are pregnant

If you marked any of these statements in this section, consult your physician or other appropriate health care provider before engaging in exercise. You may need to use a facility with a ***medically qualified staff****.*

Cardiovascular risk factors

___ You are a man ≥45 yr
___ You are a woman ≥55 yr
___ You smoke or quit smoking within the previous 6 mo
___ Your blood pressure is ≥140/90 mm Hg
___ You do not know your blood pressure
___ You take blood pressure medication
___ Your blood cholesterol level is ≥200 mg · dL^{-1}
___ You do not know your cholesterol level
___ You have a close blood relative who had a heart attack or heart surgery before age 55 (father or brother) or age 65 (mother or sister)
___ You are physically inactive (*i.e.*, you get <30 min of physical activity on at least 3 d per week)
___ You have a body mass index ≥30 kg · m^{-2}
___ You have prediabetes
___ You do not know if you have prediabetes

If you marked two or more of the statements in this section you should consult your physician or other appropriate health care as part of good medical care and progress gradually with your exercise program. You might benefit from using a facility with a ***professionally qualified exercise staff***[a] *to guide your exercise program.*

___ None of the above

You should be able to exercise safely without consulting your physician or other appropriate health care provider in a self-guide program or almost any facility that meets your exercise program needs.

[a]Professionally qualified exercise staff refers to appropriately trained individuals who possess academic training, practical and clinical knowledge, skills, and abilities commensurate with the credentials defined in *Appendix D*.

FIGURE 2.4. AHA/ACSM Health/Fitness Facility Preparticipation Screening Questionnaire. Individuals with multiple CVD risk factors should be encouraged to consult with their physician prior to initiating a vigorous-intensity exercise program as part of good medical care, and should progress gradually with their exercise program of any exercise intensity. ACSM, American College of Sports Medicine; AHA, American Heart Association; CVD, cardiovascular disease, PTCA, percutaneous transluminal coronary angioplasty. Reprinted with permission from American College of Sports Medicine. *ACSM's Guidelines for Exercise Testing and Prescription*. 9th ed. Baltimore (MD): Lippincott Williams and Wilkins; 2014; modified from American College of Sports Medicine Position Stand, American Heart Association. Recommendations for cardiovascular screening, staffing, and emergency policies at health/fitness facilities. *Med Sci Sports Exerc*. 1998;30(6):1009–18.

continued

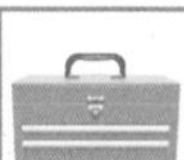

From the Practical Toolbox 2.1 *continued*

Informed Consent for an Exercise Test

1. **Purpose and Explanation of the Test**
You will perform an exercise test on a cycle ergometer or a motor-driven treadmill. The exercise intensity will begin at a low level and will be advanced in stages depending on your fitness level. We may stop the test at any time because of signs of fatigue or changes in your heart rate, electrocardiogram, or blood pressure, or symptoms you may experience. It is important for you to realize that you may stop when you wish because of feelings of fatigue or any other discomfort.

2. **Attendant Risks and Discomforts**
There exists the possibility of certain changes occurring during the test. These include abnormal blood pressure; fainting; irregular, fast, or slow heart rhythm; and, in rare instances, heart attack, stroke, or death. Every effort will be made to minimize these risks by evaluation of preliminary information relating to your health and fitness and by careful observations during testing. Emergency equipment and trained personnel are available to deal with unusual situations that may arise.

3. **Responsibilities of the Participant**
Information you possess about your health status or previous experiences of heart-related symptoms (*e.g.*, shortness of breath with low-level activity; pain; pressure; tightness; heaviness in the chest, neck, jaw, back, and/or arms) with physical effort may affect the safety of your exercise test. Your prompt reporting of these and any other unusual feelings with effort during the exercise test itself is very important. You are responsible for fully disclosing your medical history as well as symptoms that may occur during the test. You are also expected to report all medications (including nonprescription) taken recently and, in particular, those taken today to the testing staff.

4. **Benefits To Be Expected**
The results obtained from the exercise test may assist in the diagnosis of your illness, in evaluating the effect of your medications, or in evaluating what type of physical activities you might do with low risk.

5. **Inquiries**
Any questions about the procedures used in the exercise test or the results of your test are encouraged. If you have any concerns or questions, please ask us for further explanations.

6. **Use of Medical Records**
The information that is obtained during exercise testing will be treated as privileged and confidential as described in the Health Insurance Portability and Accountability Act of 1996. It is not to be released or revealed to any individual except your referring physician without your written consent. However, the information obtained may be used for statistical analysis or scientific purposes with your right to privacy retained.

7. **Freedom of Consent**
I hereby consent to voluntarily engage in an exercise test to determine my exercise capacity and state of cardiovascular health. My permission to perform this exercise test is given voluntarily. I understand that I am free to stop the test at any point if I so desire.

I have read this form, and I understand the test procedures that I will perform and the attendant risks and discomforts. Knowing these risks and discomforts, and having had an opportunity to ask questions that have been answered to my satisfaction, I consent to participate in this test.

Date	Signature of Patient
Date	Signature of Witness
Date	Signature of Physician or Authorized Delegate

FIGURE 2.5. Sample of informed consent form for a symptom-limited exercise test. Reprinted with permission from American College of Sports Medicine. *ACSM's Guidelines for Exercise Testing and Prescription*. 9th ed. Baltimore (MD): Lippincott Williams and Wilkins; 2014.

Physical Activity Readiness Questionnaire (PAR-Q)

The PAR-Q (22,23), shown in Figure 2.3, is a general screening tool that can identify factors that increase one's risk for exercise-related health problems. The assessment can be performed by means of a self-administered questionnaire, or with the assistance of a professional.

The questions can be answered with "yes" or "no" responses. Sometimes the answering option "I do not know" or "I do not remember" is also provided. The questionnaire provides direct feedback on the provided answers. If individuals answer "yes" to any items, they should see a physician prior to beginning an exercise program.

Health History Questionnaire (HHQ)

Like the PAR-Q, the HHQ (15) is a tool to screen for risk factors prior to starting physical activity. The HHQ, however, is much more detailed. The first seven items in section I: "I. Physical activity screening questions" assess risk factors with questions such as:

- "Do you know of any other reason why you should not participate in a program of physical activity?"

In section II: "II. General health history questions," 10 further questions evaluate medical conditions such as stroke, diabetes, asthma, orthopedic conditions, high blood pressure, back problems, pregnancy. The HHQ also directly assesses physical activity routines and medications:

- "Do you currently exercise less than 1 or more hour per week? If you answered yes, please describe your activities. . ."
- "Are you currently taking any medication that might impact your ability to safely perform physical activity?"

With the HHQ, feedback has to be given by the professional who is supervising the interviewed person. Thus, the professional must be fully aware of when information represents a risk factor, such as individuals with diabetes who take medication. In these situations, the individual must be advised by their physician to synchronize his or her medication and physical activity in order to prevent adverse reactions. In the case of risk factors or diseases, the professional should recommend consulting a physician for medical clearance. Objective measures to assess health are described in Table 2.5. These measures have been used and validated as objective indicators of health (18).

To illustrate, consider Case Scenario 2.3.

TABLE 2.5 Examples of Objective Measures to Assess Health

Measure	Test and Material Needed (Example)
Waist-hip-ratio, abdominal girth	Tape measure
BMI, body fat	(Normed) Weighting machine, tape measure
Resting heart rate, blood pressure	Blood measure measurement device
Grip strength	Hand grip dynamometer
Postural stability	Force platform, stop watch
Lung volume	Spirometer

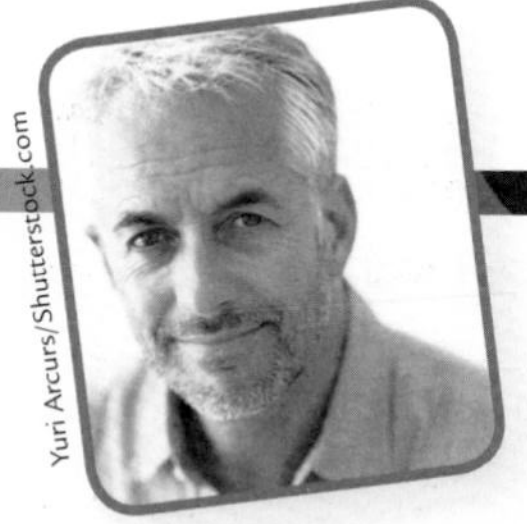

Yuri Arcurs/Shutterstock.com

Case Scenario 2.3

Professor R is over 60 years old and suffers from frequent back pain. He knows that specific physical training would be beneficial for his back. Although he experienced in the past that strength training improves his back pain and his general well-being, he is apprehensive to attend the training offered at the university recreation center. He feels he is too old, and that younger colleagues might take part in this class as well and do much better than he would do. So far, he has neither managed to participate in a class at the local sports club nor perform the exercises a physiotherapist showed him some time ago. He would be more willing to start exercising immediately if a fitness center was built on campus that is equipped with resistance training machines and personal trainers. This has materialized now, and Professor R walks straight to the center.

The personal trainer meets Professor R. What should he know about Professor R? What should he ask him, and how?

TAKE-HOME MESSAGE

Assessing medical conditions and possible contraindications for meeting general physical activity recommendations is an important step to prevent risks during exercising. Different assessment tools exist that can help professionals advise their clients. Moreover, these tools can help individuals in assessing their own challenges, and they can simplify the decision of whether or not one should talk to a physician. These approaches can make physical exercise safer, and prevent injuries and bad experiences, as well as support professionals in doing their work and improving maintenance within a program.

ASSESSING PHYSICAL ACTIVITY

CONCEPT OVERVIEW

Physical activity behavior can be performed at very different levels: mild, moderate, or vigorous. What is good for whom, and what are the recommendations in general? If we look at general guidelines for physical activity, the ACSM (3) recommends 30 minutes of moderate-intensity daily aerobic physical activity 5 days a week, or 20 minutes of vigorous-intensity daily aerobic physical activity three days a week, supplemented by 2 days a week of strength training, in order to create *health benefits*. Activity can be performed as part of daily life, in bouts of 10 minutes, or incorporated into a sports program. Recommendations differ with regard to body weight and the general aim of the physical activity (Table 2.6). These recommendations are similar to the 2008 PA Guidelines (4,8,13).

Thus, it is important to assess what the aim of the physical activity is, at what intensity level individuals perform the physical activity (it should be a moderate- or vigorous-intensity activity), and whether the recommended amount of minutes per week is achieved. As outlined in the "Assessment Modes" section of this chapter, this could be measured by observation (*e.g.*, monitoring attendance rates), by objective measures (*e.g.*, pedometers), or by directly asking the person (*i.e.*, subjective measures / perceptions). In the following subsections, we present some examples of assessment tools to measure behavior at the individual level. The following references provide a good illustration for such tools: *Godin Leisure-Time Exercise Questionnaire* (9) and the modified versions of the *Godin Leisure-Time Exercise Questionnaire* (9,17). Other examples are described in Table 2.7.

Different validated questionnaires exist, which assess physical activity behavior in comparable ways (16). Results of the questionnaire or the information gathered via questionnaire can provide useful information for developing interventions as we learn what people actually do, and where options for improvements may be (for a list of comparable tools, see reference 16, Table 2.7 and the "Web Resources" subsection in the References list).

TABLE 2.6 Recommendations for Weight Loss and Prevention of Weight Gain by the American College of Sports Medicine (4,8)

Moderate Physical Exercise should be Performed with the Aim of . . .	By. . .
. . .Preventing overweight (Body Mass Index ≥ 25)	. . .Exercising 150–250 minutes per week
. . .Reducing overweight by exercising	. . .More than 300 minutes per week
. . .Maintaining successful weight reduction	. . .Exercising more than 250 minutes per week

TABLE 2.7 Overview of Physical Activity Measures

Name of Questionnaire (Reference)	Dimensions	Number of Items / Time to Complete Questionnaire
Godin Leisure-Time Exercise Questionnaire (GLTEQ)	Leisure, sports	3 items, 2–5 min
Baecke Questionnaire (BAECKE)	Work, leisure, sports	16 items, 12–15 min
International Physical Activity Questionnaire (IPAQ long version)	Work, leisure, domestic and garden activities, sports	27 items, 15–20 min
International Physical Activity Questionnaire (IPAQ short version)	Work, leisure, domestic and garden activities, sports	7 items, 5–7 min

Source: https://sites.google.com/site/theipaq/

TABLE 2.8 Measurement of Different Intensities of Physical Activity, with Explanations

Intensity	Content/Examples
Vigorous physical activities	Heart beats rapidly, sweating
Moderate physical activities	Not exhausting, light perspiration
Mild physical activities	Minimal effort, no perspiration

Levels of Physical Activity

By means of the Godin Leisure-Time Exercise Questionnaire (GLTEQ) (see Table 2.8), one can measure how much behavior was performed during the last month. Behavior is measured in terms of the effort of activities. Clients are asked to report (a) their average number of sessions per week, and (b) the average duration of a session.

Responses for each of these three activity categories can be computed as the product of frequency and duration of physical activity. This can be done for each of the three levels, or as a sum scoring all three together: vigorous and moderate activities on one hand, or vigorous, moderate, and mild activities on the other hand. Alternatively, the three may be used as single indicators. As a result, an approximation of energy expenditure is obtained. A caveat of the GLTEQ is that it does not take different domains of physical activity into account. Physical activity can only be accounted for by means of physical exercise (Figure 2.6).

Domains and Components of Physical Activity

Since physical activity is not only performed as planned physical exercise, it may be worth considering the domain of activities: If interventions target specific subdomains, then these subdomains should be evaluated extensively as well (Figure 2.6). This can be done by assessing behavior with a rating scale that takes the four domains of physical activity shown in the next section into account.

SPECIFIC PHYSICAL ACTIVITY DOMAINS AND THEIR INTERRELATIONSHIPS

If the goal is to explain variance in behavior, domain-specific physical activity (such as physical exercise vs. active commuting) is impacted more easily by domain-specific variables. For instance, a domain specific variable that impacts physical activity is self-efficacy. This can be compared in the following ways: self-efficacy to perform fitness activities versus self-efficacy to commute to work, or motivational self-efficacy important for behavior

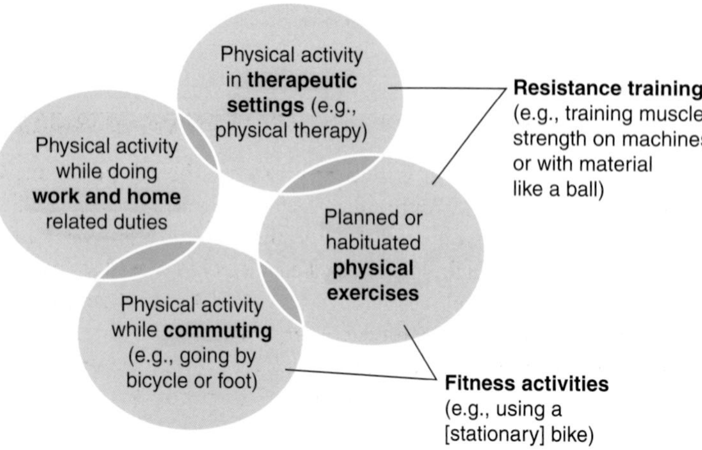

FIGURE 2.6. Domains and components of physical activity, there may be partial overlap (Please note: Physical activity while doing work- and home-related duties is typically not a target of interventions.).

initiation (starting a new behavior) and volitional self-efficacy imperative for behavior maintenance (see the "Evaluate Clients' Resources" section of this chapter). In contrast to domain-specific activity, if general physical activity (including, for example, commuting and household activities) is considered, specific variables explain less of the behavioral variance.

In clients, physical activity recommendations have to be modified accordingly. The ACSM provides specific exercise recommendations for older adults and individuals with chronic conditions (13).

For example, the recommended goal behavior is 3×40 minutes for cardiac clients per week. Clients can indicate frequency and duration of each behavior area by ticking one of the following options: "less than one time per week for 40 minutes" (1), "at least one time per week for 40 minutes" (2), "at least three times per week for 40 minutes" (3), "more than three times per week for 40 minutes" (4). Answers can then be categorized in such a way that a dichotomous variable results—for example, whether clients performed at least the recommended activity level (1) or not (0). Alternatively, such a Likert scale provides more information about the individual, as well as potential for improvements.

The two measures mentioned in the previous section (4 or 2 answering options) capture mainly:

- weekly frequency of physical activity due to leisure time physical activity, and
- weekly frequency of physical activity while commuting.

However, two other facets may also be considered. These other considerations include:

- weekly frequency of physical activity due to work, and
- weekly frequency of physical activity due to house and garden duties.

To assess these areas of activity, a questionnaire might ask the following questions: "In the last four weeks I have..."

- "...performed specific physical activities and sports (*e.g.*, at a fitness center, while playing soccer),"
- "...performed physical activity at work (*e.g.*, carrying weights, extensive walking),"
- "...performed physical activity due to commuting (*e.g.*, going by bicycle instead of using the car)," and
- "...performed physical activity due to daily chores (*e.g.*, physically exhausting care giving, garden work, climbing stairs, cutting the lawn, vacuuming)."

The items can be answered on a Likert scale (indicating the degree of agreement) or by indicating the minutes and sessions per week. Questions like those described in the preceding bullets can also guide observation (monitoring of physical activity behavior). This is illustrated in Case Scenario 2.4.

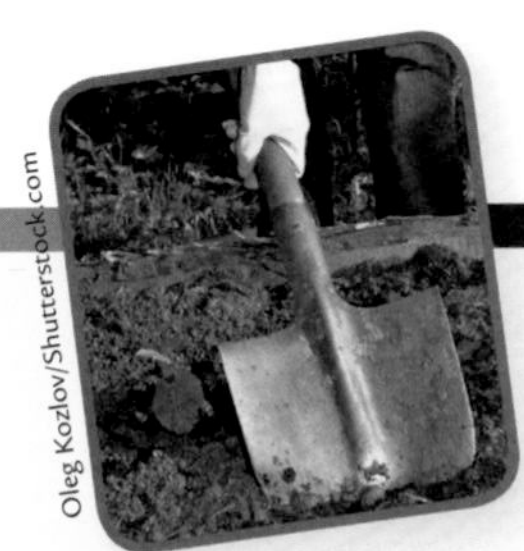

Oleg Kozlov/Shutterstock.com

Case Scenario 2.4

A group of gardeners is employed at a university to keep the campus in mint condition. They cut grass, trees, and bushes; they tear out weeds; and they care for the flowers. Some of the gardeners work as lawn mowers and transport compost with a little motorized vehicle. They carry heavy machines used for garden vacuuming and reforesting trees, and others do a lot of shoveling and cutting.

All gardeners receive the offer to join the recreation center, but no one shows interest in exercising here. How can we assess their activity level at work and in their leisure time? Should they be encouraged to work out in the recreation center? If so, how?

TAKE-HOME MESSAGE

Learning about what kind of physical activity a client is already engaged in enables the improved development of an appropriate exercise plan. Physical activity behavior can be performed in a variety of settings, and consists of very different aspects. To capture these aspects appropriately, and to evaluate whether an individual is meeting the recommendations, questionnaires and interviews should address different aspects of activities. Such questions can also guide observation (monitoring). Alternatively, objective measures like pedometers can be used to assess physical activity level. All measures can provide useful possibilities to follow up with the progress of behavior change:

- Scales to measure behavior (and other characteristics) (4)
- A collection of physical activity questionnaires for health-related research (16).

EVALUATE CLIENTS' MOTIVATIONS

CONCEPT OVERVIEW

If our goal is to know more about human behavior and what drives it, we need to know more about what exactly is going on in individuals' heads: Are they motivated to become or stay physically active? Do they intend to increase their exercising behavior? If our goal is to understand what drives human behavior, we need to appreciate the desires that lead individuals to become or stay physically active. This specific inquiry can be titled "motivation." People might be motivated to perform the recommended physical activity, which is an important prerequisite for actually adopting the behavior. Similarly, if people lack motivation, it is unlikely that a change in behavior will occur. Thus, it is essential to obtain more knowledge about the "readiness" for behavior: how close persons are to actually changing their behavior, or how far they have habituated a behavior.

Evidence

"Readiness to change" is a term typically used to capture even more than behavior and intention. "Readiness to change," also known as "stage (of change)," is conceptualized as a measurable indicator of behavior change and its psychological antecedents. People may or may not intend to change their behavior, which can be measured by intention assessments as well. Individuals could also be distinguished by whether they perform the recommended behavior, which is also measured by the behavior tools described earlier. However, we need further measures if we also want to know about the psychological characteristics: Are people performing physical activity in a *habituated* way—in other words, are they already exercising for an extended period of time? Are they at constant risk of stopping their exercise for certain periods at a time? We could use a special question measuring *habituation*, such as "How difficult is it to be physically active?", "I exercise regularly without giving much thought to it", or "How long have you currently been as physically active on a regular basis as you are now?" The main advantage of measuring stages is the ability to unite behavior, intention, and habituation into one measurement tool (see the following).

Motivation/Intention

Intention to perform behavior should be assessed in a way similar to behavior itself (Table 2.8). This could be accomplished by rating the following three items: "*I intend* to perform the following activities at least 5 days per week for 30 minutes. . ."

- "Vigorous physical activities (heart beats rapidly, sweating)";
- "Moderate physical activities (not exhausting, light perspiration)"; and
- "Mild physical activities (minimal effort, no perspiration)."

Answers can be assessed (as behavior, see earlier) on a six-point scale from *not at all true* (1) to *absolutely true* (6).

Intention should also refer to physical activity that is outside of work hours, and performed to an extent that is at least moderate. Clients can indicate at what frequency and duration they intend to exercise (see earlier). Again, answers can be categorized in such a way that a dichotomous variable results (active enough or not). Whether cardiac [orthopedic] clients intend to perform at least the recommended activity for three [two] times per week for 40 [20] minutes (1) or not (0); or whether a nonclinical person intends to perform at least the recommended activity, five times per week for 30 minutes (1) or not (0).

Stage of Change

According to stage theories (cf. Chapter 4), health behavior change consists of an ordered set of categories or "stages" into which people can be classified (14). These categories reflect psychological or behavioral characteristics such as motivation and physical activity behavior.

Classical stage assessments take time frames (*e.g.*, 30 days; half a year) into account (18). Contemporary assessments measure stages *without using a specific time frame* (10, 11). Individuals could potentially be asked to think about the last month, and then can be presented with the following question:

- "Did you engage in physical activity for at least 5 days a week for 30 minutes or more?" Replying with "yes" or "no" responses.

Further, they should be asked: "For the following month, do you intend to perform physical activities five times per week for 30 minutes or more?"—with possible answers being "yes" and "no."

Those individuals who indicate they were active in the past are then categorized as actors. People who answer that they were not active, but do intend to perform the recommended goal activity, are labeled intenders. Individuals answering that they have not been active, and are not intending to perform the recommended goal activity in the future, are classified as nonintenders. An example of a more refined stage assessment is shown in Table 2.3.

Based on their answers to the rating scale, individuals are categorized as *nonintenders*, *intenders*, or *actors*. Alternatively, people can be categorized into the following stages (see Figure 2.7):

1. precontemplation
2. contemplation
3. preparation
4. action
5. maintenance

The assessment can also be adapted to other behaviors that are relevant for health promotion (see the "Assessing Other Health Behaviors" section later in this chapter).

TABLE 2.9 Intervention Matrix for Health Action Process Approach (HAPA)-Based Stage-Specific Treatments

	Stage Group		
	Nonintender	**Intender**	**Actor**
Risk perception	x		
Outcome expectancies	x		
Self-efficacy (motivational)	x		
Goal setting/ Intention/ Motivation	x		
Action planning		x	x
Coping planning		x	x
Social support		x	x
Self-efficacy (volitional)			x

From Schwarzer R, Lippke S, Luszczynska A. Mechanisms of health behavior change in persons with chronic illness or disability: the Health Action Process Approach (HAPA). *Rehabilitation Psychology*. 2011;56(3):161–70, with permission.

With the necessary information, interventions can be tailored to psychological and behavioral characteristics of the stages. These are known as stage-specific interventions. We can capture stage movements prior to or after the actual behavior change by measuring stages, rather than just behavior (*e.g.,* development of an intention when moving from the nonintentional stage to the intentional stage). These changes might be important if we are interested in following up with changes that might not be visible in behavior change. If the stage assessment is filled out repeatedly—for instance, every half year—it could provide information as to whether individuals are moving forward or backward between stages, a success that might not be visible with behavior measures alone (cf. Figure 2.7). Sharing feedback about these changes can be an important strategy to motivate individuals, as it provides opportunities for ipsative feedback (individual frame of reference) in contrast to mere normative standards (external frame of reference).

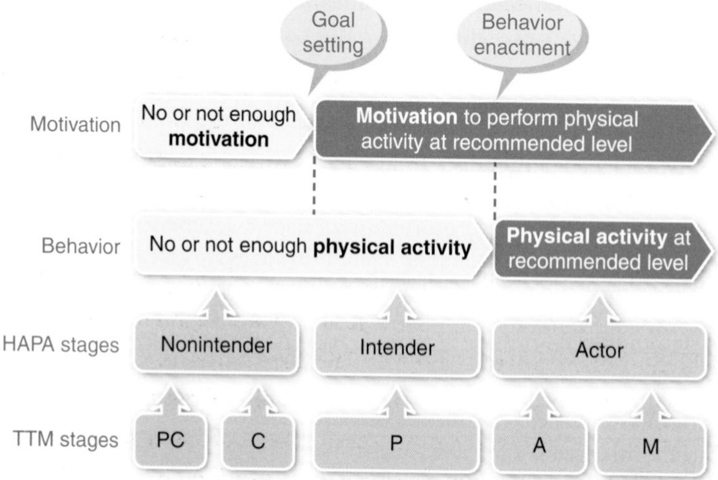

FIGURE 2.7. Motivation and behavior of individuals in different stages. HAPA=Health Action Process Approach (20); TTM=Transtheoretical Model (19); PC=Precontemplation; C=Contemplation; P=Preparation; A=Action; M=Maintenance.

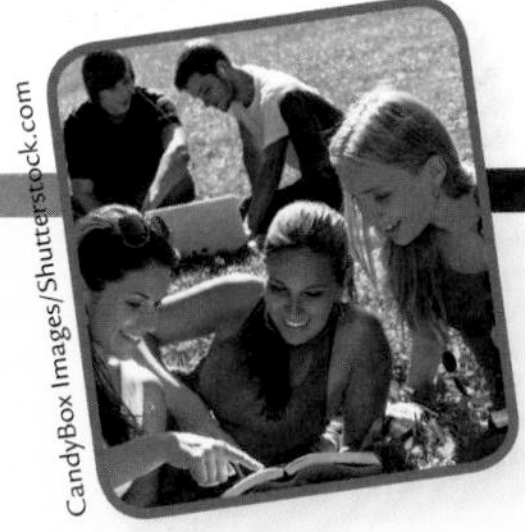
CandyBox Images/Shutterstock.com

Case Scenario 2.5

Once again, we invite you to think about the university example. This time we would like to know more about what the university members think and feel with regard to exercise—that is, their motivation to engage in exercise behavior. We therefore use the previously described questionnaires to assess the behavior of three selected people. Person A reports exercising on the campus once a week, and would like to extend her training program. Person B expresses that she is not doing anything and person C states that she is physically active every day for at least 30 minutes, but not on the campus.

If we compare the reports with the recommendations, person A and B would both be regarded as insufficiently physically active. Further, as there is a difference between A and B, what should we ask those people to learn about their motivation to exercise? Person C is meeting the recommendation, but still, is there anything that might be important to ask?

TAKE-HOME MESSAGE

If we measure motivation or assess the stage of an individual, we can gain much insight into the "readiness" of an individual to become and remain active. Intention and motivation are important determinants of behavior. Stage assessments also include behavioral aspects, which opens avenues for fast measurements of where people are in the behavior change process, and how close they are to the goal behavior. Such measurements can provide the basis for successful interventions in helping individuals to adopt and maintain their goal behavior.

EVALUATE CLIENTS' RESOURCES

CONCEPT OVERVIEW

Existing theories of such health behavior approaches are the *Social Cognitive Theory* (SCT, 5), the *Theory of Planned Behavior* (TPB, 2), and the *Health Action Process Approach* (HAPA, 20,21).

The HAPA has the advantage that it is a hybrid model, combining continuous models (like the SCT and the TPB) and stages of change (21). However, it is more parsimonious than other stage theories, which makes it easier to address the stages in interventions (21). The HAPA postulates when certain variables are imperative for stage movements (see Table 2.9).

These variables, which will be described in the following subsections, can function as resources for successful behavior change if they are high enough. If they are not high, they can be targeted in interventions to facilitate behavior change.

The HAPA distinguishes between three stages of behavior change (Nonintender, Intender, Actor). In the initial motivation phase of behavior change, known as the nonintentional stage, a person develops the intention to act. Risk perception is seen

continued

as a distal antecedent (*e.g.*, "I am at risk for cardiovascular disease"), but is itself insufficient to enable a person to form an intention or to change behavior. Instead, it serves to enable contemplation processes and further elaborates the thoughts about consequences and competencies of potential risk behaviors. Similarly, positive outcome expectancies (*e.g.*, "If I exercise five times per week, I will reduce my cardiovascular risk") are chiefly seen as being important during the motivation phase, when a person balances the pros and cons of certain behavioral outcomes. Further, one needs to believe in his or her self-efficacy, which is one's ability to perform a desired action (*e.g.*, "I am capable of performing my exercise schedule despite the temptation to watch TV"). Self-efficacy operates in concert with positive outcome expectancies, both of which contribute substantially to forming an intention.

These beliefs are needed to form intentions in order to adopt difficult behaviors, such as regular physical exercise. If the intention is successfully formed, the following phase is entered (the intentional stage). This second phase is labeled as volitional, since the regulation of behavior is under volitional control. After a person develops an inclination toward a particular health behavior, "good intentions" must be transformed into detailed instructions explaining how to perform the desired action. However, it is not sufficient to only initiate an action; maintenance of the action is important as well.

Maintenance of the action is achieved by self-regulatory skills and strategies, such as social support. Social support can be conceptualized as either a self-regulatory *barrier* or a self-regulatory *resource*. Missing social support can be a barrier to maintaining behavior, whereas instrumental, emotional, and informational social support can enable the adoption and continuation of behaviors. This was found in many exercise studies with chronically ill people, such as individuals with diabetes (17). Another important self-regulatory factor is action and coping planning, as this enables translation of intentions into behaviors, and maintenance of the behaviors in spite of potential obstacles. Measurements of these variables will be outlined in more detail in the following subsections.

Risk Perception

Risk perception can be measured by items such as "How high would you estimate the likelihood that you will ever have one of the following diseases: (a) cardiovascular diseases (*e.g.*, heart attack, stroke), or (b) diseases of the musculoskeletal system (*e.g.*, osteoarthritis, herniated vertebral disk)?" Any health risk can be added to this measurement, which is especially recommended if the clients harbor diseases / health risks. Responses should be given on a Likert scale like "*very low likelihood*" (1) and "*very high likelihood*" (6).

Outcome Expectancies

Positive outcome expectancies (pros) and *negative outcome expectancies (cons)* can be assessed with the first part of the statement:

- "If I engage in physical activity at least five times per week for 30 minutes. . ."

and a following second part of potential statements assessing pros and cons.
Pros are measured with items such as:

- "I would feel better afterward."
- "I will meet friendly people."
- "My ability to stretch would increase."

Cons can be assessed by items such as:

- "It will probably cost me a lot of money every time."
- "I would have to invest a lot (*e.g.*, into organizing my weekly schedule)."

Answers for pros and cons are assessed using six-point scales ranging from *totally disagree* (1) to *totally agree* (6). If cons outreach the pros, professionals can work with their clients on these beliefs and barriers.

Self-Efficacy

Self-efficacy can be subdivided into motivational self-efficacy and volitional self-efficacy. Motivational self-efficacy is imperative for generally getting started, while volitional self-efficacy is rather important for maintaining a routine and getting back on track.

MOTIVATIONAL SELF-EFFICACY

Motivational self-efficacy is measured with the statement "I am certain . . ." followed by one of two items: 1."...that I can be physically active on a regular basis, even if I have to mobilize myself" or 2."...that I can be physically active on a regular basis, even if it is difficult".

VOLITIONAL MAINTENANCE SELF-EFFICACY

Volitional maintenance self-efficacy is measured with the statement "I am capable of performing physical exercise on a regular basis..." followed by one of the two items:

1. "...even if it takes some time until it becomes a routine," or
2. "...even if I need several trials until I am successful"

Volitional self-efficacy on *recovery self-efficacy* can be described as: confidence to resume a physically active lifestyle, although at times physical activity was not present; or the confidence to resume regular exercise after failures and be prepared for possible failures in the future; and finally, the confidence to resume physical activity after suffering from an illness. The *items* for volitional self-efficacy on recovery self-efficacy can be worded as: "I am confident that I can resume a physically active lifestyle, even if I have relapsed several times in my life" or "I am confident that I will be able to resume my regular exercises after failures, and that I will be able to brace myself for possible failures" or "I am confident that I can resume my physical activity, even when feeling weak after suffering an illness." Answers can be assessed using six-point scales ranging from *totally disagree* (1) to *totally agree* (6).

Action Planning and Coping Planning

Action planning is making a plan to actually perform the intended behavior. Coping planning is a strategy of what to do in the face of barriers.

ACTION PLANNING

Action planning can be assessed with four items addressing the conditions of when, where, and how. The items could be worded: "for the month after rehabilitation, I have already planned..." (1) "...which physical activity I will perform (*e.g.*, walking)," (2) "...where Iwill be physically active (*e.g.,* in the park)," (3) "...on which days of the week I will be physically active," and (4) "...for how long I will be physically active." Answers can be assessed using six-point scales ranging from *totally disagree* (1) to *totally agree* (6).

COPING PLANNING

Coping planning can be measured with the statement "I have made a detailed plan regarding..." and the items (1) "...what to do if something interferes with my plans," (2) "...how to cope with possible setbacks," (3) "...what to do in difficult situations in order to act according to my intentions," (4) "...which good action opportunities to take," and (5) "...when I have to pay extra attention to prevent lapses." These items are measured with a six-point rating scale ranging from *never* (1) to *always* (6).

Social Support

Perceived social support can stem from different sources, such as family and friends. Social support regarding physical activity can be assessed with 10 items. First, individuals are asked to rate "my family..." and second, to rate "my friends..." with the following items: (1) ... encouraged me to perform my planned activities, (2) ... reminded me to engage in physical activity, (3) ... helped me to organize my physical activity, (4) ...took care of my home, giving me the possibility to engage in physical activity, (5) ...joined my physical activity program. Alternatively, friends and family can also be combined in order to gain one single item stem. The answers should be given on a six-point rating scale ranging from *never* (1) to *always* (6), or from *totally disagree* (1) to *totally agree* (6). Generally, clients appreciate if the answering options are essentially equal throughout the questionnaire or interview.

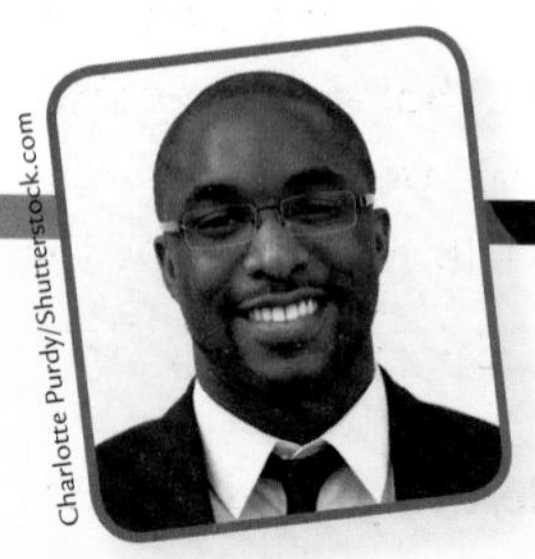
Charlotte Purdy/Shutterstock.com

Case Scenario 2.6

An employee known as Mr. S receives an invitation for a test training in a new recreation center. He was impressed by both the accessibility and high quality of the facilities. Prior to the first visit, he takes part in a personal training session. The trainer tells him "I highly recommend that you come at least three times per week and work out for 30 minutes or more, as this will improve your fitness and benefit your health." Mr. S replies "Yes, I will try to." He is actually thinking, however, that this will not be possible due to his work load and his other activities.

Over the course of the first weeks, he works out three times per week. In the subsequent six weeks, he exercises only once per week. Coincidentally, Mr. S bumps into his trainer. His trainer asks him how his workout routine is coming along, to which he replies that he enjoys working out once a week and although he realizes he should exercise more often, his busy schedule cannot allow for it and he is satisfied with his once-a-week routine

Perhaps Mr. S should be informed about risks and resources, trained to believe in his own competencies, and supported in how to manage temptations. Any of these options may work, yet a strong theory is needed in order to support individuals in a better way. A theory-and evidence-based approach is the most effective way to understand the client's problems, to develop a properly executed intervention, and to know what to evaluate after the intervention (*i.e.,* what steps should be taken at the end of the personal training session), such as what would come after the personal training session.

TAKE-HOME MESSAGE

If the goal is to increase behavior and intention, specific factors should be addressed. Risk perception and outcome expectancies are especially important for becoming motivated to change. Planning bridges the gap between intention and behavior, and self-efficacy and social support are central factors in all phases of behavior change. Thus, it is crucial to measure the level of these variables, so that any lack of such resources can then be addressed in interventions.

ASSESSING OTHER HEALTH BEHAVIORS

CONCEPT OVERVIEW

Many people hold life goals that can drive different behaviors. For instance, individuals want to socialize, and therefore may engage in activities such as an exercise class with other people, going out for a drink, or smoking. Other people strive for weight loss, and therefore engage in physical activity. At the same time, they follow a specific diet and smoke to suppress their appetite and increase metabolism. A third group might feel highly stressed, and therefore seeks relaxation by watching TV, engaging in special physical activity like yoga, or consuming chocolate.

All of the previously mentioned groups perform physical activity, but with markedly different motivations for executing the activity. All three also display other behaviors that might be beneficial for their health, like following a healthy diet, or may be counterproductive such as smoking and alcohol consumption, or TV watching. A recent study (12) demonstrated that those people who were watching more TV gained more weight within 4 years (0.31 lb more weight for 1 hour more of TV watching per day; http://www.nejm.org/doi/pdf/10.1056/NEJMoa1014296).

Different motivations result in different behaviors. For example, the socializing group X might also be fitness-oriented. Thus, drinking alcohol and smoking is conflicting with the groups' goal to become and stay fit. Perhaps they refrain from smoking, but have no further will left for abstaining from sedentary behaviors while in company.

Overall, looking at more behaviors besides physical activity might help to:

- comprehensively understand physical activity, as well as the occurrence of specific problems (Figure 2.4),
- understand why a behavior seems to be ineffective, although it should lead to a specific outcome (such as weight loss),
- make people more satisfied with thriving in their life-goals, and
- improve the healthy lifestyles of clients.

Thus, the assessment and appreciation of other health behaviors is also important (Figure 2.8). This can be done by examining the behavior as well as its determinants, such as intention toward the different physical activities, or stages of change (10,11).

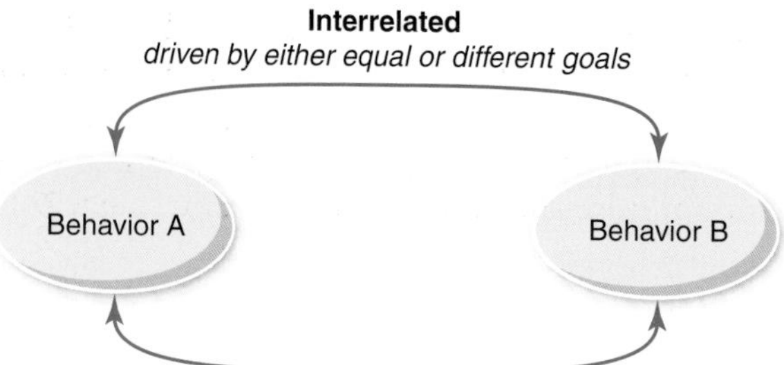

FIGURE 2.8. Interrelations between different behavior domains.

Health-Promoting Lifestyle Profile II (HPLP II)

The HPLP-II (24) measures the degree to which clients engage in an overall health-promoting lifestyle (24). It consists of 52 items, which are divided into six subscales of a health-promoting lifestyle, such as physical activity, nutrition, and stress management etc. Respondents are asked to indicate how often they engage in each behavior (never, sometimes, often, or routinely). The advantage is that the habituated lifestyle factors are assessed, not only single behaviors. Item examples are:

- "Follow a planned exercise program."
- "Choose a diet low in fat, saturated fat, and cholesterol."
- "Get enough sleep."
- "Report any unusual signs or symptoms to a physician or other health professional."
- "Expose myself to new experiences and challenges." (24)

The main advantage of this self-report questionnaire is that it covers very different aspects. Also it has been used in many previous studies. However, it is not clear whether the items measure behavior or attitudes and wishes. Thus, in the following paragraph we describe easy ways to measure different behaviors by means of stage assessment, as stages contain both behavior and motivation, and stage assessments have very few items. (See Figure 2.7 and Table 2.3.)

Dietary and Eating Habits

Regarding the *fruit and vegetable consumption stage*, the question should be "Please think about what you have consumed during the last week. Did you eat five portions of fruits and vegetables per day?"

Alternatively or additionally, a *balanced diet stage* can be measured with the instruction: "Do you eat a balanced diet on a typical day? A balanced diet consists of different aspects in addition to fruits and vegetables. Particularly, the five facets are:

1. Choice and appropriate amounts of overall calories
2. Plenty of whole grains and potatoes
3. Moderate amounts of meat, meat products, and eggs
4. Decreasing fat and fatty food intake
5. Limiting sugar and salt intake"

Moreover, a *healthy drinking stage* can be assessed with "Please think about what you typically drink. Do you drink 1.5 liters of nonalcoholic and noncaffeinated beverages (water, juice, fruit, and herbal tea) during the day?"

All behaviors can be assessed in terms of stages (12; Figure 2.7; Table 2.3). Clients can respond by means of a rating scale, with answering options being "no, and I do not intend to start" (precontemplation, PC), "no, but I am considering it" (contemplation, C), "no, but I seriously intend to start" (preparation, P), "yes, but only for a brief period of time" (action, A), and "yes, and for a long period of time" (maintenance, M). (See Figure 2.7 and Table 2.3.)

Smoking

Smoking behavior can be assessed with the standard question: "Do you currently smoke cigarettes?" with a yes/no response option. Current smokers should then be asked to indicate the amount of cigarettes they smoke per day. If clients answer the question "Do you currently smoke cigarettes?" with no, they are then asked, "Have you ever smoked cigarettes?" with a yes/no response option. Responses to these two items can be used to classify respondents as current smokers, former smokers, or never smokers.

Alternatively, some authors also suggest asking directly, and letting individuals indicate the best matching statement: "Are you a. . ."

1. "regular smoker?"
2. "occasional smoker?"
3. "ex-smoker (don't smoke anymore, but used to)?"
4. "non-smoker (don't smoke and never did)?" (33)

Alcohol Use

The *alcohol consumption* stage should be assessed with "Please think about what you typically drink. Do you avoid drinking alcoholic beverages on a daily basis (less than a glass of wine or a bottle of beer per day)?" The instruction is the same for all behaviors: "Please choose the statement that describes you best." Clients should be provided with a rating scale that has the following answering options: "No, and I do not intend to start" (Precontemplation, PC); "No, but I am considering it" (Contemplation, C), "No, but I seriously intend to start" (Preparation, P); "Yes, but this is very difficult for me" (Action, A); and "Yes, and this is very easy for me" (Maintenance, M). (See Figure 2.7 and Table 2.3.)

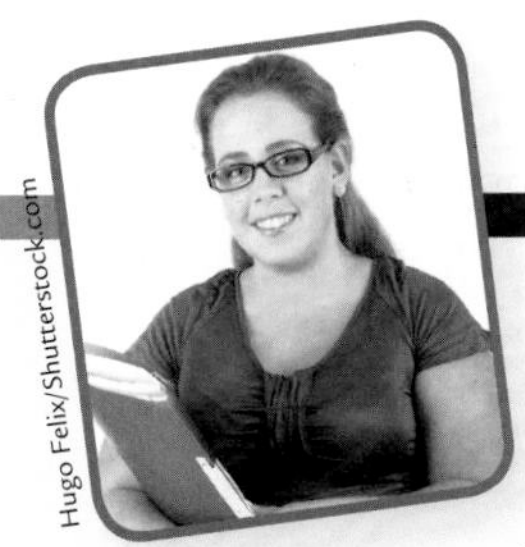

Hugo Felix/Shutterstock.com

Case Scenario 2.7

Student Y, an obese student, comes to the recreation center of the university and expresses her desire to lose weight. She has tried different strategies, including regular physical activity. Although she works out regularly, she has not managed to reduce her weight significantly. The instructor interviews her about the kind of exercises she does, and some other lifestyle factors, such as her diet, which contains a lot of fruits and vegetables, including potatoes. It turns out that student Y also has foods such as chips and French fries in mind when talking about potatoes. Student Y admits that she drinks sugar-sweetened beverages regularly. Furthermore, it becomes obvious that she gets less than 6 hours of sleep per night on most nights during the week, and that she watches television for a couple of hours every night.

Is there any chance we can provide support to reduce student Y's body weight? Can a revised training schedule help student Y? What should the trainer recommend?

TAKE-HOME MESSAGE

Physical activity and different behaviors are interrelated, not only in determining health, but also in terms of facilitating and hindering each other, in which they work in orchestration. They can be driven by equal or different goals. Other psychological mechanisms include the *transfer* of knowledge and skills from one behavior domain to another: One might have learned how to plan the goal pursuit in one behavior domain, such as how to do daily exercises for the back (regarding self-efficacy), and can now apply these skills to another behavior domain, such as managing to commute actively by getting off the bus one station early (with similar self-efficacy). People might also have severe problems with *coordinating* different behaviors, such as being exhausted by active commuting or the attempt to stop smoking, and then not feeling able to eat a healthy diet. To take this into consideration, different behaviors should be assessed.

CHAPTER TAKE-HOME MESSAGE

Assessment is central when the aim is to better understand the individual, and his or her needs and resources. Very different options for assessment exist. All have advantages and disadvantages, thus it is important to decide what to measure and for what purpose. Further, we need information about one's motivation and experiences to optimally individualize and promote health behavior. On the basis of such collected data, effective interventions can be designed, provided, and implemented. Furthermore, on the basis of proper measurement, the effectiveness of interventions can be evaluated.

REFERENCES

1. Ainsworth BE, Haskell WL, Whitt MC, Irwin ML, Swartz AM, Strath SJ. Compendium of physical activities: An update of activity codes and MET intensities. *Medicine & Science in Sports & Exercise.* 2000;32(9 Suppl.):S498–504.
2. Ajzen I. The theory of planned behavior and organizational behavior. *Human Decision Processes.* 1991;50:179–211.
3. American College of Sports Medicine. *ACSM's Guidelines for Exercise Testing and Prescription.* 9th ed. Baltimore (MD): Lippincott Williams and Wilkins; 2014.
4. American College of Sports Medicine. *Exercise recommendations specifically for different health conditions* [Internet]. [cited 2009. Available from: http://www.exerciseismedicine.org/YourPrescription.htm.
5. Bandura A. Health promotion by social cognitive means. *Health Education & Behavior.* 2004;31(2):143–64.
6. Bronfenbrenner U. *The Ecology of Human Development.* Cambridge (MA): Harvard University Press; 1979.
7. Brown WJ, Bauman AE. Comparison of estimates of population levels of physical activity using two measures. *Australia and New Zealand Journal of Public Health.* 2000;24:520–5.
8. Donnelly JE, Blair SN, Jakicic JM, Manore MM, Rankin JW, Smith BK. American College of Sports Medicine Position Stand. Appropriate physical activity intervention strategies for weight loss and prevention of weight regain for adults. *Medicine & Science in Sports & Exercise.* 2009;41:459–71.
9. Godin G, Shephard RJ. A simple method to assess exercise behavior in the community. *Canadian Journal of Applied Sport Sciences.* 1985;10:141–6.
10. Lippke S, Fleig L, Pomp S, Schwarzer R. Validity of a stage algorithm for physical activity in participants recruited from orthopedic and cardiac rehabilitation clinics. *Rehabilitation Psychology.* 2010;55: 398–408.
11. Lippke S, Nigg CR, Maddock JE. Multiple behavior change clusters into health-promoting behaviors and health-risk behaviors: Theory-driven analyses in three international samples. *International Journal of Behavioral Medicine.* 2012.
12. Mozaffarian D, Hao T, Rimm EB, Willett WC, Hu FB. Changes in diet and lifestyle and long-term

weight gain in women and men. *New England Journal of Medicine*. 2011;364:2392–404.

13. Nelson ME, Rejeski WJ, Blair SN, et al. Physical activity and public health in older adults: Recommendation from the American College of Sports Medicine and the American Heart Association. *Medicine and Science in Sports and Exercise*. 2007; 39(8):1435–45.
14. Nigg CR. There is more to stages of exercise than just exercise. *American College of Sports Medicine*. 2005; 33:32–5.
15. Pecoraro RE, Inui TS, Chen MS, Plorde DK, Heller JL. Validity and reliability of a self-administered health history questionnaire. *Public Health Rep*. 1979; 94(3):231–8.
16. Pereira MA, Fitzer Gerald SE, Gregg EW, et al. A collection of physical activity questionnaires for health-related research. *Medicine & Science in Sports & Exercise Suppl to*. 1997;29(66 Suppl):S1-205.
17. *Physical activity guidelines for Americans* [Internet]. [cited 2008. Available from: http://www.health.gov/paguidelines/ & FITT dimensions].
18. Plotnikoff RC, Lippke S, Reinbold-Matthews M, et al. Assessing the validity of a stage measure on physical activity in a population-based sample of individuals with type 1 or type 2 diabetes. *Measurement in Physical Education and Exercise Science*. 2007;11(2):73–91.
19. Prochaska JO, DiClemente CC, Norcross JC. In search of how people change: Applications to addictive behaviors. *American Psychologist*. 1992;47(9): 1102–14.
20. Schwarzer R. Modeling health behavior change: How to predict and modify the adoption and maintenance of health behaviors. *Applied Psychology*. 2008;57:1–29.
21. Schwarzer R, Lippke S, Luszczynska A. Mechanisms of health behavior change in persons with chronic illness or disability: the Health Action Process Approach (HAPA). *Rehabilitation Psychology*. 2011;56(3):161–70.
22. Shephard RJ. PAR-Q, Canadian home fitness test and exercise screening alternatives. *Sports Medicine*. 1988;5(3):185–95.
23. Thomas S, Reading J, Shephard RJ. Revision of the Physical Activity Readiness Questionnaire (PAR-Q). *Canadian Journal of Sport Sciences*. 1992; 17(4):338–45.
24. Walker SN, Sechrist KR, Pender NJ. The health-promoting lifestyle profile: development and psychometric characteristics. *Nursing Research*. 1987; 36:76–81. Tool available at: http://www.unmc.edu/nursing/docs/English_HPLPII.pdf

FURTHER WEB RESOURCES

BRFSS as an alternative questionnaire [Internet]. Available from: http://www.cdc.gov/brfss/questionnaires/english.htm.

Different validated scales to measure behavior and guide how to select a measurement [Internet]. Available from: http://toolkit.s24.net/physical-activity-assessment/.

Physical activity resource center for public health: Database of physical activity measures from (University of Pittsburg) [Internet]. Available from: http://www.parcph.org/assess.aspx.

Scales to measure different social-cognitive variables [Internet]. Available from: http://www.gesundheitsrisiko.de/docs/RACKEnglish.pdf.

Scales to measure self-efficacy, barriers, perceived severity, perceived vulnerability [Internet]. Available from: http://dccps.cancer.gov/brp/constructs/.

Scales to measure social support [Internet]. Available from: http://userpage.fu-berlin.de/~health/soc_e.htm..

Schwarzer, R et al. *Assessment and analysis of variables* [Internet] [cited 2003. Available from: http://web.fu-berlin.de/gesund/hapa_web.pdf.]

CHAPTER 3

Building Skills to Promote Physical Activity

Ryan E. Rhodes and Kristina Kowalski

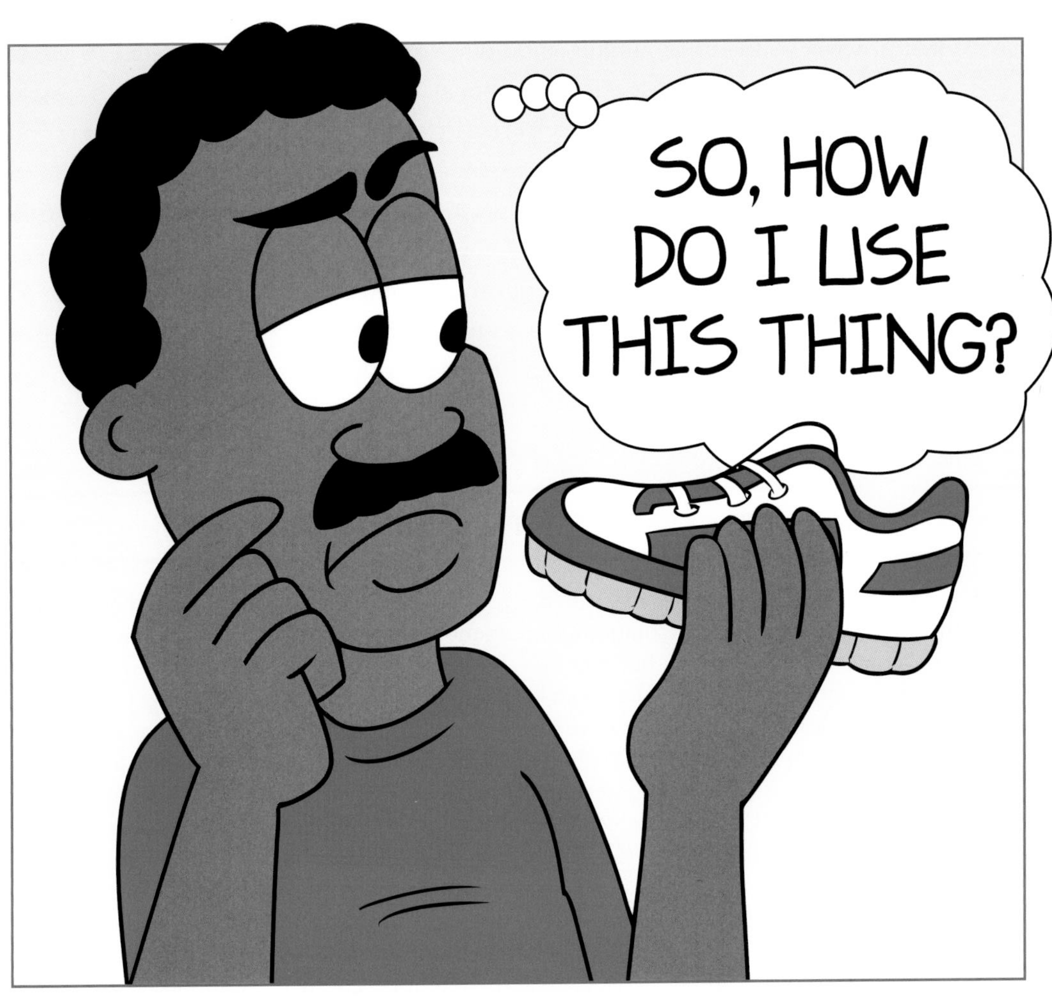

CONCEPT OVERVIEW

Our understanding of the factors that influence physical activity has shifted over the last 20 years (116). Initially, there was considerable focus on the individual-level factors responsible for why some people were active, while others were not. The reasons were considered within the realm of personal responsibility, motivation, and self-discipline. Over time, this focus for understanding physical activity has shifted to ecological models (129) that include individual, social, environmental, and policy factors that all contribute to physical activity participation. While this approach is far more likely to yield an overall accuracy in understanding physical activity, the focus on personal responsibility remains no less important. Clearly, an individual holds a great amount of agency over whether they engage in physical activity. Environmental access to exercise equipment and recreation facilities is very high in most developed countries (27,42) and the social norms regarding the benefits of physical activity are very positive across all ages (56,130,133). Indeed, personal motivation is described as the critical barrier among people who are inactive (26).

Therefore, the skills and strategies that people can use in order to promote their own physical activity is still of paramount importance to trainers and of key interest to clients. This chapter outlines the most essential personal level strategies for building and sustaining physical activity motivation from prior research efforts. We begin by outlining the findings from individual-level theories used to understand regular physical activity behavior and then apply this evidence base to guide practitioners and users with skills and strategies to improve or sustain motivation. Throughout this chapter, we refer to worksheets to assist in these approaches. These worksheets can be found in From the Practical Toolbox 3.1 through 3.6. See also Table 3.2, a decision tree for appropriate uses of these strategies, and the sample case scenarios presented toward the end of this chapter.

EVIDENCE: THE INTENTION-BEHAVIOR GAP

Most of us can immediately understand the gap between our good intentions and behavior by thinking about New Year's resolutions. Getting more exercise or eating healthier are often our most popular "self-promises," but they can also include other areas of personal improvement, such as spending more quality time with loved ones, quitting smoking, exercising restraint over spending, or learning something new. Most of us also know only too well that those initial intentions do not always pan out as planned. Psychological/behavioral theories that have been used to guide physical activity intervention initiatives and explain behavior also include an intention concept (12,46,90). Indeed, in almost all of these models, intention is viewed as the proximal determinant of action (see Figure 3.1), much like our New Year's Evening hopes.

Intention represents the decision to act on a behavior in its most modest conceptualization (96), to the motivation required to act and organizational planning in its most conservative definitions (11,104). Overall, intention has been validated as a dominant predictor of physical activity in adults (131). Clearly the intention construct is important and, in any consideration of skill building or strategy, it would be prudent to consider all critical factors that may influence intention. Our current intervention research and theoretical tests in the physical activity domain have yielded a sound understanding of intent. Thus, the first part of our chapter follows the best practice research on how to increase physical activity intentions.

From the Practical Toolbox 3.1

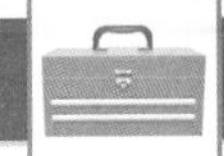

BEHAVIORAL PALATE WORKSHEET

Your belief in your ability and your attitudes toward an activity influence whether you are physically active. Belief in your ability to perform an exercise is an important part of both adopting a new activity and adhering over the long term.

Step 1: What Types of Exercise?

Instruction: Think about the physical activities you can do as part of your new exercise regime. List the type of exercises you prefer doing and your experience with each of these activities under COLUMN A. Then, list some NEW AND EXCITING MODES OF EXERCISE that you would like to try under COLUMN B, and lastly, list some CHALLENGING MODES OF EXERCISE under COLUMN C. Now that you have brainstormed activities, rate your confidence in your ability to perform/engage in each activity. Under EACH activity in EACH column also record your experience with these activities.

Please use the example provided to help you.

COLUMN A **Exercise Preferences**	**COLUMN B** **New and Exciting Modes of Exercise**	**COLUMN C** **Challenging Modes of Exercise**
Example Exercise: Walking **Confidence/experience:** Extremely confident. I walk my dog several short walks each day.	**Example Exercise:** Wii Fit **Confidence/experience:** Moderately confident. I've never been a videogamer, but it looks like fun.	**Example Exercise:** Swimming **Confidence/experience:** Slightly confident I haven't been swimming since swimming lessons when I was a kid, but I think a masters swim club would be a great way to meet new friends.
Exercise #1:	Exercise #1:	Exercise #1:
Exercise #2:	Exercise #2:	Exercise #2:
Exercise #3:	Exercise #3:	Exercise #3:

continued

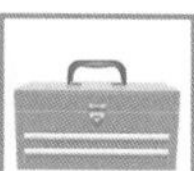

From the Practical Toolbox 3.1 *continued*

You will be more likely to persist in activities that you find enjoyable and interesting. Consider the activities you brainstormed about in the preceding chart. What factors contribute to your enjoyment of EACH OF THESE EXERCISES? How could you enhance your enjoyment of exercise? Please write down the factors that influence your enjoyment of exercise in the following table.

Step 2: Exercise Enjoyment and Strategies to Enhance Enjoyment

Instruction: Under COLUMN A, list where you will exercise and its PROXIMITY to your home. Under COLUMN B, list the AESTHETIC factors of the environment where you plan to exercise that are pleasing. Under COLUMN C, list the ways to enhance your engagement in exercise, including factors that increase your INTEREST in exercise, opportunities for SOCIAL interaction, and other aspects that provide VARIETY to your exercise routine (*e.g.*, listening to music).

COLUMN A **Proximity**	**COLUMN B** **Aesthetics**	**COLUMN C** **Interest**
Where will I exercise? Is the location where I plan to exercise close to my home?	Is the location a pleasant environment for performing exercise?	How can I. . . - make exercise more interesting/stimulating? - involve friends and family or others in exercise? - incorporate variety, and other aspects such as music to enhance my engagement in exercise?
Location #1:	Factor #1:	Interest:
Location #2:	Factor #2:	Social:
Location #3:	Factor #3:	Variety:

From the Practical Toolbox 3.2

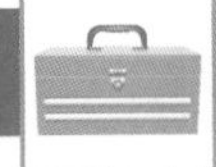

DECISIONAL BALANCE WORKSHEET

A helpful strategy when considering behavior change is to think about the benefits and the costs of your current behavior and of changing your behavior. Record the costs and benefits of your current behavior and of changing your behavior in the following table. Then, compare the costs and benefits of your current behavior and the new behavior. Ask yourself: Why do I want to change my behavior and become more active? What are the most important reasons?

Step 1: Costs and Benefit Analysis		
	Current Behavior ___________	**Behavior Change**___________
Benefits		
Costs		

Step 2. Take a look at your decisional balance worksheet. Ask yourself. . .

1. Why do I want to change my behavior and become more active?

2. What are the most important reasons for changing your behavior?

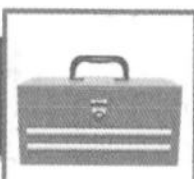

From the Practical Toolbox 3.3

GOAL SETTING WORKSHEET

Step 1: Think about your goals.

Think about what you want to achieve for your physical activity and fitness. Brainstorm a few goals that you want to get out of your new physical activity program. Write down the two or three goals that come to mind on the lines below.

1.
2.
3.

If you want to increase your chances of being successful, you should:

1. **Set goals that you personally value and that reflect your personal interests.** Strive to do something that you like doing and/or are interested in doing.
2. **Set goals that are not only challenging, but are also achievable.** Your goals should not be too hard or too easy.
3. **Set goals that are clear and specific.** Research shows that people are less successful when their goals are vague.
4. **Set both short- and long-term goals.** Make short-term goals along the way to reaching your long-term goals.

To help you set goals that meet these guidelines, make them SMART.
SMART goals are **specific (S; describe when, where, how, what), measurable (M; quantifiable), achievable/realistic (AR),** and include **time frame considerations (T).**

Step 2: Evaluate your goals.

Instruction: Take a look at your above goals. Are these goals SMART? Use the form below to help you evaluate your goals.

	Is your goal specific, measurable, and achievable/realistic, and does it include time frame considerations? Why? Why not? How so?
Goal 1	

From the Practical Toolbox 3.3 *continued*

	Is your goal specific, measurable, and achievable/realistic, and does it include time frame considerations? Why? Why not? How so?
Goal 2	
Goal 3	

Step 3: Reframe your goals using the SMART technique.

Instruction: Revise your goals below using the SMART technique. Remember SMART goals are **specific (S; describe when, where, how, what), measurable (M; quantifiable), achievable/realistic (AR),** and include **time frame considerations (T).** Design both short- and long-term goals.

		Short-Term Goals	Long-Term Goals
Goal 1	S		
	M		
	A/R		
	T		
Goal 2	S		
	M		
	A/R		
	T		
Goal 3	S		
	M		
	A/R		
	T		

Still, there are several advances in intention research within the physical activity domain that suggest some modifications to our theoretical and practical use of intention may be necessary. Though intention is a powerful predictor of physical activity, at least 70% of physical activity is not explained by intent. The intention-behavior gap so well known to students of New Year's resolutions is also present in our current theories. Some of this gap may be due to the waxing and waning of intention strength. A recent review of the moderators of the physical activity intention-behavior relationship showed that the temporal consistency of intention is the most reliable and largest moderator (111). Thus, many people don't really hold fast to their intentions and have a strong sense of resolve. More problematic to the intention-behavior relationship proposed in current theories, however, is the experimental evidence. For example, Web and Sheeran (141) conducted a meta-analysis of experimental evidence

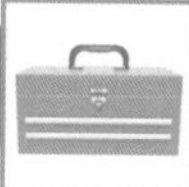

From the Practical Toolbox 3.4

PLANNING WORKSHEET

Most people fall short of achieving their goals because they don't establish an adequate ***plan of action***. Research tells us that people who plan out how they will reach their goal are more likely to succeed. This means that after you set a SMART goal you must then plan ***what you will do, how you will do it, where you will do it, and when you will take action.***

Step 1: ACTION PLANNING – What, where, and when will you engage in exercise?

Instruction: List the SPECIFIC EXERCISES you plan on doing under COLUMN A. Describe the LOCATION where this exercise will be performed under COLUMN B, and then describe WHEN you will perform that exercise under COLUMN C.

Please use the example provided to help you.

COLUMN A **Exercise Activity**	**COLUMN B** **Where I will engage in this activity?**	**COLUMN C** **When I will engage in this activity?**
Example Exercise: Walking	**Where?:** The park in my community	**When?:** Monday, Wednesday, and Friday evenings between 6:00 and 7:00
Exercise #1:	Where?	When?
Exercise #2:	Where?	When?
Exercise #3:	Where?	When?

Now that you have established an action plan, it is important that you anticipate and manage situations associated with performing unwanted behaviors and overcome barriers to the desired behavior using effective coping strategies. Effective problem solving and coping strategies are essential for translating intention into action and for maintaining a desired behavior or activity over the long term.

Step 2a: Coping Planning – Exercise Barriers and Strategies to Overcome Them

General Instructions:

Please think about ***each exercise activity*** you listed in Step 1: Action Planning. Which obstacles or barriers might interfere with the implementation of ***each of your exercise plans***? How could you successfully cope with these barriers? Please write down your ***strategies to overcome EACH exercise barrier*** in the following table.

From the Practical Toolbox 3.4 *continued*

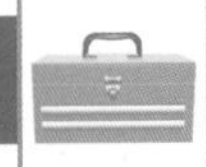

Instructions:

1. In COLUMN A, list the exercise activities you identified in Step 1: Action Planning.
2. For EACH ACTIVITY you listed in column 1, identify EXERCISE BARRIERS that may prevent you from performing the exercise activity under COLUMN B and STRATEGIES TO OVERCOME the exercise barriers under COLUMN C. Try to think of the main barriers that could get in the way of each activity and then strategies to overcome them.

COLUMN A Exercises/Activities	COLUMN B Exercise Barrier	COLUMN C Strategy to Overcome Exercise Barrier
1.		
2.		
3.		

Having trouble deciding how to reach your goal? There are a number of ways to reach a goal. Try brainstorming as many ways to reach your goal as you can. Don't worry about coming up with the perfect plan. Instead, just get those creative juices flowing and write down all the options that come to mind. You can use the following worksheet to eliminate options and to choose the method that is most suitable for you.

Step 2b. Coping Planning: Substituting Alternatives

Instruction: There is more than one method to reach your goals, each with its own advantages and disadvantages. Record your SMART GOAL below and generate a list of ways to meet this goal in COLUMN A. Brainstorm the advantages and disadvantages for each option in COLUMNS B and C. Compare the advantages and disadvantages for each option and assign a rank for each (*e.g.*, 1 = most likely to be successful, 3 = least likely to be successful).

continued

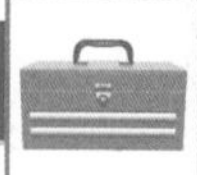

From the Practical Toolbox 3.4 *continued*

What is your goal?

COLUMN A Options	COLUMN B Advantages	COLUMN C Disadvantages	COLUMN D Rank
1.			
2.			
3.			

in 47 studies linking intention and behavior. The findings demonstrated that a large change in intention subsequently resulted in a small change in behavior. This demonstrated that while intentions and physical activity are correlated, a change in intention does not always create a change in behavior. This meta-analysis was recently replicated with physical activity behavior exclusively (112), and the results showed that changes in behavior, from changes in intention, may be even smaller than other health behaviors. The results cast considerable doubt that raising intention alone will result in increases in physical activity behavior.

Recent research that has separated the intention-behavior relationship into quadrants provides an explanation for the discordance (52,122); see Table 3.1. Specifically, intention-behavior relations are asymmetrical. Only three of the four possible quadrants yield ample sample sizes: those who did not intend to be active and subsequently are not active (nonintenders), those who intended to be active yet failed to meet these intentions (unsuccessful intenders) and those who intended to be active and succeeded in following through with their intentions (successful intenders) (109). These results demonstrate that intention is a pivotal construct but not sufficient to explain behavioral action on its own.

With this evidence in tow, the second half of our chapter is dedicated to the skills and strategies of translating good intentions into behavior. Several recent theories have been postulated and tested for closing the intention-behavior gap (53,54,98,126). We draw upon those findings to illustrate the best practice for translating strong physical activity intentions into actual behavior.

BUILDING INITIAL INTENTIONS

Understanding critical determinants of intention to exercise and subsequent exercise behavior is essential in helping clients maintain their positive intentions. Current research clearly identifies significant correlations between many psychological constructs and intentions to exercise (17,66,134,136). Most of these variables, however, are well represented under different names by two constructs contained within Social Cognitive Theory (self-efficacy, outcome expectancy), the Transtheoretical Model (self-efficacy, decisional balance), and the Theory of Planned Behavior (perceived behavioral control, attitudes) (11). For the purpose of this chapter, these overlapping behavioral determinants of exercise will be

From the Practical Toolbox 3.5

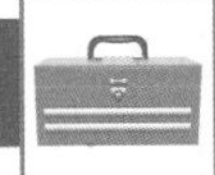

EXERCISE CONTRACT

For each SMART GOAL you create, complete the following contract to show your commitment to your goal. Refer to the contract regularly to remind yourself of your commitment.

1. Goal

My goal is to ______________________________.

2. How will I know if I have successfully reached my goal? List specific measurable behaviors necessary to reach my goal. Also, describe when and how often these behaviors will be measured.

- *To achieve this goal, I will* ______________________________.
- *To achieve this goal, I will* ______________________________.
- *To achieve this goal, I will* ______________________________.

3. Support Team or Resources

I will do this with the support of ______________________________

______________________________.

4. Rewards and Time Frame

As a reward for accomplishing the above goal by ____________________, *I will*

Insert date

____

______________________________.

This contract and my progress toward it will be revised on ____________________.

Insert date

5. Signature

By signing below, I, ____________________, *commit to*

____

Rewrite the details of above commitment here.

____

____

____________________ ____________________

Signature and date Witness signature and date

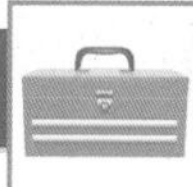

From the Practical Toolbox 3.6

SELF-MONITORING WORKSHEET

Journal and Tracking Log

Instruction: Each time you participate in your exercises, write down WHEN you did them in COLUMN A, WHAT you did in COLUMN B, WHERE and WITH WHOM you did them in COLUMN C, and HOW it felt in COLUMN D. In COLUMN E, write down any other important comments or observations you made while exercising. Use the example provided to help you.

COLUMN A Date and Time	COLUMN B What did you do (type of activity, intensity)?	COLUMN C Where did you do it? Who did you do it with?	COLUMN D How did it feel (before, during, after)?	COLUMN E Other Comments/ Observations
Example: September 23 7:00–8:00pm	**Example:** I went for a brisk walk.	**Example:** Around the park by my house.	**Example:** I felt less anxious afterward about work and it gave me a boost of energy.	**Example:** Walked by a group participating in a boot camp in the park. It looked like fun. It was sunny out. The beautiful weather made me smile.

TABLE 3.1 Intention-Behavior Relationship

		No Intention of Being Active	Intention of Being Active
Active?	N	Nonintenders	Unsuccessful intenders
	Y	N/A	Successful intenders

TABLE 3.2 Decision Tree for Choices of Worksheets and Strategies

Type of Client	Choose Course of Action	Useful Worksheets	Other Useful Strategies	Example of Appropriate Client for These Tools
Low intention / resistant	Major focus on building intent; minor focus on goal setting and action planning	Behavioral palate worksheet (FTPT 3.1); decisional balance worksheet (FTPT 3.2); goal setting worksheet (FTPT 3.3); planning worksheet (FTPT 3.4), focusing on Step 1: Action Planning	• Review benefits of exercise with focus on affective experience • Behavior modification (contingency management, reinforcement) • Self-monitoring	See Case Scenario 3.1 at the end of this chapter
High intention / problems translating intention into action	Major focus on goal setting, action planning, and coping planning	Goal setting worksheet (FTPT 3.3); planning worksheet (FTPT 3.4), focusing on all steps	• IDEA approach to problem solving • Building automaticity • Building social and environmental support • Self-monitoring	See Case Scenario 3.2 at the end of this chapter
Moderate intention / problems main-taining behavior	Focus on planning, especially coping planning; minor focus on building intent	Planning worksheet (FTPT 3.4), focusing mostly on Steps 2a and 2b; behavioral palate worksheet (FTPT 3.1)	• Review benefits of exercise with focus on affective experience • Behavior modification (contingency management, reinforcement) • Consideration of cross-behavioral conflict • Self-monitoring	See Case Scenario 3.3 at the end of this chapter

FTPT, From the Practical Toolbox.

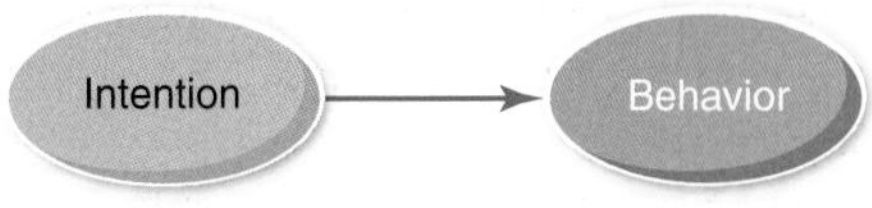

FIGURE 3.1. Intention is viewed as the proximal determinant of behavior.

grouped into the following two key constructs: (1) the expected outcomes of exercise, and (2) perceptions of control over exercise. Related evidence-based strategies or skills that the fitness and health professional can use with their clients to help them maintain their positive intentions to be physically active will also be discussed.

EXPECTED OUTCOMES OF EXERCISE

A recent review among nonclinical populations demonstrated that one of the most common approaches for promoting physical activity is to focus on increasing expected outcomes (117). The client's expected outcomes toward physical activity may represent a variety of factors, such as the expected outcomes/consequences of participating in physical activity behaviors, the advantages and disadvantages (pros/cons) associated with engaging in physical activity, and the anticipated benefits and barriers to participation (46). The value or significance the individual places on that desired outcome may also be important (*i.e.,* if improving fitness is highly valued by the individual, they will be more likely to engage in that behavior).

The construct, in various guises, is present in most of the theoretical models used in physical activity promotion and explanation. For example, in the theory of planned behavior (5), the attitude construct represents the summary thinking of expected outcomes of performing physical activity (*e.g.,* good vs. bad). According to meta-analyses of the theory of planned behavior, attitude is the strongest predictor of exercise intention (Symons Downs & Hausenblas, 41,60). This provides some evidence that our intentions may be influenced by what we expect to occur from being regularly physically active. Recent research also suggests that expected outcomes can be reliably distinguished in terms of either instrumental or affective properties (48,79,103,106), and these affective properties may have greater impact on physical activity intentions than instrumental properties. Affective expected outcomes refer to judgments about the pleasure/displeasure, enjoyment, and feeling states expected from engaging in a behavior, while instrumental expected outcomes refer to judgments about the costs and benefits of engaging in physical activity (79,114). Outcomes from regular exercise that do not directly involve feeling states, such as improvements in fitness and physical appearance, and reduced risk of chronic disease are instrumental; whereas outcomes that involve feeling states derived directly from the exercise experience such as enjoyment, boredom, pain, exhilaration, stress-relief, and satisfaction are affective. These two domains are also divided generally as proximal (affective) and distal (instrumental) in terms of their derived outcomes (11,58). In support of this distinction, recent studies have shown that affective attitude has better predictive ability than instrumental attitude in the physical activity domain (48,100,114).

CHANGING EXPECTED OUTCOMES TOWARD PHYSICAL ACTIVITY

Best Practice Strategies

Expected outcomes are thought to derive most of their foundation from the individual's knowledge base via education or a cost-benefit weighing process. Decisional balance, a construct from the Transtheoretical Model (96), is a decision making behavioral change strategy that may best encompass the weighting strategy. It involves having the client weigh the pros and cons of changing their physical activity behavior (25,86) and evaluate their beliefs about the benefits and barriers to becoming physically active.

Generally, weighing the pros and cons of engaging in a new behavior is particularly important in the initial stages of engaging in an activity when an individual is likely to perceive greater costs and barriers to physical activity than benefits. In support of the view that individuals are more likely to initiate a behavior if they perceive favorable outcomes associated with it, a recent review found that providing information to participants about the costs and benefits of engaging in physical activity produced significantly greater improvements in physical activity than those that did not (143). Being satisfied and valuing these favorable outcomes likely plays a greater role in sustaining physical activity behavior over time than the mere presence of positive outcomes.

A decisional balance worksheet (see From the Practical Toolbox 3.2) is one tool that can be drawn upon to help clients change their expected outcomes toward physical activity. Specifically, a decisional balance worksheet can be used to help individuals identify their perceptions about the pros and cons of adopting a physical activity behavior and the barriers (actual and perceived) to engaging in physical activity. Decisional balance worksheets, in which the benefits and costs of physical activity are written down, have been found to significantly increase exercise class attendance (*e.g.,* 62,89). Once benefits and barriers are identified, possible strategies aimed at enhancing benefits and minimizing barriers and shifting decisional balance in favor of physical activity (*i.e.,* so the benefits outweigh the costs) can be implemented.

When working through the benefits and barriers to engaging in physical activity with a client, it is recommended that affective properties of physical activity are the focus. Focusing on instrumental/distal outcomes such as weight loss, reduced risk of chronic conditions, improved function, fitness, and health will likely have more limited influence on whether the client chooses to adopt physical activity into his or her routine. Despite the negligible effects of instrumental attitude on physical activity (73,117), briefly educating clients on the benefits of regular physical activity is an appropriate course of action and is typically a more accepted approach than focusing on the hazards of inactivity. In fact, messages that are framed positively (*i.e.,* benefits of regular physical activity) are typically better received than those with negative framing (65,72,92). A handout briefly outlining the benefits of physical activity has been found to be effective in changing instrumental expected outcomes toward physical activity (68). See Chapter 3 for an example of such a handout.

When taking on the challenge of changing a client's expected outcomes toward physical activity, place more effort on helping clients to consider and focus on the exercise experience and the positive affective properties associated with the exercise experience (*e.g.,* enjoyment, intellectual stimulation, pleasant body states, mental health). Despite the reliable and robust association between affective attitude and physical activity, few studies have focused on modifying affective attitudes and the impact of these changed attitudes on physical activity intention and behavior (83,114). Several recent studies found that, in participants randomly allocated to either a control (no message), an affective message group, or a cognitive message group, individuals in the affective message group reported greater self-reported physical activity than other groups (34). Interestingly, the impact of affective messages on self-reported physical activity was greatest in those with a high need for affect or a low need for cognition suggesting that individual characteristics like preference for emotion or thinking may be important when targeting attitude change. In addition, a recent study with adolescents found that in inactive participants only, the affective message group had significantly greater increases in physical activity compared to the instrumental messages, combined messages, and control groups (124). Although confirmation of this finding and further exploration with different populations is needed, it appears that interventions targeting affective expected outcomes may have a greater impact on physical activity in inactive individuals.

In addition, print materials including messages targeting the stress-relieving and anti-depressive qualities of physical activity has been effective in changing affective attitude and exercise behavior (33,92). Parrott et al. found that print material targeting exercise enjoyment and mental health benefits of exercise was successful for improving exercise among those individuals with higher baseline levels of affective expected outcomes (in this case, attitude) but not effective for those with lower baseline levels. Caution needs to be exercised when choosing to use print materials to persuade clients to exercise. Personality characteristics and previous experience with physical activity should be considered. Focusing on the affective properties of physical activity (*e.g.,* enjoyment) may work as a useful prime or reminder for those who have found it fun and appealing in the past, but it may be a futile approach with individuals whose affective experience with physical activity has been negative (*e.g.,* boring, unpleasant, tiring).

Substantial evidence points to the importance of enjoyment and psychological well-being in motivating people to exercise (17,19,20). As such, creating opportunities for positive experiences with exercise, where people can learn to reinterpret physical activity as enjoyable and good for mental health may represent a more effective means to change expected outcomes. A second means of creating positive experiences with exercise is through manipulating the physical activity environment. Research also suggests that individuals should engage in physical activity in an environment that is aesthetically pleasing (*e.g.,* exercising outdoors (93)). Environmental aesthetics have been associated with both physical activity (64) and affective expected outcomes (105,108). Having the client focus on environment, rather than on the affective experience (*e.g.,* boredom, fatigue), may also improve the exercise experience through distraction. The behavioral palate worksheet found in From the Practical Toolbox 3.1 can help you with this task.

A third means to improve affective expected outcomes toward physical activity is through the introduction of novel, enjoyable, and engaging exercise activities. Rhodes and colleagues have demonstrated that interactive videogame bikes result in better adherence to exercise prescription than standard exercise due to an increase in affective expected outcomes (118,119). Thus, the selection of fun activities is paramount when possible. The behavioral palate worksheet found in From the Practical Toolbox 3.1 can also be used to help guide the choice of enjoyable activities.

Behavior modification strategies, including reinforcement control and contingency management, represent additional methods to motivate individuals to become active through short-term modification of expected outcomes (40). Reinforcement control involves increasing the frequency of the target behavior through positive reinforcement (adding something positive) and negative reinforcement (removing something negative (25)). This process introduces changes to the expected short-term outcomes of performing the act. Carefully structuring the exercise prescription at the client's level will be an important consideration in managing the client's immediate affective experience and increasing the likelihood that a client will perceive the exercise experience as rewarding (21). Intensity of exercise is one means of influencing experiences with exercise, and in choosing a starting intensity level a client's past history with exercise and current fitness levels need to be considered. High-intensity activities for clients who are resuming activity and are unfit are often deemed less enjoyable (43). Early on in the stage of exercise adoption, the affective experience of exercise may be negative (*e.g.,* soreness, pain, discomfort, fatigue) and it may take time for the positive affective benefits of physical activity to become reinforcing in themselves. In the interim, more immediate extrinsic rewards (*e.g.,* praise, concert tickets) and incentives may be required to help support engagement in the new behavior via the placement of external expected outcomes. Thus, creation of sought-after rewards for adherences and contingency structures are important strategies to help manage the consequences of physical activity. For example, participation in other preferred leisure activities could be made contingent on performance of exercise. Some caution should be applied to the utility of expected outcomes, more specifically external rewards, and their effect on overall behavior change.

TAKE-HOME MESSAGE

In summary, the expected outcome of physical activity is a well-demonstrated construct that has a potential impact on building the intention to be physically active. Consideration of the affective expected outcomes (*e.g.*, pleasure, enjoyment) may be even more important than the instrumental outcomes (*e.g.*, reducing risk of chronic disease, improved fitness). The best strategies to improve and change expected outcomes include decisional balance worksheets, information about the benefits of regular activity, and choices of pleasant physical activities and exercise environments. It is also possible that building in short-term expectations in the form of rewards or contingency scenarios may help increase initial intentions, although caution should be employed when using these extrinsic sources because they are unlikely to be sustaining.

PERCEPTIONS OF CONTROL OVER PHYSICAL ACTIVITY

A second major construct that the fitness and health professional needs to consider when helping their clients increase positive intentions is perceptions of control (*i.e.*, their degree of confidence) over engaging in regular physical activity. Almost all theories of human behavior include a construct related to control over behavior (12,46). For instance, self-efficacy is a construct from social cognitive theory, which is defined as one's belief in his or her capacity to perform a skill or behavior successfully (10,12). Similarly, perceived behavioral control, a construct from the theory of planned behavior, represents a person's perception of their capability (*i.e.*, perceived ease or difficulty) to perform the behavior, assuming he or she wants to (4,103). This perception of control reflects beliefs regarding past experiences and current skills. Perceived behavioral control/self-efficacy is one of the most reliable correlates of intention, comparable to expected outcomes of physical activity (57,128,131). The challenge, however, is often to separate real control issues from motivation, values, or affective expected outcomes (99,107). The best example of this difficulty may be with a consideration of the most common barrier to control over exercise: lack of time (26). Most people cite lack of time as the reason they cannot exercise, but actual leisure-time hours are not reliably linked to exercise (exercisers have just the same amount of time in a day as non-exercisers), thus the statement appears to be more of an excuse or cover for different values than a real control issue (22).

BUILDING PERCEPTIONS OF CONTROL OVER PHYSICAL ACTIVITY

Best Practice Strategies

Bandura (8,10) highlights the importance of four sources of information for self-efficacy:

1. Mastery experiences
2. Social modeling/vicarious experience (observing others similar to oneself experience success/cope with challenges)
3. Verbal persuasion (*e.g.*, praise, encouragement)
4. Judgments/interpretations of physiological/affective responses to exercise

These four sources, in diminishing value, are considered the important skills to build upon control perceptions of physical activity.

Mastery experiences are probably best created through shaping (*e.g.*, 25). Shaping is a strategy where reinforcement is used to help the client gradually increase his or her physical activity levels and feelings of competence. Begin by having the client participate in a behavior that he or she is capable of doing and then gradually increasing intensity, duration, and frequency of activity (*i.e.*, principle of progression). Choosing the appropriate starting level is a tricky balancing game of managing interest and difficulty. Failure to consider the principle of progression in exercise prescription may result in early attrition. The concept of mastery is considered the most powerful influence on self-efficacy, so negative experiences and failure to achieve the program can have deleterious consequences on self-efficacy. Thus, careful consideration of an achievable program is important.

It is essential that clients feel confident in their capability to perform their physical activity program. To enhance the client's sense of control, ownership, and confidence in their behavior change, and to ensure their physical activity program is matched with their own preferences and lifestyle, the health professional should get their client's input in the development of the program or have clients write their own program with guidance and support. With the help of the health professional, generating detailed instructions on the specifics of how, when, and where to engage in the behavior is a useful additional means to enhance feelings of control (67). Moreover, we suggest creating the opportunity for the client to have at least one positive mastery experience in a setting chosen by the client (*e.g.*, meeting at the local gym and working through the prescribed exercises). Providing positive reinforcement—that is positive and specific—for small behavioral successes and progress toward the desired goal may enhance initial self-efficacy and is consistent with Bandura's (8) initial tenets.

While mastery experiences are considered essential for improving control, social modeling (by people similar to the client) may also be important. The principle underlying this approach is to gain self-efficacy via vicarious learning. In the absence of personal experience, people look to similar others in order to gain information about whether a behavior is controllable (73). Thus, it may be important to ensure that participants see others successfully engaged in the target activity. This might be achieved through videotapes, demonstrations, or by having the participants themselves model the activity. The challenge for the physical activity promoter is to have modeling relevant to the client. Trainers often do not resemble the demographics and experiences of their clients, so choosing locations and times with others who are similar to the client becomes critical.

The principal strategy that underlies the enhancement of self-efficacy through verbal persuasion is that participants are provided with considerable information about the "why," "what," and "where" of physical activity. This might be achieved through orientation sessions, pamphlets, articles, newsletters, and so on, or through media presentations (*e.g.*, videotapes, television, newspapers). Information about the ease of performing certain physical activities may help build positive intentions in the short term. A concentration on the affective benefits of physical activity, similar to that recommended in improving expected outcomes may also benefit short- and long-term control perceptions. Convincing evidence is available to show that people who do not feel confident in their performance of a task subsequently perceive it as less enjoyable (63,87). Methods described earlier for increasing positive affective experiences with exercise are equally applicable here.

Finally, the principal strategy underlying the enhancement of self-efficacy through physiological states is ensuring that participants understand the body's response to activity. Physical activity produces increases in heart rate and sweating, for example. The meaning the individual attaches to those physiological changes is important. Individuals who are frequently active expect and understand the body's response to a physical load. Participants new to physical activity may not. Therefore, they must be helped to interpret what the physiological changes mean and how those physiological responses to activity changes with training. Educating beginners about the normal physiological consequences of exercise, post-exercise soreness, and the recovery timeline should help clients understand their body states and build their confidence around what can be expected from an exercise program.

TAKE-HOME MESSAGE

In summary, control over the act of physical activity is an extremely well-validated correlate of intention and a construct that resides in most theories of human motivation. Shaping the act in achievable bouts that successively move toward a larger behavioral repertoire (*i.e.,* small, achievable steps) is considered the best strategy to improving a sense of control. Short-term improvements in control may also be fostered by displays of similar others performing physical activity and information that attempts to persuade the client about the ease of the act. Finally, consideration of the affective properties (feeling states of physical activity) and education about some of the short-term negative body states, such as muscle soreness, should improve assessments of behavioral control.

While control over the act of physical activity may be important to fostering intentions, maintaining intention in the face of challenges and barriers over the long-term also requires an improved sense of control. Developing self-regulation skills is critical to developing perceived control over exercise, especially in translating positive intention into action and for long-term adherence. As such, these skills are described in the next section.

TRANSLATING INTENTIONS INTO ACTION

Most of our established theories used to aid in physical activity promotion and adherence have their main focus on the antecedents of intention. As demonstrated earlier, a robust level of evidence is present to suggest that building upon expected outcomes of the behavior and control over physical activity will result in increased intention. More recently, theories are being proposed to suggest that the translation of intention into behavior needs the same attention as building those initially strong intentions (53,54,97,126). Overall, these approaches suggest that behavior change from strong intentions depends primarily on self-regulatory skills, followed by partial automaticity of the act, environmental support for exercise, and the reduction of cross-behavioral conflict. The following subsections outline these factors and provide suggestions for successful intention translation.

Self-Regulatory Skills

According to Bandura's Social Cognitive Theory, self-regulation is defined as the strategies that an individual uses to regulate his or her goal-directed behavior or performance (9,12). A critical piece of goal-directed self-regulation is "the attempt to reduce discrepancies between current states and desired end states" (61, p. 1281). Although the term self-regulation is typically used to describe how a person regulates his or her own behavior when pursuing conscious intents or goals (*e.g.,* to lose 10 pounds), it can also occur outside of conscious awareness or "active" regulation on the part of that individual (*e.g.,* being surrounded with people who value physical activity and healthy living, 18,45). In other words, the environment, including the people surrounding the client, is also a strong shaper of his or her physical activity behaviors.

When working with clients to help them build the skills to facilitate their translating their intentions to become physically active into action, targeting self-regulatory skills is an excellent place to begin. Interventions targeting self-regulatory skills are among the most frequently used in the domain of physical activity behavior change and they also have the most convincing research support for their effectiveness in changing exercise behavior of all behavioral interventions (55,117,135).

Self-regulatory skills include, but are not limited to, *goal setting, planning,* and *self-monitoring* (84). Self-regulation can also involve skills such as *enlisting the support* of others and *creating environmental support* to promote physical activity behaviors. The following section will provide health and fitness professionals with the necessary tools to help their clients build skills in goal setting, planning, and self-monitoring. Building these skills with clients is an important step in helping clients translate their intention into action and to adopt and maintain a healthy lifestyle. There are many curricula available for both youth and adults—using these self-management skills—and research to support them. See "fitness for life" among others.

Goal Setting and Planning

Goal setting is a process by which an individual evaluates his or her current state or performance, creates a goal (*i.e.,* what the individual is aiming to achieve; the desired end state), and outlines the actions to be taken to reach that goal, 74,75,76–78,80,123). Goals can be described in terms of their properties:

1. difficulty (*i.e.,* difficult goals require more effort to be achieved)
2. specificity (*i.e.,* goals can vary on a continuum of specific to vague; specific goals are clearly defined, have a narrow focus, and outline the type and effort required to realize the goal)
3. proximity (*i.e.,* short vs. long term, 78,123)

Goals can also be considered process (*i.e.,* focused on the behavior being conducted, such as jogging for 30 minutes, three times weekly) and outcome (*i.e.,* focused on the end result of a behavior such as weight loss). Setting achievable, process-focused short-term goals fosters feelings of control more so than equally achievable long-term goals due to the frequency of feedback or cues regarding competence (13). Process-focused short-term goals are also valuable to avoid setting clients up for failure or disappointment by focusing only on long-term goals. Moreover, Shilts et al. (123) suggest that setting short-term goals rather than long-term goals mobilizes energy, while setting long-term goals may help with keeping the big picture in mind but they increase the likelihood of postponing efforts. Short-term goals can be used as one method of helping achieve long-term goals (13,75,80,125). Goal setting using the SMART framework is a popular approach to self-regulation (74,76,123) that incorporates many of the important properties of goal setting described earlier. SMART goals are specific (S; when, where, how, what), measurable (M; quantifiable), achievable/realistic (AR), and include time frame considerations (T).

Other important considerations when helping clients with their physical activity goals and plans are persistence (*i.e.,* "the tenacity people show in their endeavors to overcome difficulties and master challenges" (3, p. 285)) and commitment to change (*i.e.,* "the degree to which the individual is attached to the goal, considers it significant or important, is determined to reach it, and keeps at it in the face of setbacks and obstacles (71)). People have a tendency to set goals that they perceive as both desirable and feasible; however, this perception does not guarantee commitment to the goals (15). One means to enhance commitment is creating and signing an exercise contract, which serves to hold the individual accountable and is a visual reminder (*i.e.,* an extrinsic motivator) of the goal and required behavioral response (25,80). The exercise contract (*i.e.,* contingency contract, behavioral contract) should include the exercise (frequency, intensity, time, and type) the individual is committing to, how success (or lack thereof) will be measured, the consequences of not meeting the goal, and a reward (positive reinforcer) for successful completion of the desired behavior.

An individual must not only set desirable and feasible goals, but must also actively strive to achieve these strategies' goals in the face of challenges by employing effective coping responses. Goal setting is not sufficient on its own: In the absence of careful planning, many goals fail to be achieved (3). The distinction between two types of planning relevant to translating initial intentions into action can be made: action planning and coping planning (126,127). Action planning is a plan aimed at performing goal-directed behavior that specifies the when, where, and how to turn intention into action.

Coping planning, in contrast to action planning, involves anticipating and managing the risky situations associated with performing undesired behaviors and overcoming barriers to translating the intention into action by using effective coping responses (80,126,127). Coping planning is thought important not only in translating initial intentions into action, but also in maintaining long-term behavior change. Problem solving and substituting alternatives are coping responses that can be employed to manage risky situations. Problem solving is a means of brainstorming solutions to problems that may arise. The IDEA approach is a simple problem-solving framework that can be used to generate a solution to a problem behavior or barrier. The IDEA approach to problem solving involves:

1. Identifying a barrier to being active (I).
2. Developing a list of creative solutions (D).
3. Evaluating the solutions by choosing a solution and determining how the solution will be carried out (E).
4. Analyzing how well the plan worked and revising when necessary (A; 85).

Substituting alternatives involves brainstorming alternative options for achieving a goal, evaluating the advantages and disadvantages associated with each method of reaching one's goal, and then choosing the option that is most likely to lead to successful behavior change.

BEST PRACTICE STRATEGIES

Evidence for the use of goal setting strategies for fostering physical activity and dietary behavior change with adults is moderate (69,123); however, there is a need for further research to establish the efficacy with children and adolescents (123). Research has consistently demonstrated that setting goals that are specific, concrete, and challenging rather than vague and easy to achieve results in better performance (71,77). A meta-analytic review of the domain of sports and exercise found that short-term and combined short-term and long-term goals are more effective than long-term goals alone (69). Research has also demonstrated that tenacity/persistence is a good predictor of goal attainment (3). Moreover, when commitment to goals is high, individuals are more likely to act in accordance with their goals than when their commitment to goals is low (71). In one study, frequency of goal setting, which may reflect a higher commitment to behavior change goals or possibly may reflect more provision of feedback/cues regarding performance, was found to be positively associated with use of behavioral strategies for physical behavioral change (91). To assist in goal setting with your client, you can use the goal setting worksheet provided in From the Practical Toolbox 3.3.

In the domain of physical activity research, convincing evidence continues to emerge that planning is critical to translating intention into action (*e.g.*, 7,28,81,121,143). However, research also suggests that intention moderates the planning-behavior relationship, such that an individual with high intention is more likely to act on their plans than an individual with low intention (121,142). Evidence also supports the idea that action coping is more important at early stages of behavior change; whereas, coping planning is more important for adherence to behavior change (121,127). Moreover, accumulating evidence suggests planning interventions that include coping planning or both coping and action planning are effective in promoting adherence to health behavior change (6,126,144). In addition, in a recent meta-analysis, action planning was associated with increases in both self-efficacy and physical activity (143). It has also been found that people with higher self-efficacy benefit more from planning interventions than individuals who lack self-efficacy (81). A planning worksheet outlining how to make effective action and coping plans is provided in From the Practical Toolbox 3.4.

Self-Monitoring and Feedback

Self-monitoring refers to "paying attention to one's own thoughts, feelings, and behaviors, and gauging them against a standard" (80, p.154). Self-monitoring, typically through activity logs or journals (see the self-monitoring worksheet in From the Practical Toolbox 3.6), is an excellent way of keeping record of the dimensions of physical activity (frequency, intensity, type, time) and the context of physical activity behavior. Self-monitoring is a means to increase the client's awareness of their physical activity, the cues and consequences of the behavior, and the barriers standing in the way of successfully engaging in the desired behavior (25). It also provides the individual with feedback about their progress and may increase the individual's confidence in their ability to be active. According to goal setting theory, feedback regarding progress toward a goal is key to effective goal setting (77). Comprehensive psychological and exercise testing can also serve as a useful baseline for setting goals, monitoring progress/movement toward goals, and for evaluating and revising goals and the plans implemented to reach those goals (24). A more affordable tool is the pedometer/step counters, which also allows for goal setting, self-monitoring, and feedback. Ample research has shown that physical activity interventions that include self-monitoring are more effective in changing physical activity behavior than those that do not include self-monitoring (31,32,88).

Although behavior change from strong intentions depends primarily on the self-regulatory skills discussed earlier, there is emerging evidence that partial automaticity of the act, environmental and social support for exercise, and the reduction of cross-behavioral conflict also play a role. These concepts and preliminary evidence are presented next.

Automaticity

The automaticity construct has been controversial in human behavior models for almost 40 years (132), but its utility in predicting exercise has been established (49). Automaticity, in this context, refers to the performance of physical activity behavior without decision or formal thought. This automaticity is thought to develop from decisional/intended behaviors that were once conscious and motivation-based, but now are partially acted upon through environmental cues (1,2,137–139). Thus, automaticity is not random, thoughtless, action. Instead, automaticity develops from repeated, practiced, and highly motivated actions. The best example of automaticity may be in cases of driving behavior. Many people can drive to work and home without thinking about it. The behavior has become so practiced that it is essentially automatic. Indeed, when we attempt to alter this route—say to go to a store on the way home—we sometimes find ourselves home even though our initial intention was to stop at a different destination first! Certainly, in the case of physical activity, we are not suggesting that we want to build skills that create exercise robots (82); however, it does stand to reason that an efficient physical activity routine that can be performed without a constant motivational struggle is highly desirable. Based on prior theorizing and research (37,110), it has been shown that those who can act without conscious deliberation or rumination increase their chances in translating intentions into behavior. For example, it is proposed that someone who is so used to an exercise routine that they begin the act without deliberation via simple cues has a much better chance of action control than a person who has to engage in self-talk, planning, and decision making to act each time (139).

Automaticity is thought to be affected by prior history with the behavior and occur with behaviors that are highly practiced (14). Therefore, individuals with a more meager exercise history are proposed as at-risk for having low automaticity when initiating an intention into behavior. While prior physical activity experience may be an intractable determinate, skill building and prescriptions that involve exercise repetition in terms of time, acts, location, and other characteristics may help in habit formation (70). Another intervention with considerable utility to automaticity formation may be planning via implementation intentions (53). Implementation intentions, the act of setting plans about where, when, how, and what behaviors will be performed, are proposed to partially act as mini mental links between the behavior and environmental cues (53,54). It has been proposed and supported by research that implementation intentions may foster automaticity (54).

Environmental and Social Support

While we intend to make desirable changes like adopting regular physical activity, sometimes we need help to realize the goal. In this capacity, when one views exercise as a means for maintaining or improving friendships over the long term, it increases the likelihood that exercise outcome expectations are strengthened beyond our own individual goals. Similarly, other social outcomes such as building a sense of commitment or responsibility have shown supportive findings. Research on social affiliation among friends/partners (130), children (29,56), and even dogs (23,36,59) has supported this conjecture. Therefore, it is recommended that social interventions should focus on the broader social exchange and social meaning behind the regular physical activity if possible.

The enjoyment and distractions from exertion or monotony caused by exercising with others may also aid in translating strong intentions into behavior (113). If the exercise experience can fulfill socialization (38), it should strengthen the expectations of the experience (30,44,47). Opportunities to socialize during exercise also provide a type of multitasking by combining social needs and personal health and wellness needs (38). In this sense, it can increase the opportunities to act on exercise because one can combine these objectives within a single act. Relatedly, organizing times to exercise with someone introduces a sense of accountability toward the other person. Also, social support, specifically the tangible aid from others so one can create time to exercise (35,115), is a likely influence on the opportunity to act. Others who can free up time by helping with daily chores will increase the time available to exercise and make it easier to translate intentions into behavior (30,44,47). Health and fitness professionals can also serve as a means of social support, especially at the outset of a program, by providing their clients with verbal support and encouragement. This support may increase their client's motivation and confidence in their ability to initiate physical activity.

Adjustments to the environment around people with the intention to change may also help. A focus on improving a client's opportunities for physical activity needs to be considered. Specific characteristics of the environment, such as proximity to facilities, serve as cues to action that facilitates or inhibits successful intention translation. This effect has been demonstrated consistently in past research (95,105,108). This probably aids in the ease of access of performing physical activity and helps shrink the distance between initial intentions and the time to act.

Cross-Behavioral Conflict

The successful translation of good intentions into a behavior may be determined, in part, by the amount of motivation and commitment one has placed on other leisure-time pursuits. This cross-behavioral conflict serves to thwart physical activity by acting as a negative determinant. The basis for this determinant resides in the concept of time displacement (101), whereby motivation and planning for other behaviors compete in the behavioral choices made during free time. Specifically, under the limits of free time, investments of time spent on one behavior may affect the time that can be spent on another behavior. In this capacity, one behavior can impede another. Cross-behavioral conflict has been validated in physical activity (50,51,94,100–02,120) and it is a central tenet of a theory known as behavioral economic theory (140). Television viewing, due to its high prevalence, is the most noteworthy candidate as a cross-behavioral regulation that may thwart physical activity, but any leisure-time activity other than exercise can serve in the capacity.

In order to build the skills to decrease cross-behavioral conflict, it is suggested that increasing the knowledge base about the detriments of prolonged sedentary behavior and lowering ease/ability and scheduling/planning of these behaviors would be of benefit (100). For example, in the context of TV viewing behavior, an intervention should focus on educating clients about the health risks of continuous sitting and public health guidelines around anti-sedentary behavior. Lessening the ease of access (*e.g.*, removal of multiple TVs, removal of cable), and opportunity (*e.g.*, by keeping a schedule of very specific viewing times when it is less convenient to do other activities such as 9–10:30 pm) may also be effective. Another means of reducing sedentary behavior involves educating and having clients consider ways to accumulate active lifestyle activities into their daily routine (*e.g.*, climbing stairs instead of the escalator, walking to work/nearby store), rather than scheduling a session of continuous exercise (*e.g.*, strength training at the gym). Incorporating competing activities such as exercising while watching TV may also be a strategy to increase exercise without asking the client to give up things they like and does not require extra time in the day. Early research in these sedentary reduction behaviors has shown success with these strategies (39).

TAKE-HOME MESSAGE

In summary, to facilitate a client's initial intentions to be physical active, it is essential that the fitness and health professional help their clients be active in their exercise prescription. The exercise professional should aim to facilitate the self-regulatory process for the client but not to simply create the self-regulatory plan for them. The development of the client's self-regulation skills and toolbox is more important than the plan itself because goals and plans change over time and life context. Further, a plan created for the client without their input and collaboration will not result in adherence to an exercise program and is typically no different than the absence of a plan (16). The preceding section suggested that building skills for goal setting, self-monitoring, and planning are crucial to self-regulation, with the additional consideration of automaticity, social and environmental support, and lowering cross-behavioral conflict.

To assist you in selecting strategies for use with your clients, the next section provides step-by-step instructions and worksheets demonstrating how to implement these approaches. For ways to model the appropriate selection of strategies and tools to implement with your client, see Table 3.2 and, at the end of this chapter, several sample case scenarios.

STEP-BY-STEP

Follow these steps to implement the approaches discussed in the previous section:

1. Conduct a brief informal interview with your new client and establish rapport (see Chapter 5).
2. Get to know who your client is and what is important to them, as well as their history related to physical activity, fitness, and health and wellness (see Chapter 2).
3. Determine where your client lies on the intention behavior continuum. Are they. . .
   - Low intent? High intent?
   - Having difficulty translating their intention into action?
   - Having difficulty adhering over the long term?

   Take a look at Case Scenarios 3.1, 3.2, and 3.3 for examples of clients who vary on the intention behavior continuum.

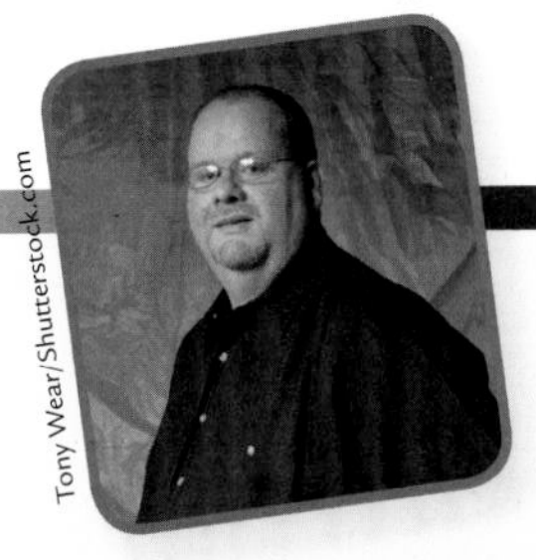
Tony Wear/Shutterstock.com

Case Scenario 3.1

LOW INTENTION TO EXERCISE; HIGH RESISTANCE

Paul is a 50-year-old overweight man who has never been interested in his health and fitness. He has always been naturally slim and has never regularly engaged in a physical activity routine. However, in recent years he has put on considerable weight. He has fallen into a sedentary lifestyle. During his nonworking hours, he and his wife spend their time eating large unhealthy meals, watching television, and surfing the Web. His wife has recently taken an interest in their health as a couple, feels frustrated by their unhealthy routine, and has been pushing Paul to engage in a healthier lifestyle. In pursuit of this goal, his wife decided to buy them both gym memberships and personal training sessions with you for a Christmas present. She is determined to start living a healthy lifestyle and to age successfully; however, Paul is resistant to change and quite anxious about becoming active and finding his way around the gym. He complains that he is already tired after work and has no interest in getting hot, sweaty, and experiencing discomfort and muscle soreness.

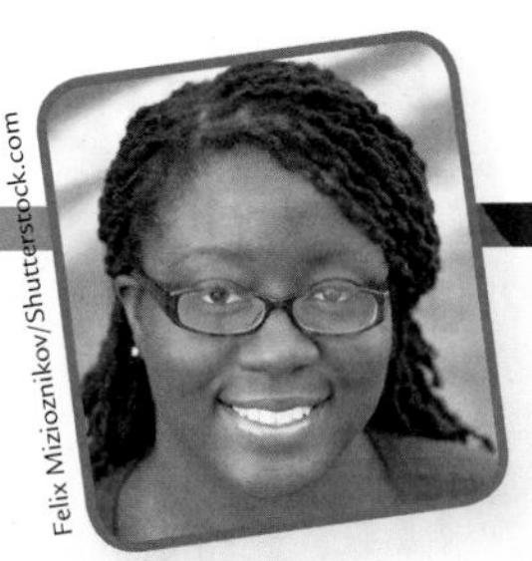
Felix Mizioznikov/Shutterstock.com

Case Scenario 3.2

HIGH INTENTION TO EXERCISE: "LOST IN TRANSLATION"

Andrea is a 25-year-old woman with two young children aged 3 and 5 years of age. She works full time in an administrative position for the government, while her husband works long, irregular hours as a manager in the restaurant business. She was active in her youth, when physical education was mandatory and her parents had her enrolled in several extracurricular sports after school. She has found it very difficult to focus on her physical activity and fitness level after having children and returning to work. Although she is highly motivated to get active and stay healthy so she can keep up and have fun with her kids, she is having trouble translating her intention into practice. Without the structure provided by school and her parents and the demands of working and parenthood, she feels lost and has no idea where to begin. She recently signed up for the corporate gym membership at the local gym. She has come to you with a strong desire to become active and is looking for guidance on how to adopt a healthier lifestyle.

4. Based on your answers to Step 2, prioritize which physical activity skills building activities you will need to work through with your client. Possible worksheets to choose from include the:
   - Behavioral palate worksheet (see From the Practical Toolbox 3.1)
   - Decisional balance worksheet (see From the Practical Toolbox 3.2)
   - Goal setting worksheet (see From the Practical Toolbox 3.3)
   - Planning worksheet (see From the Practical Toolbox 3.4)
   - Exercise contract (see From the Practical Toolbox 3.5)
   - Self-monitoring worksheet (see From the Practical Toolbox 3.6)

   For guidance in choosing appropriate worksheets for your clients, use Table 3.2, Decision Tree for Choices of Worksheets and Strategies. The decision tree

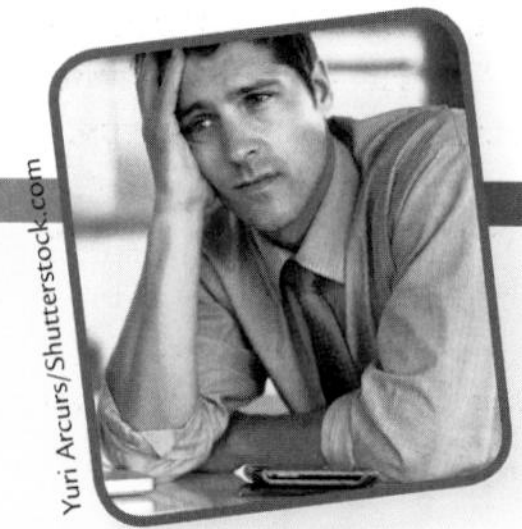
Yuri Arcurs/Shutterstock.com

Case Scenario 3.3

INTENTION BUT NO SUCCESS: STRUGGLES IN LIMBO

Cameron is a 35-year-old who recently graduated from Law school and got hired on at a major law firm. He is trying to make a good name for himself, and work is a high priority. He has been putting in long hours at work, is experiencing high levels of stress, his mood is poor, and he is having trouble sleeping. He makes time for physical activity infrequently and often cancels workouts for work engagements. Although he grew up in a household that valued health and physical activity and he played on many sports teams throughout his elementary and secondary school years, this is not the first time he has fallen off track. He first had difficulty engaging in regular physical activity when he went away to college at 19 years of age. He recalls being highly motivated to keep physically active when he was away at school, and intended on going to the gym regularly. He even joined a volleyball team for his first semester. During his first few weeks of school, he kept to his intention to be physically active, but then things began to unravel. He had considerable difficulty balancing his heavy course load and study schedule with his social life. He quit his recreational volleyball team in the first semester of school and he put on the "frosh fifteen." He is beginning to see a pattern and has come to you for help to break it and learn how to maintain a healthy lifestyle in the long term.

provides appropriate strategy and worksheet selection for Case Scenarios 3.1, 3.2, and 3.3. For a client who has low intention or is resistant to engaging in exercise (Case Scenario 3.1), appropriate tools include the behavioral palate worksheet, the decisional balance worksheet, and the planning worksheet (focusing on Step 1: Action Planning). Additional strategies appropriate for a client who has little intention for exercising include reviewing the benefits of exercise with an emphasis on the affective experience (*e.g.*, enjoyment, improved mood) or creating contingency structures (*e.g.*, creating rewards for engaging in physical activity). See Table 3.2 for solutions to the other sample scenarios.

5. Work collaboratively with your client on the selected worksheets. Notice that each worksheet includes steps and instructions for you to work through with your clients.
6. Sign an exercise contract based on the activities developed from the worksheets to help increase commitment to the exercise (see the sample exercise contract in From the Practical Toolbox 3.5).
7. Monitor progress using the self-monitoring worksheet (see From the Practical Toolbox 3.6).
8. Schedule regular follow-ups to evaluate progress, and revise program and sign new exercise contracts when necessary.

REFERENCES

1. Aarts H, Dijksterhuis A. Habits as knowledge structures: Automaticity in goal-directed behaviour. *Journal of Personality and Social Psychology*. 2000;78:53–63.
2. Aarts H, Paulussen T, Schaalma H. Physical exercise habit: On the conceptualization and formation of habitual health behaviours. *Health Education Research*. 1997;12:363–74.
3. Achtziger A, Gollwitzer RM. Motivation and volition in the course of action. In: Heckhausen J, Heckhausen H, editors. *Motivation and Action*. 2nd ed. New York: Cambridge University Press; 2008. p. 272–95.
4. Ajzen I. The theory of planned behavior. *Organizational Behavior and Human Decision Processes*; 1991;50:179–211.

5. Ibid.
6. Araujo-Soares V, McIntyre T, Sniehotta FF. Predicting changes in physical activity among adolescents: The role of self-efficacy, intention, action planning and coping planning. *Health Education Research*. 2009;24: 128–39.
7. Armitage CJ, Sprigg CA. The roles of behavioral and implementation intentions in changing physical activity in young children with low socioeconomic status. *Journal of Sport & Exercise Psychology*. 2010;32(3): 359–76.
8. Bandura A. Self-efficacy: Toward a unifying theory of behavioral change. *Psychological Review*. 1977;84: 191–215.
9. Bandura A. Social cognitive theory of self-regulation. *Organizational Behavior and Human Decision Processes*. 1991;50(2):248–87.
10. Bandura A. *Self-efficacy, the Exercise of Control*. Editor. New York: Freeman; 1997.
11. Bandura A. Health promotion from the perspective of social cognitive theory. *Psychology and Health*. 1998;13:623–49.
12. Bandura A. Health promotion by social cognitive means. *Health Education and Behavior*. 2004;31: 143–64.
13. Bandura A, Simon KM. The role of proximal intentions in self-regulation of refractory behavior. *Cognitive-Therapy-and-Research*. 1977;1(3):177–93.
14. Bargh JA. The four horsemen of automaticity: Awareness, intention, efficiency, and control in social cognition. In: Wyler RS, Srull TK, editors. *Handbook of Social Cognition*. Hillsdale (NJ): Erlbaum; 1994. p. 1–40.
15. Bargh JA, Gollwitzer PM, Oettingen G. Motivation. In: Fiske ST, Gilbert DT, Lindzey G, editors. *Handbook of Social Psychology, Vol 1*. (5th ed). Hoboken (NJ): John Wiley & Sons Inc; 2010. p. 268–316.
16. Bassett S, Petrie KJ. The effect of treatment goals on patient compliance with physiotherapy programs. *Physiotherapy*. 1999;85:130–7.
17. Bauman AE, Sallis JF, Dzewaltowski DA, Owen N. Toward a better understanding of the influences on physical activity – The role of determinants, correlates, causal variables, mediators, moderators, and confounders. *American Journal of Preventive Medicine*. 2002;23(2):5–14.
18. Baumeister RF, Schmeichel BJ, Vohs KD. Self-regulation and the executive function: The self as controlling agent. In: Kruglanski AW, Higgins ET, editors. *Social Psychology: Handbook of Basic Principles*. 2nd ed. New York: Guilford Press; 2007. p. 516–39.
19. Biddle SJH, Fuchs R. Exercise psychology: A view from Europe. *Psychology of Sport and Exercise*. 2009; 10(4):410–9.
20. Biddle SJH, Mutrie N. Psychological well-being. Does physical activity make us feel good? editors. *Psychology of Physical Activity: Determinants, Well-Being and Interventions*. New York: Routledge; 2001. p. 163–98.
21. Biddle SJH, Mutrie N. Stage-based and other models of physical activity, editors. *Psychology of Physical Activity: Determinants, Well-Being and Interventions*. New York: Routledge; 2001. p. 118–36.
22. Brawley LR, Martin KA, Gyurcsik NC. Problems in assessing perceived barriers to exercise: Confusing obstacles with attributions and excuses. In: Duda JL, editor. *Advances in Sport and Exercise Psychology Measurement*. Morgantown, WV: Fitness Information; 1998. p. 337–50.
23. Brown SG, Rhodes RE. Relationships among dog ownership and leisure time walking amid Western Canadian adults. *American Journal of Preventive Medicine*. 2006;30:131–6.
24. Buckworth J. Exercise determinants and interventions. / Les determinants de l'activite physique et les interventions visant a elever le niveau d'activite physique de la population generale. *International Journal of Sport Psychology*. 2000;31(2):305–20.
25. Buckworth J, Dishman RK. Interventions to change physical activity behavior, editors. In: Buckworth, J, editor, *Exercise Psychology*. Champaign, IL: Human Kinetics, c2002, p. 229–253.
26. Canadian Fitness and Lifestyle Research Institute. 2002 Physical Activity Monitor. 2002 [cited August]. Available from: http://www.cflri.ca/cflri/pa/surveys/2002survey/2002survey.html.
27. Canadian Fitness and Lifestyle Research Institute. Increasing physical activity: Trends for planning effective communication. 2004 [cited February 24]. Available from: http://www.cflri.ca/eng/statistics/surveys/capacity2004.php.
28. Carraro N, Gaudreau P. The role of implementation planning in increasing physical activity identification. *American Journal of Health Behavior*. 2010;34(3):298–308.
29. Casiro N, Rhodes RE, Naylor PJ, McKay HA. Correlates of intergenerational and personal physical activity of parents. *The American Journal of Health Behavior*. 2011;35:81–91.
30. Cerin E, Taylor LM, Leslie E, Owen N. Small-scale randomized controlled trials need more powerful methods of mediational analysis than the Baron-Kenny method. *Journal of Clinical Epidemiology*. 2006;59:457–64.
31. Conn VS, Isaramalai S, Banks-Wallace JA, Ulbrich S, Cochran J. Evidence-based interventions to increase physical activity among older adults. *Activities, Adaptation & Aging*. 2002;27(2):39–52.
32. Conn VS, Valentine JC, Cooper HM. Interventions to increase physical activity among aging adults: A meta-analysis. *Annals of Behavioral Medicine: A Publication of the Society of Behavioral Medicine*. 2002; 24(3):190–200.
33. Conner M, Rhodes RE. Instrumental and affective interventions to change exercise behaviour. In: *Instrumental and affective interventions to change exercise behaviour*. Editor (Ed.)^(Eds.) City: British Psychological Society, 2007.
34. Conner M, Rhodes RE, Morris B, McEachan R, Lawton R. Changing exercise through targeting affective or cognitive attitudes. *Psychology and Health*. 2011;26:133–49.
35. Courneya KS, Plotnikoff RC, Hotz SB, Birkett N. Social support and the theory of planned behavior in the exercise domain. *American Journal of Health Behavior*. 2000;24:300–8.

36. Cutt H, Giles-Corti B, Knuiman M, Timperio A, Bull F. Understanding dog owners' increased levels of physical activity: Results from RESIDE. *American Journal of Public Health*. 2008;98:66–9.
37. de Bruijn GJ. Exercise habit strength, planning and the theory of planned behaviour: An action control approach. *Psychology of Sport and Exercise*. 2011;12:106–14.
38. Deci EL, Ryan RM. *Intrinsic motivation and self-determination in human behavior*. Editors. New York: Plenum Press; 1985.
39. DeMattia L, Lemont L, Meurer L. Do interventions to limit sedentary behaviours change behaviour and reduce childhood obesity? A critical review of the literature. *Obesity Reviews*. 2006;8:69–81.
40. Dishman RK, Buckworth J. Increasing physical activity: A quantitative synthesis. In: Smith D, Bar-Eli M, editors. *Essential Readings in Sport and Exercise Psychology*. Champaign (IL): Human Kinetics; 2007. p. 348–55.
41. Downs DS, Hausenblas HA. The theories of reasoned action and planned behavior applied to exercise: A meta-analytic update. *Journal of Physical Activity & Health*. 2005;2(1):76–97.
42. Duncan M, Spence JC, Mummery WK. Perceived environment and physical activity: A meta-analysis of selected environmental characteristics. 2005. Available from: http://www.ijbnpa.org/content/2/1/11.
43. Ekkekakis P, Lind E. Exercise does not feel the same when you are overweight: The impact of self-selected and imposed intensity on affect and exertion. *International Journal of Obesity*. 2006; 30:652–60.
44. Fahrenwald NL, Atwood JR, Johnson DR. Mediator analysis of moms on the move. *Western Journal of Nursing Research*. 2005;27:271–91.
45. Finkel EJ, Fitzsimons GM. The effects of social relationships on self-regulation. In: Vohs KD, Baumeister RF, editors. *Handbook of Self-regulation: Research, Theory, and Applications*. 2nd ed. New York: Guilford Press; 2011. p. 390–406.
46. Fishbein M, Triandis HC, Kanfer FH, Becker M, Middlestadt SE, Eichler A. Factors influencing behavior and behavior change. In: Baum A, Revenson TA, editors. *Handbook of Health Psychology*. Mahwah (NJ): Lawrence Erlbaum Associates; 2001. p. 3–17.
47. Fortier MS, Sweet SN, O'Sullivan TL, Williams GC. A self-determination process model of physical activity adoption in the context of a randomized controlled trial. *Psychology of Sport and Exercise*. 2007;8:741–57.
48. French DP, Sutton S, Hennings SJ, et al. The importance of affective beliefs and attitudes in the theory of planned behavior: Predicting intention to increase physical activity. *Journal of Applied Social Psychology*. 2005;35:1824–48.
49. Gardner B, de Bruijn GJ, Lally P. A systematic review and meta-analysis of applications of the Self-Report Habit Index to nutrition and physical activity behaviors. *Annals of Behavioral Medicine*. In press.
50. Gebhardt WA, Maes S. Competing personal goals and exercise behaviour. *Perceptual and Motor Skills*. 1998;86:755–9.
51. Gebhardt WA, Van Der Doef MP, Maes S. Conflicting activities for exercise. *Perceptual and Motor Skills*. 1999;89:1159–60.
52. Godin G, Shephard RJ, Colantonio A. The cognitive profile of those who intend to exercise but do not. *Public Health Reports*. 1986;101:521–6.
53. Gollwitzer PM. Implementation intentions: Strong effects of simple plans. *American Psychologist*. 1999; 54:493–503.
54. Gollwitzer PM, Sheeran P. Implementation intentions and goal achievement: A meta-analysis of effects and processes. *Advances in Experimental Social Psychology*. 2006;38:69–119.
55. Greaves CJ, Sheppard KE, Abraham C, et al. Systematic review of reviews of intervention components associated with increased effectiveness in dietary and physical activity interventions. *BMC Public Health*. 2011;11:119.
56. Gustafson S, Rhodes RE. Parental correlates of child and early adolescent physical activity: A review. *Sports Medicine*. 2006;36:79–97.
57. Hagger M, Chatzisarantis NLD, Biddle SJH. A meta-analytic review of the theories of reasoned action and planned behavior in physical activity: Predictive validity and the contribution of additional variables. *Journal of Sport and Exercise Psychology*. 2002;24:1–12.
58. Hall PA, Fong GT. Temporal self-regulation theory: A model for individual health behavior. *Health Psychology Review*. 2007;1:6–52.
59. Ham SA, Epping J. Dog walking and physical activity in the United States. *Preventing Chronic Disease*. 2006;3:1–7.
60. Hausenblas HA, Carron AV, Mack DE. Application of the theories of reasoned action and planned behavior to exercise behavior: A meta-analysis. *Journal of Sport and Exercise Psychology*. 1997;19:36–51.
61. Higgins ET. Beyond pleasure and pain. *American Psychologist*. 1997;52(12):1280–300.
62 Hoyt MF, Janis IL. Increasing adherence to a stressful decision via a motivational balance-sheet procedure: A field experiment. *Journal of Personality and Social Psychology*. 1975;31(5):833–9.
63. Hu L, Motl RW, McAuley E, Konopack JF. Effects of self-efficacy on physical activity enjoyment in college-aged women. *International Journal of Behavioral Medicine*. 2007;14:92–6.
64. Humpel N, Owen N, Leslie E. Environmental factors associated with adults' participation in physical activity: A review. *American Journal of Preventive Medicine*. 2002;22:88–199.
65. Jones LW, Sinclair RC, Rhodes RE, Courneya KS. Promoting exercise behaviour: An integration of persuasion theories and the theory of planned behaviour. *British Journal of Health Psychology*. 2004; 9:505–21.
66. King AC. Interventions to promote physical activity by older adults. *Journals of Gerontology Series A – Biological Sciences and Medical Sciences*. 2001;56: 36–46.
67. Kirk A, Barnett J, Mutrie N. Physical activity consultation for people with type 2 diabetes: Evidence and guidelines. *Diabetes Medicine*. 2007;24:809–16.

68. Kliman A, Rhodes RE. Do government brochures affect physical activity cognition? A pilot study of Canada's Physical Activity Guide to Healthy Active Living. *Psychology, Health and Medicine*. 2008;13:415–22.
69. Kyllo LB, Landers DM. Goal setting in sport and exercise: A research synthesis to resolve the controversy. / Fixation d' objectifs en sports et exercices physiques, une synthese pour resoudre la controverse. *Journal of Sport & Exercise Psychology*. 1995;17(2):117–37.
70. Lally P, van Jaarsveld CHM, Potts HWW, Wardle J. How are habits formed: Modelling habit formation in the real world. *European Journal of Social Psychology*. 2009;40:998–1009.
71. Latham GP, Locke EA. Self-regulation through goal-setting. *Organizational Behavior and Human Decision Processes*. 1991;50(2):212–47.
72. Latimer AE, Brawley LR, Bassett RL. A systematic review of three approaches for constructing physical activity messages: What messages work and what improvements are needed? *International Journal of Behavioral Nutrition and Physical Activity*. 2010.
73. Lewis BA, Marcus B, Pate RR, Dunn AL. Psychosocial mediators of physical activity behavior among adults and children. *American Journal of Preventive Medicine*. 2002;23(2S):26–35.
74. Locke EA. Towards a theory of task motivation and individual performance. *Organizational Behavior and Human Performance*. 1968;3:157–80.
75. Locke EA, Latham GP. The application of goal setting to sports. *Journal of Sport Psychology*. 1985;7(3): 205–22.
76. Locke EA, Latham GP. *A theory of goal setting performance*. Editors. Englewood Cliffs (NJ): Prentice Hall; 1990.
77. Locke EA, Latham GP. Building a practically useful theory of goal setting and task motivation: A 35-year odyssey. *American Psychologist*. 2002;57(9):705–17.
78. Locke EA, Shaw KN, Saari LM, Latham GP. Goal setting and task performance: 1969–1980. *Psychological Bulletin*. 1981;90(1):125–52.
79. Lowe R, Eves F, Carroll D. The influence of affective and instrumental beliefs on exercise intentions and behavior: A longitudinal analysis. *Journal of Applied Social Psychology*. 2002;32:1241–52.
80. Lox CL, Ginis KAM, Petruzzello SJ. *The psychology of exercise: Integrating theory and practice*. 2nd ed. Editors. Scottsdale, (AZ): Holcomb Hathaway, Publishers; 2006.
81. Luszczynska A, Schwarzer R, Lippke S, Mazurkiewicz M. Self-efficacy as a moderator of the planning-behaviour relationship in interventions designed to promote physical activity. *Psychology & Health*. 2011;26(2):151–66.
82. Maddux JE. Habit, health, and happiness. *Journal of Sport and Exercise Psychology*. 1997;19:331–46.
83. Maio GR, Haddock G. Attitude change. In: Kruglanski AW, Higgins ET, editors. *Social Psychology: Handbook of Basic Principles*. 2nd ed. New York: Guilford Press; 2007. p. 565–86.
84. Marcus BH, Ciccolo JT, Whitehead D, King TK, Bock BC. Adherence to physical activity recommendations and interventions. In: Shumaker SA, Ockene JK, Riekert KA, editors. *The Handbook of Health Behavior Change*. 3rd ed. New York: Springer Publishing Co; 2009. p. 235–51.
85. Marcus BH, Forsyth L. *Motivating people to be physically active*. 2nd ed. Editors. Champaign (IL): Human Kinetics; 2009.
86. Marcus BH, Rakowski W, Rossi JS. Assessing motivational readiness and decision making for exercise. *Health Psychology*. 1992;11(4):257–61.
87. McAuley E, Talbot HM, Martinez S. Manipulating self-efficacy in the exercise environment in women: Influences on affective responses. *Health Psychology*. 1999;18:288–94.
88. Michie S, Abraham C, Whittington C, McAteer J, Gupta S. Effective techniques in healthy eating and physical activity interventions: A meta-regression. *Health Psychology*. 2009;28:690–701.
89. Nigg CR, Courneya KS. Maintaining attendance at a fitness center: An application. *Behavioral Medicine*. 1997;23(3):130.
90. Noar SM, Zimmerman RS. Health behavior theory and cumulative knowledge regarding health behaviors: Are we moving in the right direction? *Health Education Research*. 2005;20:275–90.
91. Nothwehr F, Yang J. Goal setting frequency and the use of behavioral strategies related to diet and physical activity. *Health Education Research*. 2007;22(4):532–8.
92. Parrott MW, Tennant LK, Olejnik S, Poudevigne MS. Theory of planned behavior: Implications for an email-based physical activity intervention. *Psychology of Sport and Exercise*. 2008;9:511–26.
93. Plante TG, Gores C, Brecht C, Carrow J, Imbs A, Willemsen E. Does exercise environment enhance the psychological benefits of exercise for women? *International Journal of Stress Management*. 2007;14: 88–98.
94. Presseau J, Sniehotta FF, Francis JJ, Gebhardt WF. With a little help from my goals: Integrating intergoal facilitation with the theory of planned behaviour to predict physical activity. *British Journal of Health Psychology*. 2010;15:905–19.
95. Prins RG, van Empelen P, te Velde SJ, et al. Availability of sports facilities as moderator of the intention–sports participation relationship among adolescents. *Health Education Research*. 2010;25:489–97.
96. Prochaska JO, DiClemente CC. Transtheoretical therapy: Toward a more integrative model of change. *Psychotherapy: Theory, Research & Practice*. 1982;19:276–88.
97. Rhodes RE. Action control theory of exercise behaviour. In review.
98. Rhodes RE. Action control theory of exercise behaviour. *International Journal of Behavioural Nutrition and Physical Activity*. In review.
99. Rhodes RE, Blanchard CM. What do confidence items measure in the physical activity domain? *Journal of Applied Social Psychology*. 2007;37: 753–68.
100. Rhodes RE, Blanchard CM. Do sedentary motives adversely affect physical activity? Adding cross-behavioural cognitions to the theory of planned behaviour. *Psychology and Health*. 2008;23: 789–805.

101. Rhodes RE, Blanchard CM. Time displacement and confidence to participate in leisure-time physical activity. *International Journal of Behavioral Medicine*. In press.
102. Rhodes RE, Blanchard CM, Bellows K. Exploring cues to sedentary behavior as processes of physical activity action control. *Psychology of Sport and Exercise*. 2008;9:211–24.
103. Rhodes RE, Blanchard CM, Matheson DH. A multi-component model of the theory of planned behavior. *British Journal of Health Psychology*. 2006; 11:119–37.
104. Rhodes RE, Blanchard CM, Matheson DH, Coble J. Disentangling motivation, intention, and planning in the physical activity domain. *Psychology of Sport and Exercise*. 2006;7:15–27.
105. Rhodes RE, Brown SG, McIntyre CA. Integrating the perceived neighbourhood environment and the theory of planned behaviour when predicting walking in Canadian adult sample. *American Journal of Health Promotion*. 2006;21:110–8.
106. Rhodes RE, Conner M. Comparison of behavioral belief structures in the physical activity domain. *Journal of Applied Social Psychology*. 2010;40(8):2105–20.
107. Rhodes RE, Courneya KS. Differentiating motivation and control in the theory of planned behavior. *Psychology, Health and Medicine*. 2004;9:205–15.
108. Rhodes RE, Courneya KS, Blanchard CM, Plotnikoff RC. Prediction of leisure-time walking: An integration of social cognitive, perceived environmental, and personality factors. *International Journal of Behavioral Nutrition and Physical Activity*. 2007;4:51.
109. Rhodes RE, Courneya KS, Jones LW. Translating exercise intentions into behavior: Personality and social cognitive correlates. *Journal of Health Psychology*. 2003;8:447–58.
110. Rhodes RE, de Bruijn GJ, Matheson DH. Habit in the physical activity domain: Integration with intention temporal stability and action control. *Journal of Sport and Exercise Psychology*. 2010;32(1):84–98.
111. Rhodes RE, Dickau L. Moderators of the intention-behaviour relationship for physical activity: A systematic review. *Journal of Sport and Exercise Psychology*. 2010;32:S213–S4.
112. Rhodes RE, Dickau L. Meta-analysis of experimental evidence for the intention-behavior relationship in the physical activity domain. In preparation.
113. Rhodes RE, Fiala B, Conner M. Affective judgments and physical activity: A review and meta-analysis. *Annals of Behavioral Medicine*. 2009;38:180–204.
114. Rhodes RE, Fiala B, Conner M. A review and meta-analysis of affective judgments and physical activity in adult populations. *Annals of Behavioral Medicine*. 2009;38(3):180–204.
115. Rhodes RE, Jones LW, Courneya KS. Extending the theory of planned behavior in the exercise domain: A comparison of social support and subjective norm. *Research Quarterly for Exercise & Sport*. 2002;73:193–9.
116. Rhodes RE, Nasuti G. Trends and changes in research on the psychology of physical activity across 20 years: A quantitative analysis of 10 journals. *Preventive Medicine*. 2011;53:17–23.
117. Rhodes RE, Pfaeffli LA. Mediators of physical activity behaviour change among adult non-clinical populations: A review update. *International Journal of Behavioral Nutrition and Physical Activity*. 2010;77(37), 1–11.
118. Rhodes RE, Warburton DER, Bredin SS. Predicting the effect of interactive video bikes on exercise adherence: An efficacy trial. *Psychology, Health & Medicine*. 2009;14:631–41.
119. Rhodes RE, Warburton DER, Coble J. Effect of interactive video bikes on exercise adherence and social cognitive expectancies in young men: A pilot study. *Annals of Behavioral Medicine*. 2008;35:S62.
120. Riediger M, Freund AM. Interference and facilitation among personal goals: Differential associations with subjective well-being and persistent goal pursuit. *Personality and Social Psychology Bulletin*. 2004; 30: 1511–23.
121. Scholz U, Schüz B, Ziegelmann JP, Lippke S, Schwarzer R. Beyond behavioural intentions: Planning mediates between intentions and physical activity. *British Journal of Health Psychology*. 2008;13(3):479–94.
122. Sheeran P. Intention-behaviour relations: A conceptual and empirical review. In: Hewstone M, Stroebe W, editors. *European Review of Social Psychology*. Chichester, UK: John Wiley & Sons; 2002. p. 1–36.
123. Shilts MK, Horowitz M, Townsend MS. Goal setting as a strategy for dietary and physical activity behavior change: A review of the literature. *American Journal of Health Promotion*. 2004;19(2):81–93.
124. Sirriyeh R, Lawton R, Ward J. Physical activity and adolescents: An exploratory randomized controlled trial investigating the influence of affective and instrumental text messages. *British Journal of Health Psychology*. 2010;15(4):825–40.
125. Smith JA, Hauenstein NMA, Buchanan LB. Goal setting and exercise performance. *Human Performance*. 1996;9(2):141–54.
126. Sniehotta FF. Towards a theory of intentional behaviour change: Plans, planning, and self-regulation. *British Journal of Health Psychology*. 2009;14:261–73.
127. Sniehotta FF, Schwarzer R, Scholz U, Schüz B. Action planning and coping planning for long-term lifestyle change: Theory and assessment. *European Journal of Social Psychology*. 2005;35(4):565–76.
128. Spence JC, McGannon KR, Poon P. The effect of exercise on global self-esteem: A quantitative review. *Journal of Sport and Exercise Psychology*. 2005;27:311–34.
129. Stokols D. Translating social ecological theory into guidelines for community health promotion. *American Journal of Health Promotion*. 1996;10: 282–98.
130. Symons Downs D, Hausenblas HA. Elicitation studies and the theory of planned behavior: A systematic review of exercise beliefs. *Psychology of Sport and Exercise*. 2005;6:1–31.
131. Symons Downs D, Hausenblas HA. Exercise behavior and the theories of reasoned action and planned behavior: A meta-analytic update. *Journal of Physical Activity and Health*. 2005;2:76–97.

132. Triandis HC. *Interpersonal Behavior.* Editor. Monterey (CA): Brooks/Cole; 1977.
133. Trost SG, Owen N, Bauman A, Sallis JF, Brown W. Correlates of adults' participation in physical activity: Review and update. *Medicine and Science in Sports and Exercise.* 2002;34:1996–2001.
134. Trost SG, Owen N, Bauman AE, Sallis JF, Brown W. Correlates of adults' participation in physical activity: Review and update. *Medicine and Science in Sports and Exercise.* 2002;34(12):1996–2001.
135. Umstattd MR, Wilcox S, Saunders R, Watkins K, Dowda M. Self-regulation and physical activity: The relationship in older adults. *American Journal of Health Behavior.* 2008;32(2):115–24.
136. Van der Horst K, Paw MJCA, Twisk JWR, Van Mechelen W. A brief review on correlates of physical activity and sedentariness in youth. *Medicine and Science in Sports and Exercise.* 2007;39(8): 1241–50.
137. Verplanken B. Beyond frequency: Habit as a mental construct. *British Journal of Social Psychology.* 2006; 45:639–56.
138. Verplanken B, Aarts H. Habit, attitude, and planned behaviour: Is habit an empty construct or an interesting case of goal-directed automaticity? In: Stroebe W, Hewstone M, editors. *European Review of Social Psychology.* New York: John Wiley & Sons; 1999. p. 101–34.
139. Verplanken B, Melkevik O. Predicting habit: The case of physical exercise. *Psychology of Sport and Exercise.* 2008;9:15–26.
140. Vuchinich RE, Tucker JA. Behavioral theories of choice as a framework for studying drinking behavior. *Journal of Abnormal Psychology.* 1983;92:408–16.
141. Webb TL, Sheeran P. Does changing behavioral intentions engender behavior change? A meta-analysis of the experimental evidence. *Psychological Bulletin.* 2006;132:249–68.
142. Wiedemann AU, Schüz B, Sniehotta F, Scholz U, Schwarzer R. Disentangling the relation between intentions, planning, and behaviour: A moderated mediation analysis. *Psychology & Health.* 2009; 24(1):67–79.
143. Williams SL, French DP. What are the most effective intervention techniques for changing physical activity self-efficacy and physical activity behavior – and are they the same? *Health Education Research.* 2011;26(2):308–22.
144. Ziegelmann JP, Lippke S, Schwarzer R. Adoption and maintenance of physical activity: Planning interventions in young, middle-aged, and older adults. *Psychology & Health.* 2006;21(2):145–63.

CHAPTER 4

Building Motivation: How Ready Are You?

Sara S. Johnson and Brian Cook

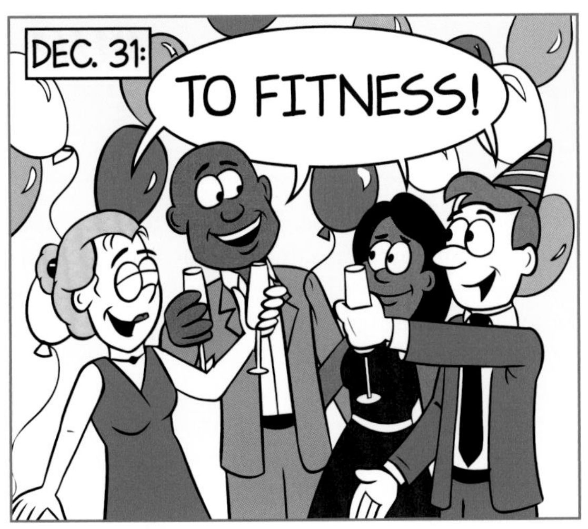

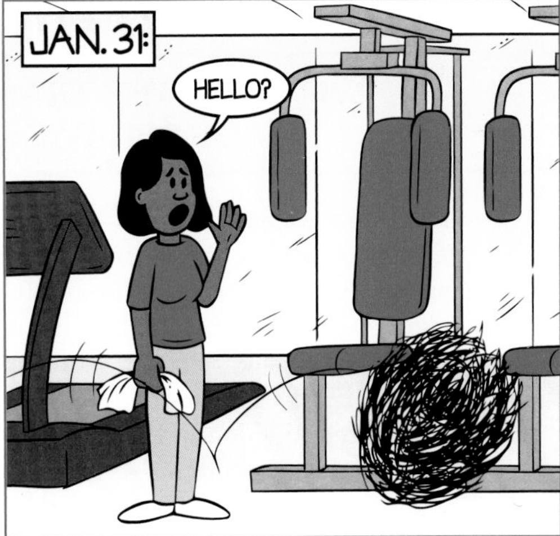

CONCEPT OVERVIEW

Promoting the adoption and maintenance of regular exercise is undoubtedly a significant behavior change challenge. A mere 30% of adults are exercising in accordance with the current American College of Sports Medicine guidelines (2), and nearly 40% engage in no leisure-time physical activity (6). The question is: What can motivate people to exercise?

The answer depends in part on where they start: Often, what motivates people to begin thinking about starting to exercise is different than what motivates them to actually begin, which in turn differs from what motivates them to continue once they are exercising regularly. For those reasons, ACSM (2) reports that effective exercise interventions are often individually tailored on constructs from a health behavior change theory and incorporate behavioral strategies such as goal setting, social support, and relapse prevention.

EVIDENCE: THE TRANSTHEORETICAL MODEL OF BEHAVIOR CHANGE (TTM)

The Transtheoretical Model of Behavior Change (TTM), also known as the Stages of Change model, is one of the most commonly employed health behavior change theories within exercise interventions (20,23). Reviews of interventions matched to individuals' readiness to change (13,22) have demonstrated that tailoring messages is an extremely effective way to change behavior. Furthermore, multiple studies (5,9,12,14–19,32) revealed that tailored, TTM-based exercise interventions, including those delivered by health coaches (27), increase the adoption and maintenance of regular exercise. The success of these interventions underscore an important lesson for fitness professionals: It is crucial to assess each client's readiness to engage in regular exercise and tailor your interventions to his or her stage of change. Recognizing the unique needs of individuals in early stages and reconceptualizing progress as movement to the next stage can significantly increase the impact of your work with a client. Given the utility of the TTM for assisting clients in adopting and maintaining regular exercise, this chapter will provide an overview of the TTM and illustrate its practical application to assisting individuals in adopting and maintaining regular exercise.

The Five TTM Stages

The TTM conceptualizes change as a process that unfolds over time in a series of five stages of readiness to change (see Figure 4.1).

PRECONTEMPLATION

Precontemplation is the stage of change in which individuals are not intending to exercise regularly in the foreseeable future (typically defined as the next 6 months). Individuals in this stage are often unaware or under-aware of the benefits of adopting exercise and overestimating the costs of changing. They are often characterized by one or more of the three Ds: defensiveness, denial, or demoralization. Often they are described by the health professionals with whom they interact as nonadherent, unmotivated, or difficult. It is important, however, not to confuse lack of readiness to adopt exercise with lack of desire to exercise: Individuals

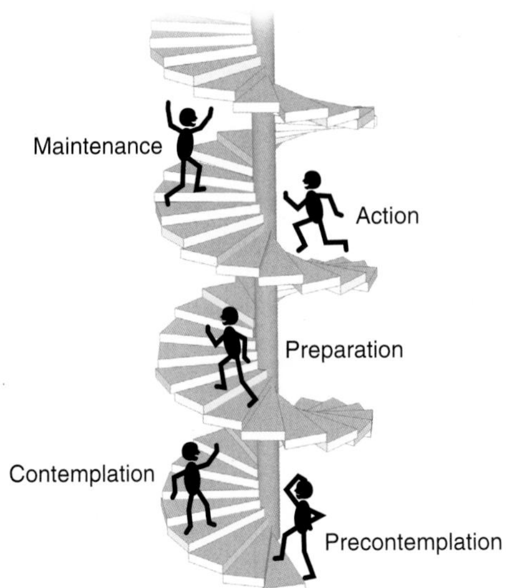

FIGURE 4.1. Stages of change.

in Precontemplation may want to begin exercising regularly or wish they would, but are not ready to do so because of perceived barriers, have low self-efficacy (*i.e.,* confidence—or the belief that they can engage in regular exercise), or lack of information on how to get started.

CONTEMPLATION

Individuals in *Contemplation* are intending to exercise regularly within the next 6 months. They are more aware of the numerous benefits of exercise, but are also acutely aware of the cons, or drawbacks. As a result, they may be ambivalent about exercise. At times, the ambivalence is so profound that individuals get "stuck" in Contemplation, which is referred to as "chronic Contemplation." These individuals often lack the confidence and commitment they need to adopt regular exercise.

PREPARATION

Individuals in *Preparation* are ready to exercise regularly in the next 30 days and have often taken some steps closer to their goal, such as exercising on some days or exercising less than 30 minutes per day. They are creating a plan for how to move forward and are the perfect candidates for traditional messaging and programs that encourage people to take action to exercise regularly (*e.g.,* Just Do It!). They are also more committed and confident about their ability to exercise regularly.

ACTION

Individuals in *Action* have adopted regular exercise within the past six months and are actively using behavioral strategies to create a new habit. They are likely to experience a setback when they experience a challenge (*e.g.,* bad weather, injuries, schedule conflicts) unless they have planned ahead.

MAINTENANCE

Individuals in *Maintenance* have been exercising regularly for quite some time (typically defined as more than six months) and are significantly more confident about their ability to maintain the behavior change. Recent research indicates that low confidence or self-efficacy is the single best predictor of discontinuing exercise while in the Maintenance stage (11).

Moving Individuals Forward in the Stages of Change

As will be illustrated in the following text, an individual's stage of change has important implications for selecting intervention strategies and messaging. Equally important, though, are the implications the stage paradigm has for reconceptualizing what "success" means in working with clients to help them adopt or maintain exercise. A reasonable goal for each client is to help them move forward one stage of change, as forward stage movement is an important predictor of later success. In fact, assisting individuals in moving forward at least one stage of change (*e.g.,* from Precontemplation to Contemplation) can as much as double the probability that they will take effective action in the following 6 months. Helping them move two stages can triple their chances of taking action (29). How can you help clients achieve that goal? By encouraging them to use behavior change strategies matched to their stage of change.

Those strategies are derived from other behavior change constructs included in the TTM, such as decisional balance, self-efficacy, and the 10 processes of change.

PROS (BENEFITS) AND CONS (DRAWBACKS)

Decisional balance represents an individual's relative weighting of the pros (*i.e.,* benefits) and cons (*i.e.,* hassles, barriers, or drawbacks) of changing (31). An extensive review of the pros and cons for 48 health behaviors (10) revealed a consistent pattern of the pros and cons across the stages for 48 health behaviors. The cons are higher than the pros in the Precontemplation stage, while the pros outweigh the cons in the Action stage. The relationship between the pros and cons across the stages has important implications for intervention strategies. The key take-away messages for fitness professionals and other health care providers are that:

1. Raising the pros is twice as important as reducing the cons.
2. It is crucial to raise the pros for individuals in the early stages.
3. Contemplation is the time to begin addressing the barriers.

SELF-EFFICACY

Self-efficacy is defined as an individual's belief about his or her ability to do or achieve a specific behavior (3). Within TTM-based exercise interventions, it is operationalized as confidence to make and sustain changes. Confidence is low in the Precontemplation stage and increases across the stages (8). Given the importance of self-efficacy, it needs to be raised early by assisting individuals in setting and achieving small goals that will build their confidence for taking on increasingly difficult challenges. If, for example, someone is not exercising at all but is intending to do so in the next 6 months, it would be helpful to have them set a reasonable and achievable goal to begin exercising slowly (*e.g.,* 10 minutes, three times a week) and increase the frequency and intensity once that goal has been mastered.

THE PROCESSES OF CHANGE

The *processes* of change (25;26) (see Table 4.1) represent both the covert and overt behavior change strategies that individuals use to progress through the stages of change (26). Research demonstrates that experiential (*i.e.,* cognitive, affective, and evaluative) processes of change are typically emphasized by individuals in the earlier stages, whereas individuals in later stages rely more on the behavioral processes (*i.e.,* social support, commitments, and behavior management techniques) (28). Additional research demonstrates that process use differs significantly across the stages of change for exercise (4,18,21,30,33). Each process can be activated by various techniques. Consciousness raising, for example, can be accomplished by reading articles or listening to news stories about the importance of exercise, talking with a health care provider or trainer about what modes of exercise best suit a person given their health history and physical limitations (if any), asking friends what types of exercises they enjoy, checking out the website of a local gym or fitness facility to see what types of

TABLE 4.1 Processes of Change

Processes of Change	Description	Strategy Examples
Experiential Processes		
Consciousness Raising (Become Informed)	Learning new facts, ideas, and tips that support exercise	Read books, magazines, or visit Web sites that focus on exercise and health.
Dramatic Relief (Pay Attention to Feelings)	Experiencing negative emotions (fear, anxiety) that go along with the health consequences of not exercising or the positive emotions (*e.g.*, inspiration) that go along with regular exercise	Think about somebody close to you that has had severe health problems that may have been prevented by regularly exercising. Does their inactivity and subsequent health problem upset you?
Environmental Reevaluation (Notice your Effect on Others)	Realizing the negative impact not exercising has on others and our society—and the positive impact that exercising could have	Consider the example your inactivity sets for your children, family, friends, and coworkers.
Self-Reevaluation (Create a New Self-Image)	Realizing that regular exercise is an important part of one's identity	Ask yourself, "How do I think and feel about myself as someone who is not exercising regularly? How might I feel differently if I was exercising regularly?"
Social Liberation (Notice Social Trends)	Realizing that social norms are changing to support exercise	Name some social changes that support exercise (*e.g.*, walking paths).
Behavioral Processes		
Self-Liberation (Make a Commitment)	Believing in one's ability to exercise regularly and making a commitment to change based on that belief	Set a date to start exercising regularly and tell your friends, family, and coworkers your plan.
Helping Relationships (Get Support)	Seeking and using social support to start and/or continue exercising	Join an adult sports league or ask a friend to walk around the neighborhood with you every evening after dinner.
Counterconditioning (Use Substitutes)	Substituting healthy alternative behaviors and thoughts for unhealthy ones	Ride your bike to work instead of driving your car.
Reinforcement Management (Use Rewards)	Increasing the intrinsic and extrinsic rewards for exercise and decreasing the rewards for being sedentary	Buy a new set of workout clothes after you have met an exercise goal.
Stimulus Control (Manage your Environment)	Removing reminders or cues to be sedentary and using cues to exercise	Leave your running shoes and clothes in a bag by the door to remind you to run during your lunch break.

programs they offer, or keeping a diary (paper or a mobile app) of how much physical activity a person is getting during the week. The first column of Table 4.1 includes both the official and (parenthetically) a more informal name of each process of change. Figure 4.2 illustrates the stages in which various processes of change are most relevant.

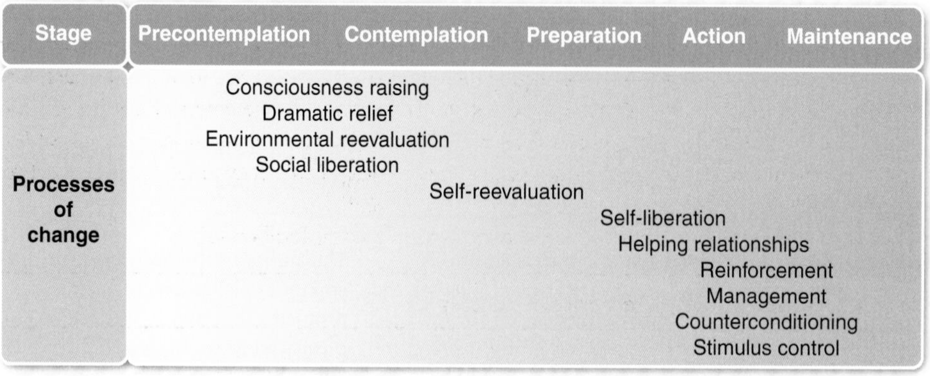

Stage | Precontemplation | Contemplation | Preparation | Action | Maintenance

Processes of change

Consciousness raising
Dramatic relief
Environmental reevaluation
Social liberation
Self-reevaluation
Self-liberation
Helping relationships
Reinforcement
Management
Counterconditioning
Stimulus control

FIGURE 4.2. Processes by stage of change.

Step-by-Step

The basic assumption of traditional action-oriented interventions is that everyone is ready to change. The stage paradigm, however, operates under a fundamentally different assumption—that the majority of individuals are not ready to change. This difference in perspective allows exercise professionals to assist clients in employing the most effective strategies at the right time to help them get ready to initiate and maintain an exercise routine. Thus, encouraging the use of specific processes at the appropriate time facilitates forward stage movement.

1. **Step 1. Assess Readiness to Change:** Matching the intervention program or message to the needs of your client increases the likelihood that she or he will successfully adopt and maintain regular exercise. To begin, you will first need to assess how ready each client is to exercise to guidelines (*i.e.*, in accordance with the ACSM guidelines for 30 minutes per day on 5 or more days per week of moderate exercise, or 20 minutes on 3 or more days per week of vigorous exercise, or some combination (2). It is crucial to know how ready he or she is to meet the public health recommendation, which is the ultimate goal. If a client has physical limitations that prevent him or her from achieving that level of exercise, you can assess readiness to engage in whatever level of physical activity is safe for them based on their health care provider's recommendations. You can separately assess readiness to engage in resistance exercises for each major muscle group and neuromotor exercise 2 to 3 days per week or flexibility exercises on at least 2 to 3 days per week (1).
2. **Step 2. Target Interventions to Individual's Readiness to Change:** Once you have assessed each individual's readiness to exercise regularly, you can employ the suggestions on the following pages to assist them in moving to the next stage. If, for example, your client is in the Contemplation stage, you can employ the intervention strategies described in the Contemplation section. We've also provided sample activities you can use with clients in each stage (25). These activities are handouts for the client, so they are written as if the client is reading them. For more guidance about how to apply the TTM successfully, you can participate in an e-learning module developed by Pro-Change Behavior Systems on using the TTM for coaching (details at www.prochange.com/e-learning) or refer to *Mastering Change, A Coach's Guide to Using the Transtheoretical Model with Clients* (24).

PRECONTEMPLATION

The goal in Precontemplation is to encourage clients to view success as progress to Contemplation. They are not ready to take action, so encouraging them to do so is likely to lead to dropout or demoralization. Providing information is a great way to initiate the behavior change process. Keep in mind that although they are not ready to begin exercising regularly, they may be willing to set a small goal (*e.g.*, adding a few minutes of exercise to their day once a week). If they aren't ready to set that goal, see if you can arrive at one that feels reasonable to them.

For a sample Precontemplation activity, see From the Practical Toolbox 4.1.

Precontemplation: Key Intervention Strategies

Increase the Pros

- Encourage clients to list their own "pros" of exercise–How will they benefit from exercising regularly? What's in it for them?
- Reinforce what they came up with and point out additional benefits, including some that are specific to them.
- Provide a list of over 75 benefits.
- Encourage clients to create a Top Ten List of the most personally relevant benefits.

Raise Consciousness—Help Clients Become Informed

- Increase their awareness of consequences of sedentary behavior (e.g., ask their health care provider about how being sedentary is affecting their health).
- Make observations (e.g., "You're saying that you have less energy since you stopped exercising. . .").
- Encourage the client to be more open to information from media, health care providers, friends, etc. (e.g., ask them to notice headlines related to exercise).

Social Liberation-Notice Social Trends

- Encourage the client to name some social changes that support exercise; provide examples to add to what they mention.
- Ask them to notice other social trends that are making it easier to exercise, including:
  - Walking paths
  - Free or low-cost exercise programs and fitness classes offered through towns or worksite wellness programs
  - Fund-raising groups (e.g., The Leukemia Society's Team-In-Training) designed to train clients for exercise while raising money for a great cause
  - Increasing opportunities to work out at home (e.g., fitness DVDs from Netflix, video games like Dance, Dance Revolution, Wii Sports, and Wii Fit)
  - Mobile wireless technology is making it easier to work out and track physical activity by downloading fitness programs and trackers to cell phones or MP3 players (e.g., work out apps such as Nike + or mapmyrun.com).

Environmental Reevaluation—Notice Your Effect on Others

- Encourage the client to consider the effect of not exercising on others, including children, spouse, friends, and family.
- Ask if the client is setting the example he or she wants to set for those people.
- Ask whether someone else will have to deal with the potential consequences of their sedentary behavior (*e.g.*, chronic diseases, physical limitations, early death).

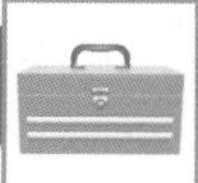

From the Practical Toolbox 4.1

SAMPLE ACTIVITY FOR PRECONTEMPLATORS: RAISE THE PROS

People in Precontemplation usually don't focus enough on all of the good reasons to exercise regularly. The more good reasons, or "Pros" you have, the easier it will be to take the next step—when you are ready.

The following are 75 benefits of exercising regularly.

Which benefits are most important to you? Be sure to check them off as you go.

Exercise will improve your health in many ways:

- ❑ You will manage your weight better.
- ❑ You will lower your risk of an early death.
- ❑ You will improve your quality of life.
- ❑ You may lose weight, particularly if you also reduce calories.
- ❑ You will improve heart, lung, and muscle fitness.

You can reduce your risk of many illnesses:

- ❑ Coronary heart disease
- ❑ Diabetes
- ❑ High blood pressure
- ❑ Osteoporosis (brittle bones)
- ❑ Stroke
- ❑ Depression
- ❑ Dementia
- ❑ Diverticulitis
- ❑ Gallstones
- ❑ Colon cancer
- ❑ Breast cancer
- ❑ Endometrial cancer
- ❑ Lung cancer
- ❑ Hip fracture

It's good for your overall well-being:

- ❑ Exercise increases your energy.
- ❑ Regular exercise helps you cope with stress.
- ❑ Exercising regularly relaxes you.
- ❑ Regular exercise improves your sleep.
- ❑ Regular exercise controls your appetite.
- ❑ Exercising regularly makes you stronger.
- ❑ Exercise improves your mood.
- ❑ Exercise increases your endurance.
- ❑ Exercise can reduce pain.
- ❑ Exercise can reduce body fat.

It's good for your heart:

- ❑ Helps raise levels of "good" cholesterol (HDL)
- ❑ Decreases levels of "bad" cholesterol (LDL)
- ❑ Increases your chance of surviving a second heart attack
- ❑ Decreases risk of clogged blood vessels
- ❑ Lowers your resting heart rate

From the Practical Toolbox 4.1 *continued*

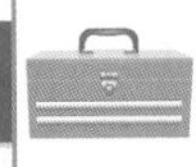

❑ Decreases irregular heart rhythms
❑ Improves circulation

It improves your self-image:
❑ Increases confidence
❑ Improves self-esteem
❑ Helps you look better
❑ Improves your posture
❑ Helps you be more productive
❑ Increases your joy in life
❑ Increases your sense of well-being
❑ Improves your self-worth

It improves your overall health:
❑ Helps your immune system work better
❑ Helps your body use insulin
❑ Increases your metabolism
❑ Helps muscles burn more energy all day
❑ Strengthens joints
❑ Makes your bones stronger
❑ Lowers the risk of erectile dysfunction
❑ Improves bowel regularity
❑ Strengthens muscles

You'll notice changes in your everyday life:
❑ You'll feel less nervous or anxious.
❑ You'll have increased stamina.
❑ You'll be more alert and focused.
❑ You'll improve your memory.
❑ You'll be more flexible.
❑ You'll become better coordinated.
❑ You'll help relieve the pain of tension headaches.
❑ You'll reduce your risk of falling.
❑ You'll reduce and prevent low back pain.
❑ You'll have less muscle tension.
❑ You'll better tolerate heat and cold.
❑ You'll have increased sex drive and improved sexual performance.
❑ You'll have fewer illnesses and absences from work.
❑ You can challenge yourself in new and different ways.
❑ You'll be able to better manage your anger.
❑ You'll find that exercise takes your mind off other things for a while.
❑ Your balance will improve.
❑ You will function better.
❑ Your clothes may fit better.

Others will benefit, too!
❑ Your loved ones would worry less about your health.
❑ You will set an example about making healthy choices.
❑ You would be a healthy role model for your own children, family, and friends.

CONTEMPLATION

The goal in Contemplation is to encourage clients to view success as progress to Preparation. They are getting ready to take action, so encouraging them to rush to adopt regular exercise before they are ready is likely to be ineffective. The real risk for a Contemplator is that they will get stuck in "chronic" Contemplation because they are ambivalent. They see the value of adopting regular exercise, but are still acutely aware of the barriers or drawbacks. To help them keep moving forward, encourage them to take small steps. Being successful with those small steps will build their confidence and help them see the benefits of exercise more clearly.

For a sample Contemplation activity, see From the Practical Toolbox 4.2.

Contemplation: Key Intervention Strategies

Make the Pros Outweigh the Cons

- Ask client to name his or her most significant con(s).
- Acknowledge changing does have costs, but avoid debate about whether change is "worth it."
- Ask clients to shrink cons by:
  - Comparing them to their growing list of pros.
  - Asking how important cons are relative to pros.
  - Challenging themselves to overcome the cons.

Consciousness Raising—Become Informed

- Encourage clients to keep an exercise log or wear a pedometer so they can see how much, if any, exercise they are getting and when.
- Encourage clients to ask questions and search for more information (*e.g.*, explore alternatives for exercise venues that are well matched to preferences and schedules, talk to friends about how they fit exercise into their schedule).
- Ask clients what headlines or news stories they have seen recently about exercise (*e.g.*, a story on National Public Radio about exercise increasing memory capacity among older adults, etc.) and challenge them to look for more.

Self-Reevaluation—Create a New Self Image

- Encourage the client to ask him or herself about self-image: "How do I think and feel about myself as someone who is not exercising regularly?"
- Challenge the client to describe the kind of person he or she wants to be.
- Ask the clients to describe how their self-image might improve if they were exercising regularly.
- Provide a checklist of adjectives for the client to endorse (*e.g.*, energetic, sluggish, fit, out of shape, etc.).

Dramatic Relief—Pay Attention to Feelings

- Ask the client to share an inspirational story about someone they knew who improved their health and well-being by starting to exercise regularly (a friend, family member, celebrity, etc.).
- If she or he cannot think of an example, share one from your experience–convey the impact of beginning to exercise on someone who had been in the stage where this client is now.
- Ask the client to describe how she or he would feel if they were diagnosed with a chronic disease like diabetes or heart disease due in part to an unhealthy lifestyle–would they regret not exercising? Would she or he be worried about premature death? How can taking small steps toward regular exercise help him or her deal with those feelings?

From the Practical Toolbox 4.2

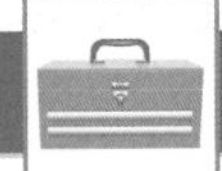

SAMPLE CONTEMPLATION ACTIVITY: OVERCOME THE ROADBLOCKS

There is a good chance you are wondering whether regular exercise is worth the effort. It can be challenging to change old habits, especially at first. We have three strategies to help reduce the drawbacks or roadblocks you might be facing. Jot down your three biggest roadblocks in the table below. Which of the following strategies will you use to overcome each barrier?

1. Create a list of the benefits, or pros, of exercising regularly. (The Sample Activity for Precontemplators: Raise the Pros, found in From the Practical Toolbox 4.1, can be used here, as well, if you have not already done so.) As you add to your list, the drawbacks, or cons, may seem less important.
2. Consider the cons as the hassles they are, compared to the serious consequences of not exercising regularly. For example:
   - How does the cost of an exercise class or a new pair of sneakers compare to the risk of diabetes or heart disease?
   - How does finding the time to exercise compare to the time you could be adding to your life by doing it?
   - How does the temporary discomfort of starting to exercise compare to the chance you will have less strength and endurance over time if you don't exercise?
3. Counter the cons, or drawbacks, with practical alternatives or challenges. For example:
   - If I lack a 30-minute block of time to exercise, I can do three, 10-minute blocks during the day.
   - I can watch a favorite show while I am on a treadmill to make the time pass more quickly.
   - If I am embarrassed to exercise in front of others, I can exercise at home, go to a class for beginners, or hit the gym when it is not crowded. I will feel less self-conscious.
   - If I cannot afford a gym membership, I can walk outside for free, sign up for a low-cost class at my community center, or ask if the gym offers a sliding scale membership fee.

List Your Three Biggest Roadblocks Here:	List Three Practical Alternatives Here:

- Encourage Small Steps (to Build Self-Efficacy)
  - Provide clients with options for a small step they can take toward their goal (*e.g.*, a 10-minute walk each day, going to one exercise class each week, taking the stairs instead of the elevator, making an appointment with their health care provider to get clearance to begin exercising).
  - Ask clients to choose among the small steps suggested or provide their own examples. Check in with them again to see how they did.

PREPARATION

The goal in Preparation is to encourage clients to be successful when they adopt regular exercise. Help them set a date, make a concrete plan, and build a support team. Encourage them to anticipate potentially difficult situations (*e.g.,* travel, upcoming busy times at work, bad weather) and make contingency plans so they do not get off track. Having a plan will build clients' confidence that they can achieve their goals. Your encouragement and support will also be crucial.

For a sample Preparation activity, see From the Practical Toolbox 4.3.

Preparation: Key Intervention Strategies

Self-Liberation—Make a Commitment

- Encourage client to make a strong commitment to start exercising regularly by:
  - Setting a specific start date, rather than waiting for a magic moment
  - Sharing commitment with others (tell others, post on Facebook or other social networking sites, etc.)
  - Creating a specific "Action Plan" and gathering any information they need
  - Writing down their commitment, start date, and action plan

Helping Relationships—Get Support

- Ask clients to identify others who can support their change efforts
  - A friend trying to make similar change
  - Loved ones, family, friends, neighbors, coworkers
  - Facebook friends
  - You or other staff at their gym, provider's office, etc.
  - Encourage clients to be as specific as possible about the type and amount of support and encouragement they need.
- Assist client by:
  - Role-playing requests for support
  - Identifying additional sources of support
  - Tapering support if it appears he or she is becoming dependent on you (*e.g.,* by meeting less often).

Self-Reevaluation—Keep Creating a New Self-Image

- Encourage clients to think about how they will think and feel about themselves after they have started making changes.
- Utilize visualization exercises (*i.e.,* client imagining themselves in 3 to 6 months or a year)
  - How they think about themselves
  - How their image of themselves has shifted
  - How their health has changed
  - How their outlook has changed
- Here are some additional guidelines for visualization (6):
  - Find a quiet place free of distractions. Relax and take deep breaths.
  - Visualize color–first as large blue circles. See them shrink to small dots and then disappear. Blue is a relaxing color.
  - Fill the scene with exercise images. Be as specific and detailed as possible.
  - Progressively add specific details including the client seeing themselves in great detail.
  - Have the client imagine themselves in the exercise setting. Imagine in detail how regular exercise will change their self-image. Have the client imagine the tasks and motor skills in vivid detail.
  - End by guiding them to breathing deeply, slowly opening their eyes, and adjusting to the real external environment.

From the Practical Toolbox 4.3

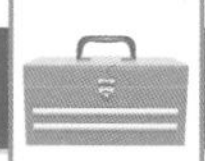

SAMPLE PREPARATION ACTIVITY: MAKE A COMMITMENT

Before beginning any exercise program, it is important to check with your doctor to make sure he or she does not have any concerns or recommendations for you.

Once you have gotten the green light, it is full steam ahead.

1. Set a Goal

Choose the specific goal you will work on by checking one of the following boxes.

- ❑ 150 minutes of moderate exercise (at least 30 minutes on at least 5 days per week)
- ❑ 75 minutes of vigorous exercise (at least 20 minutes a day on 3 or more days)
- ❑ A combination of moderate and vigorous activity that adds up to those targets (assuming 1 minute of vigorous exercise = 2 minutes of moderate)
- ❑ 8 to 12 repetitions of resistance exercises that include all major muscle groups, 2 to 3 days per week
- ❑ Exercises to improve balance, coordination, and agility, 2 to 3 days per week
- ❑ Flexibility exercises (60 seconds per exercise) for each major muscle-tendon group, at least 2 days per week

2. Find an Exercise

Making exercise a habit is a lot easier if you find something that matches your exercise goals, and that you really enjoy doing.

The most popular form of exercising in America is walking. However, you may prefer using a stationary bike, swimming, doing Zumba, taking a fitness class, doing yoga, playing basketball, or lifting weights.

The key is to think about what you want to gain from exercise, and then find the right type of exercise for you.

The exercise I choose is:_______________.

3. Set Your Start Date

When will you start to exercise regularly? Studies have shown that it helps to:

- Pick a date in the next month.
- Choose a day that you have some control over.
- Select a day that will not be too stressful.
- Mark your date where you will be reminded (in your planner or phone, etc.).

I will start exercising regularly on:

4. Tell Others about Your Commitment

Public commitments are stronger than private ones. Every time you tell someone about your promise to start exercising regularly, you make your commitment stronger.

Start to strengthen your determination to exercise by:

- Deciding who you will tell about your commitment, and
- Telling them about your plans.

Who will you tell about your plan?

I will tell:

_______________ _______________

_______________ _______________

How will you tell people? Consider these ideas:

- *Update your Facebook or Twitter status to:* "I am starting an exercise program!"
- *Say to your friends, family, and coworkers:* "I wanted to let a few people know that I'm planning to start exercising regularly. Telling people will help me stick with it. I plan to start on ________. Look for me at the gym/pool/on the road/walking path!"

continued

From the Practical Toolbox 4.3 *continued*

- *Send an email, text message, or instant message stating:* "I am committing to an exercise plan!"
- *Put a note on your refrigerator:* Exercise plan starts __________!
- *Download a smartphone app:* Apps like Runkeeper will not only track your workout for you, but will upload your workouts and results to Facebook or Twitter.

Do not wait! Let as many people as possible know that you are going to be exercising regularly.

5. Make an Action Plan

You will be more successful if you plan your strategy in advance. Be as specific as possible, keeping in mind how you will tackle any roadblocks that occur. For example, have a backup plan for bad weather.

My Action Plan
Start Date:
Days of the week I will exercise:

My Exercise Plan

	Time of Day	Activity	Location	Duration/Distance	Backup Plan
Monday					
Tuesday					
Wednesday					
Thursday					
Friday					
Saturday					
Sunday					

To make sure I exercise, I need to: (register for gym classes, pack exercise clothes the night before, etc.)

____

Before starting, I need to: (buy new sneakers, get gym schedule, etc.)

____

What else do I need to get started?

____

Counterconditioning—Use Substitutes

- Encourage clients to substitute healthy thoughts for unhealthy ones that might hold them back. You can share these examples:
  - If you are feeling tired, tell yourself how much energy you will have after you exercise.
  - "On stressful days, think of exercise as a time away from the day's worries."
  - "When you think you're too busy, remind yourself that exercise is an important part of being healthy."

ACTION

The goal in Action is to help the client continue exercising regularly. Encourage them to plan ahead to prevent slips: Remind them that failing to plan is planning to fail. Having a specific plan to deal with any potentially difficult situation (*e.g.,* holidays, stressful times at work, gym closures) will keep their confidence high, which is crucial in Action. At the same time, reassure them if they have a slip that they need not get discouraged. It is common to slip. Educate them that the most important thing is to evaluate what went wrong, create a plan for dealing with the situation in the future, and get back on track as quickly as possible.

For a sample Action activity, see From the Practical Toolbox 4.4.

Action: Key Intervention Strategies

Counter Conditioning—Use Substitutes

- Assist clients in replacing negative behaviors with positive behaviors (*e.g.,* "Instead of waiting until the end of the day to exercise (when I might not get to it), I will exercise in the morning").
- Teach clients to challenge negative thoughts by substituting positive alternatives (*e.g.,* "Instead of thinking of exercise as a chore, I will think of it as a gift I give to myself").
- Problem-solve with clients to identify behavioral alternatives that will work for them.

Stimulus Control—Take Control of Your Environment

- Help the client identify and avoid people, places, and things that increase the likelihood of being sedentary (*i.e.,* sitting down to watch "just one" show at night, busy days, friends who do not exercise, travel) and plans to work around those.
- Encourage clients to use reminders to exercise, like notes, scheduling exercise in their calendar, or signing up for a class so they have a specific time to exercise.
- Assist clients in identifying ways to restructure their environment to make it easier to exercise regularly (*e.g.,* exercise at lunch time with coworkers, leave their gym bag and sneakers in the car so they do not have to go home after work first, etc.).

Helping Relationships—Get Support

- Encourage clients to seek support from others, especially those who are regular exercisers.
- Encourage clients to be as specific as possible about the type and amount of support and encouragement they need.
- Point out that support can come from professionals as well as personal sources (*e.g.,* trainers, health care professionals, etc.).
- Remind clients that they may need to adjust their support team over time.

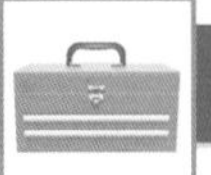

From the Practical Toolbox 4.4

SAMPLE ACTIVITY FOR ACTION: USE SUBSTITUTES

Replacing old habits and ways of thinking with new ones is one of the secrets to continuing to exercise regularly. The following examples will show you how others have made healthy substitutes.

Name	Old Way of Thinking	Healthy Substitute
Paul	"I used to get frustrated when I got to the gym and the machines were taken. So I'd just turn around and leave—without exercising."	"Now, I go to the gym early in the morning when it's not so busy. When I can't do that, I go for a jog outside or do squats, sit-ups, push-ups, lunges, and use free weights at home. That way, I'm certain to get a daily workout."
Jake	"I always found it difficult to set aside time for exercise because I let all my other priorities come first."	"I had to schedule a time to exercise to be sure I did it. It has worked really well—so now, I treat that time like an appointment. On the rare times when I don't feel like going, I tell myself that I can go for a few minutes and stop if I want. I've never stopped—once I get moving, I'm fine."
Danielle	"I used to skip exercising when I felt stressed."	"Now I remind myself that exercising is one of the best ways to manage my stress. I always feel better after I work out. Plus, it makes me more productive."
Lila	"I used to watch a lot of TV in the evenings.	"Now I tell myself that I can trade one of my half-hour shows for a brisk walk. I read last year that watching too much TV can actually make you gain weight. Watching TV for a half hour burns 36 calories—brisk walking burns about 148."
Terry	"I get bored easily."	"To keep myself interested in exercise, I add variety to my exercise program. Two days a week I walk, 2 days I swim, and 2 days I use the stair climber or elliptical machine at the gym. Cross-training has also given me the confidence to try new things. I feel stronger overall."

Now give some thought to the old thoughts and behaviors you might need to replace with healthier substitutes. Come up with at least one alternative for each.

Instead of. . .	I will. . .

Reinforcement Management—Use Rewards

- Encourage the client to notice the intrinsic rewards of exercising regularly (more energy, lower blood pressure, more self-confidence, higher self-esteem, higher productivity, etc.).
- Encourage clients to reinforce themselves with positive self-statements.
- Ask the client if they want to use tangible rewards for meeting various short- and long-term goals or milestones (*e.g.*, new sneakers or workout clothes after 3 months of regular exercise).

Self-Liberation—Make a Commitment

- Encourage the client to reaffirm their commitment to exercising regularly and to believe in his or her ability to do so.

MAINTENANCE

The goal in Maintenance is to help the client make regular exercise a life-long habit. Assist your clients in planning ahead to prevent slips in times of unusual distress (major stressors). Encourage them to get back on track quickly if they happen to have a slip to prevent that slip from turning into a major backslide.

For a sample Maintenance activity, see From the Practical Toolbox 4.5.

Maintenance: Key Intervention Strategies

Stimulus Control—Continue to Control

- Help client identify any people, places, or situations that they need to avoid to stay on track.
- Encourage clients to continue to use reminders to exercise.
- Ask clients if they have restructured their environments enough to ensure that they will keep exercising.

Counterconditioning—Continue to Substitute

- Encourage the client to keep his or her thinking positive (rule of thumb—three positive thoughts for each negative thought).
- Help clients to plan ahead to deal with difficult situations so confidence is high.
- Remind clients that a majority of relapses occur at times of distress and that although distress cannot be prevented, relapse can be.
- Remind clients that one of the best stress relievers and mood elevators is exercise. Other alternatives for dealing with distress include seeking support and using relaxation.

Reinforcement Management—Use Rewards

- Encourage clients to reward themselves for reaching various goals and overcoming any slips they might have.

Get Support

- Encourage the client to seek support as needed.
- Remind them they can now offer support to others to consolidate their own gains.

Recycling

- Many clients relapse before reaching permanent Maintenance.
- Encourage clients to view setbacks/lapses as an opportunity to learn and move ahead better prepared.
  - Encourage the view of a setback as temporary.
  - Help clients analyze slips and problem-solve about what can be done differently the next time.

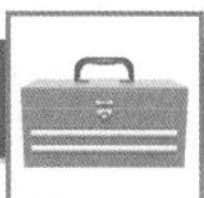

From the Practical Toolbox 4.5

SAMPLE MAINTENANCE ACTIVITY: PLAN AHEAD TO KEEP CONFIDENCE HIGH

Having been a regular exerciser for so long, you're probably pretty confident in your ability to keep exercising.

During the coming years, though, you might face new situations that could challenge your confidence. Read the following stories to learn how others have dealt with difficult situations and answer the questions that follow each one.

Difficult Situation: Stacey

Stacey had been walking as a way to stay healthy and maintain her weight for just over a year. During winter, though, she slipped on the ice, fell, and sprained her ankle.

By the time her injury had healed, it was spring. Though there was no ice on the ground, she still didn't want to head outside for a walk. She knew she needed to exercise—especially after she tried on her spring clothes and discovered that they were tight.

It took a while, but one day she just put on her sneakers and went for a walk. "I can't believe how good it felt! I don't know why I waited so long. My body needs this!"

Since then, she's back to walking regularly, and is feeling better than ever. She's even been saving up to buy a treadmill when winter hits. This winter there will be no ice to slip her up!

Imagine that you couldn't perform your regular exercise. What would you do instead?

____

Difficult Situation: Brian

Brian has been working toward a promotion at work. He is very good at his job, and has been putting in extra hours to stay in the race for the position.

He was stressed, feeling like he needed to be there all the time to show his commitment. This meant he stopped running. . .for the first time in years. Not running affected Brian pretty quickly. By the second week, he was less focused, could not sleep well, his stress was building, and he was grouchy all the time. On the tenth day of his "all work, no play" routine he took a run during lunch. "When I got back from that run, I had so much more energy and was so focused that I had a really productive afternoon and evening. It's easy to take exercise for granted once you're used to doing it regularly. But after stopping for a couple of weeks, I realized that getting out for a run helped me clear my head and stay balanced. I had to keep it up to be able to focus on my work."

After that, Brian made sure to get a run in every day during lunch, rain, or shine. He had learned a lesson about moderation—all work and no play is often less productive. And because he showed his boss he was able to dedicate himself to work in a healthy way, he got the promotion!

Brian discovered that he could not function well without exercising regularly. How would you function without your regular exercise?

____

How does exercise help you achieve your goals?

____

From the Practical Toolbox 4.5 *continued*

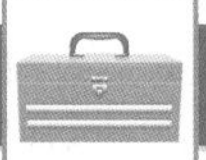

What other unexpected situations could derail you (*e.g.*, extended travel, change in daily routine like a new longer commute, or change in family demands, such as a sick parent)?

How will you handle those unexpected situations?

- Encourage clients to maintain an image of who they are working to be and an image of themselves as someone who is succeeding in the process.
- Ask clients to reassess their current stage if they slip out of exercising regularly.

Avoiding Boredom

Maintaining an exercise routine is a daunting task that involves continuously motivating choice in performing a behavior. Thus, it is not surprising that many individuals often focus on performing one, or only a few, different types of physical activities when beginning or maintaining an exercise routine. For this and any number of other potential reasons, people may become bored with their routine. To avoid boredom, you could encourage your clients to:

- Incorporate a variety of physical activity into their exercise routines
- Keep their usual routine interesting by varying their route
- Change the music they listen to
- Inviting different friends to join them.

The following strategies will also help your client to avoid boredom and relapsing to sedentary behavior. It will be most helpful to engage in nondirective problem solving with your client to generate solutions for avoiding boredom using the suggestions that follow. In other words, engage them in an active discussion in which you are facilitating their creation of a plan to incorporate variety into their routine.

For a sample form for monitoring workouts to avoid boredom, see From the Practical Toolbox 4.6.

Strategies to Avoid Boredom

- Have your client reconceptualize boredom with their current routine as an opportunity rather than a hindrance. This is a good time to finally attempt a sport, activity class, or new exercise routine that they have wanted to try.
- Challenge your client to identify what they hope to get out of exercise and to identify what types of activities could provide that feeling or outcome. If, for example, they want to build strength, they can lift weights, try white water rafting, or take Zumba. If they want creativity, they can try skateboarding, snowboarding, freestyle dance, mountain biking, urban hip hop, or inline skating. If they want to build stamina, they can try hiking, distance running, or swimming, or to boost a mind-body connection they could try yoga, Tai Chi, Pilates, or martial arts.
- Encourage them to look for helpful information while exploring other types of exercise.
- Help them to internalize their motivation to exercise by focusing on how good it feels to try other forms of physical activity and experience the sensations of participating in a new physical activity.

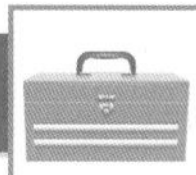

From the Practical Toolbox 4.6

SAMPLE MONITORING FORM

Date: ______________________ Location of workout: ________________________________

Type of Activities	Intensity/Effort Expended	Duration of Workout

Did today's workout keep me on track for my **short-term** goals? Yes No

Did today's workout keep me on track for my **medium-range** goals? Yes No

Did today's workout keep me on track for my **long-term** goals? Yes No

How did I feel before today's workout?

How did I feel during today's workout?

How did I feel after today's workout?

Which (if any) parts of my workout could I change to help me stay motivated, enthusiastic, and on track to accomplish all of my goals?

Any additional notes or comments:

- Encourage your client to get help from others. Good examples include joining a new gym, activity group, recreational sports team, or community recreation league. Encourage them to ask different friends, family members, and/or coworkers to join them to exercise.
  - Recognize that many clients are looking to exercise professionals for this type of helping relationship. Encourage them to become their own coach by determining what exactly they are bored with in their routine (*e.g.*, lack of enjoyment; lack of satisfaction with performance/results) and problem-solving about other ways to achieve the desired outcome.

- Help them to realistically evaluate their goals and expectations. Give them information about which other activities may help accelerate progress toward appropriate short-, medium-, and long-term goals.

- Have your client track their progress daily. Carefully monitoring all aspects of their workouts allows you (and them) to see exactly which aspect(s) are contributing to boredom. Be sure to monitor:
  - What types of exercise are being performed, and their level of interest while performing it
  - Feelings of perceived exertion
  - Satisfaction with each workout
  - If short-, moderate-, and long-term goals are being met. Are these goals realistic to begin with? Can they be adjusted?

Relapse Prevention

Understanding that slips and setbacks will happen is the first step in not letting those slips derail all of the hard work an individual has done to become physically active. In terms of exercise, this means avoiding relapse to sedentary behaviors. Thus, strategies for preventing relapse must focus on addressing the temptations to be sedentary.

Strategies to Help Avoid Relapse

- Encourage your client to recognize the times when they are tempted to skip a workout. Come up with a strategy to avoid succumbing to this temptation. For example:
  - Get a gym membership or treadmill for the home if they enjoy running, but do not like running outside in bad weather.
  - Call a friend when they are not in the mood to exercise and need a little extra social support to stay on track.
  - Focus on the mood improvements that result from exercising to avoid skipping a workout when they feel down.

- Assist your client to recognize all of their previous accomplishments, successes, and new knowledge they have about exercise and health. Help them realize the barriers they have overcome to get where they are now, and remember the experiences that they had while becoming a regular exerciser.

- Encourage your client to reward themselves for all of their accomplishments. It may seem obvious to reward behavioral milestones such as working out 4 days in one week, or reaching a new performance goal, but remind them to reward other accomplishments, even if the reward is a positive self-statement (Good job! I knew I could do it!). For example, reward small steps such as joining a gym, subscribing to a fitness magazine, or scheduling appointments with a trainer or a group exercise class.

- Help your client identify other people and/or groups that they may turn to for help and support. Provide them with a list of websites that post exercise classes, recreational sports leagues, local road races, and physical activity meet-up groups.
- Identify the cues in your client's life that are triggering sedentary behaviors. Can they, for example, leave some workout equipment (*e.g.*, light weights/dumbbells, DVDs, or therabands) in places where they would normally be sedentary (*i.e.*, living room, bedroom, home office, etc.)?
- Encourage your client to substitute negatives with positives. For example, help them:
  - Have walking meetings at work.
  - Ride a stationary bike while watching TV instead of sitting on the couch.
  - Ask a friend to catch up and talk while walking around the neighborhood instead of talking over coffee.
- Help your client stay up to date on exercise strategies, opportunities, and benefits by encouraging them to subscribe to fitness-oriented magazines, bookmark their favorite physical activity–oriented Web sites, and talk to people about specific issues and/or questions about staying on track.
- Encourage your client to monitor their exercise routines, progress, goals, and setbacks. Daily monitoring is key in identifying where and when setbacks are likely to occur.

The Action section earlier in this chapter provides additional tips on avoiding relapse.

RESOURCES FOR CLIENTS

To provide clients with additional assistance navigating the behavior change process, you can refer them to a variety of free resources with behavior change tips.

Behavior Change Resources for Clients

Web Sites

Centers for Disease Control: http://www.cdc.gov/physicalactivity/index.html

National Institutes of Health: http://health.nih.gov/topic/ExercisePhysicalFitness; older adults can also find guidance at http://health.nih.gov/topic/ExerciseforSeniors.

Computer-Tailored Intervention

You can also refer them to an evidence-based computer-tailored intervention for exercise within the LifeStyle Management Suite of programs available at www.prochange.com/myhealth. Participants can interact with the fully tailored intervention, which gives individualized feedback on the behavior change processes they are using and suggestions about what they need to use more or less to move forward. A demo of the program is available at www.prochange.com/exercisedemo. The suite also contains a Personal Activity Center that includes interactive activities designed to activate the most appropriate strategies for change. A nominal fee grants access for 1 year. Participants can print and share their computer-tailored intervention report with you or other health professionals.

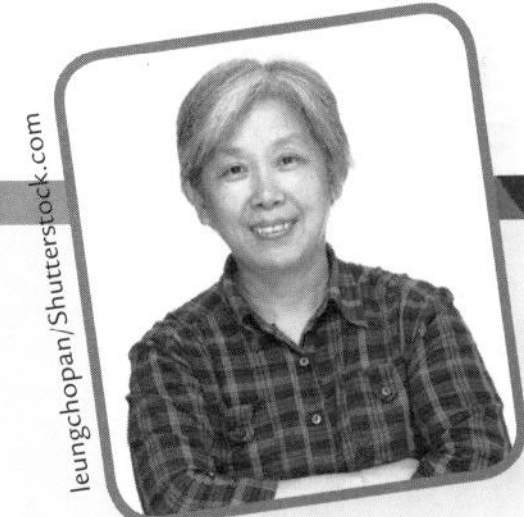
leungchopan/Shutterstock.com

Case Scenario 4.1

Marianne is a 56-year-old woman with hypertension, high cholesterol, and a body mass index of 27. She was referred through a worksite wellness program to a session with a health coach, who can see from her Health Risk Assessment that she is not currently exercising.

During their first call, Marianne reports that she has no intention to begin exercising regularly in the next 6 months. She explains that she has no time for exercise given her busy work schedule. She also reports that she does not need to exercise because she is "pretty healthy." She attributes her weight gain in the past 5 years to menopause.

What stage of change is Marianne likely in, and what interventions do you suggest?

____

____

____

Intervention Suggestions:

- Raise the Pros
- Decrease defenses—Marianne is blaming her weight gain on menopause, rather than recognizing the role a sedentary lifestyle could be playing. She is potentially denying the role her sedentary lifestyle and overweight status is playing in her chronic illnesses, both of which increase her risk of cardiovascular disease. It will be helpful to point out that we often use defenses, and to assist Marianne in recognizing hers, so she can use them less.
- Ask Marianne if she has spoken with her health care provider about the role exercise could play in managing her hypertension and high cholesterol. If she has not, ask her if she will. Would it be possible to get off the medication she is now taking if she exercised more? Would exercise also lower her risk of other conditions, such as diabetes?
- Does she pay attention to news stories and headlines about exercise? Could she find one between now and your next call?
- Does Marianne have children or other young family members (*e.g.*, nieces or nephews)? Is she concerned about living as long as she can for them or seeing important milestones in their lives (*e.g.*, weddings, first babies)? Could exercising help her be there for those special people? Ask her if she has thought about what type of example she would be setting for them if she were to start exercising someday.

What else might be an effective intervention for Marianne?

Marianne is in the Precontemplation stage because she is not intending to exercise regularly in the next 6 months. Another effective intervention strategy for those in Precontemplation is to encourage them to look for inspiration from others who have adopted regular exercise. Ask if she knows anyone who has improved his or her health and well-being by beginning to exercise regularly. How did that person do it? Does that person's success inspire her to want to exercise?

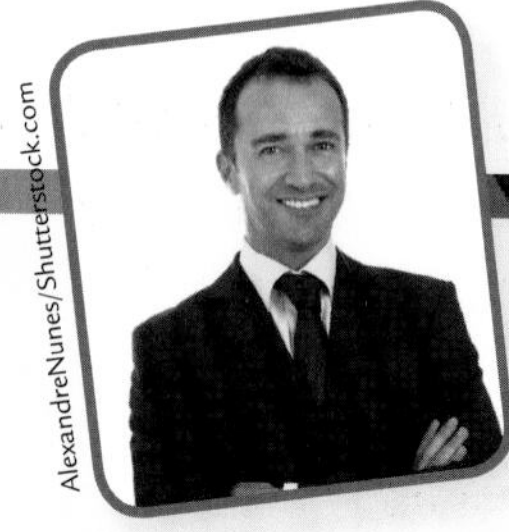

Case Scenario 4.2

Bill is a 33-year-old with no notable medical history and a body mass index of 22. He played basketball in high school and college, but has little time now that he has a new demanding position as a supervisor at work and a new baby at home. He reports that he is "thinking about" beginning to exercise again sometime in the next 6 months or so, but has no specific plans. He also reports that he "feels guilty" spending time exercising after work since his wife seems more overwhelmed when he comes home later.

What stage of change is Bill likely in, and what interventions do you suggest?

____

____

____

Intervention Suggestions:

- Stress, a demanding schedule, and feeling guilty over taking time away from his new family are big cons for Bill. Assist him in overcoming those cons by coming up with practical ways around them (*e.g.,* Can he exercise on his lunch hour at the company's fitness facility? Can he ride his bike to and from work so his transportation is his exercise and he will not be hassled with traffic? Can he find some way to give his wife a break and exercise by taking the baby for a walk or jog in the stroller?) and/or comparing them to the advantages he is familiar with (*e.g.,* he will feel less stressed if he exercises, he is likely to be more productive, and he will live longer for his new baby).
- Can Bill talk to coworkers and friends to figure out how they are fitting exercise into their schedules? Are there any alternatives that might fit into his schedule (*e.g.,* a gym that opens up early enough for him to go on his way to work so he can still be home in the evening)?
- Ask Bill to list his values and what is important to him. Is his sedentary lifestyle consistent with those values? Is that the image he wants his new son to have of him?
- Has he been inspired by anyone who manages to fit exercise in and has benefited as a result? Has he heard any stories of colleagues who had health problems because they did not take care of themselves by exercising and eating well?
- Are there any small steps he can take to start to reincorporate exercise into his life?

What else might be an effective intervention for Bill?

Bill is in the Contemplation stage. Another effective intervention strategy for individuals in Contemplation is to ask him to consider the effect of his inactivity on the important people in his life. Could he be a better role model to his child, and other people in his life, if he were exercising regularly?

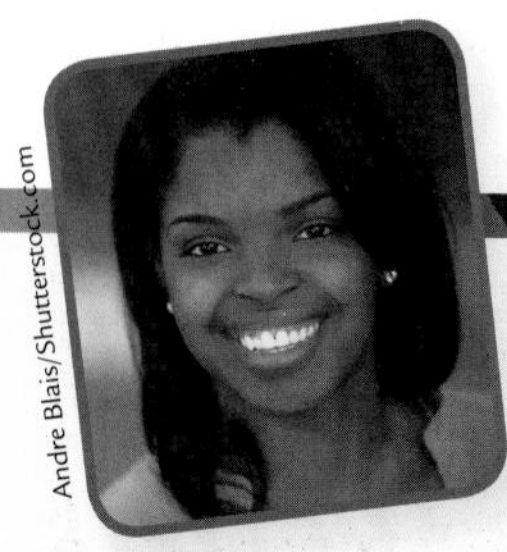

Case Scenario 4.3

Michelle is a 25-year-old recent college graduate with a body mass index of 25. She is in good health overall, but would like to drop a few pounds. Her typical workout routine has included 30 minutes a day on the elliptical machine at the gym in her apartment complex or walking around the neighborhood. Recently her motivation and adherence to this routine has waned

Case Scenario 4.3 *continued*

because she is frustrated with her slowing weight loss. She now reports that she has a hard time consistently exercising because of work and social obligations. She also seems to be overestimating how many calories are burned during exercise and the intensity level of her workouts. She reports that she is going to get back on track in the next week or so, but wants some tips.

What stage of change is Michelle likely in, and what interventions do you suggest?

____

____

____

Intervention Suggestions:

- Encourage Michelle to renew her commitment to exercising regularly and encourage her to focus on all of the benefits, rather than just on the potential to lose weight. Ask her if exercise will make her feel more energetic, confident, and healthy.
- Encourage Michelle to share her commitment to get started again with her friends, family, and coworkers.
- Assist Michelle with making detailed plans for how and when she will exercise, anticipating potential challenges. What will she do when she has to work late or when the weather is bad?
- Help Michelle find accurate information about the intensity of her exercise and educate her about the duration and intensity needed to burn calories. Does she need to increase the intensity of her exercise to see the results she wants?
- Encourage Michelle to employ substitutes for negative thoughts that could be getting in her way (*e.g.*, If she is busy with work, can she walk or bike there to add more activity to her day or get off public transportation a few stops earlier? If she feels like she is missing out on social obligations when she is exercising, can she involve friends in her activity—going for hikes or bike rides? If she is bored with the elliptical and not getting the results she wants, can she add more variety to her routine?)

What else might be an effective intervention for Michelle?

Michelle is in the Preparation Stage. She had been in Action and is planning to get back on track. To help Michelle reach her goal, you could suggest that she turn her social network into a support network. Suggest that she ask for the encouragement of important people in her life and talk with her about how specifically she can do that. Does she want to challenge her friends informally or formally in apps like Nike+? If you sense reluctance, ask if a closed social network like LoseIt! might work for her.

TAKE-HOME MESSAGES

Other behavior theories and models are described in Chapter 1. This chapter further details the TTM as a useful intervention framework for assisting clients in adopting and maintaining regular exercise. It is crucial to assess each client's readiness to engage in regular exercise and tailor your interventions to his or her stage of change. Recognizing the unique needs of individuals in early stages and reconceptualizing progress as movement to the next stage can significantly increase the impact of exercise interventions. Adequate preparation prior to taking action has the potential to decrease relapse rates and assist individuals in recycling more quickly if they do relapse to an earlier stage. The suggestions and sample activities provided here will assist you in using stage-appropriate strategies for the entire population of clients with whom you come into contact, rather than the minority who are prepared to take action.

REFERENCES

1. American College of Sports Medicine. *ACSM's Guidelines for Exercise Testing and Prescription*. 9th ed. Baltimore (MD): Lippincott Williams and Wilkins; 2014.
2. American College of Sports Medicine. Quantity and quality of exercise for developing and maintaining cardiorespiratory, musculoskeletal, and neuromotor fitness in apparently healthy adults: Guidance for prescribing exercise. *Med Sci Sports Exerc*. 2011;1334–59.
3. Bandura A. Self-efficacy. In: Ramachaudran VS, editor. *Encyclopedia of Human Behavior*. New York: Academic Press; 1994. p. 71–81.
4. Blaney C, Robbins M, Paiva A, et al. Validation of the TTM processes of change measure for exercise in an adult African American sample. In: *Proceedings of the 31st Annual Conference of the Society of Behavioral Medicine*, 2010, Seattle WA.
5. Butterworth SW. Influencing patient adherence to treatment guidelines. J Manage Care Pharm. 2008;14(6 suppl b):21.
6. Centers for Disease Control and Prevention. *Health Behaviors of Adults: United States 2005–2007. Vital Health Stat Series 10*, Number 24, 2010.
7. Cox RH. *Sports Psychology*. 7th ed. New York: McGraw-Hill; 2012.
8. DiClemente CC, Prochaska JO, Fairhurst SK, Velicer WF, Velasquez MM, Rossi JS. The process of smoking cessation: an analysis of precontemplation, contemplation, and preparation stages of change. *J Consult Clin Psychol*. 1991 Apr;59(2):295–304.
9. Dunn AL, Marcus BH, Kampert JB, Garcia ME, Kohl III HW, Blair SN. Comparison of lifestyle and structured interventions to increase physical activity and cardiorespiratory fitness. *JAMA*. 1999;281(4):327–34.
10. Hall KL, Rossi JS. Meta-analytic examination of the strong and weak principles across 48 health behaviors. *Prev Med*. 2008;46(3):266–74.
11. Johnson S, Paiva A, Castle PH. Cluster analysis within the Maintenance stage: Profiles predicting relapse from regular exercise. In: *Proceedings of the 31st Annual Conference of the Society of Behavioral Medicine*, 2010, Seattle WA.
12. Johnson SS, Paiva AL, Cummins CO, et al. Transtheoretical Model–based multiple behavior intervention for weight management: Effectiveness on a population basis. *Prev Med*. 2008 Mar;46(3):238–46.
13. Krebs P, Prochaska JO, Rossi JS. A meta-analysis of computer-tailored interventions for health behavior change. *Prev Med*. 2010 Sep;51(3–4):214–21.
14. Marcus BH, Emmons KM, Simkin-Silverman LR, et al. Evaluation of motivationally tailored vs. standard self-help physical activity interventions at the workplace. *Am J Health Promot*. 1998;12(4):246–53.
15. Marcus BH, Lewis BA, Williams DM, et al. A comparison of Internet and print-based physical activity interventions. *Arch Intern Med*. 2007;167(9):944.
16. Marcus BH, Lewis BA, Williams DM, et al. Step into motion: A randomized trial examining the relative efficacy of Internet vs. print-based physical activity interventions. *Contem Clin Trials*. 2007;28(6): 737–47.
17. Marcus BH, Napolitano MA, King AC, et al. Telephone versus print delivery of an individualized motivationally tailored physical activity intervention: Project STRIDE. *Health Psych*. 2007;26(4):401.
18. Marcus BH, Rossi JS, Selby VC, Niaura RS, Abrams DB. The stages and processes of exercise adoption and maintenance in a worksite sample. *Health Psych*. 1992;11(6):386.
19. Mauriello LM, Ciavatta MMH, Paiva AL, et al. Results of a multi-media multiple behavior obesity prevention program for adolescents. *Prev Med*. 2010;51(6):451–6.
20. Neville LM, O'Hara B, Milat A. Computer-tailored physical activity behavior change interventions targeting adults: A systematic review. *Int J Behav Nutr and Phys Act*. 2009;6(1):30.
21. Nigg CR, Courneya KS. Transtheoretical Model: Examining adolescent exercise behavior. *J Adolesc Health*. 1998;22(3):214–24.
22. Noar SM, Benac CN, Harris MS. Does tailoring matter? Meta-analytic review of tailored print health behavior change interventions. *Psychol Bull*. 2007 Jul;133(4):673–93.
23. Norman GJ, Zabinski MF, Adams MA, Rosenberg DE, Yaroch AL, Atienza AA. A review of eHealth interventions for physical activity and dietary behavior change. *Am J Prev Med*. 2007;33(4):336–45.
24. Pro-Change Behavior Systems, Inc. *Mastering Change: A Coach's Guide to Using the Transtheoretical Model with Clients*. Kingston (RI): Pro-Change Behavior Systems, Inc.; 2004.
25. Pro-Change Behavior Systems, Inc. *Roadways to Healthy Living: A Guide for Exercising Regularly*. Kingston (RI): Pro-Change Behavior Systems, Inc.; 2009.
26. Prochaska JO, DiClemente CC, Norcross JC. In search of how people change: Applications to addictive behaviors. *Am Psychol*. 1992 Sep;47(9):1102–14.
27. Prochaska JO, Evers KE, Castle PH, et al. Enhancing multiple domains of well-being by decreasing multiple health risk behaviors: A randomized clinical trial. *Popul Health Manag*. 2012 Oct;15(5):276–86.
28. Prochaska JO, Velicer WF, DiClemente CC, Fava J. Measuring processes of change: Applications to the cessation of smoking. *J Consult Clin Psychol*. 1988 Aug;56(4):520–8.
29. Prochaska JO, Velicer WF, Fava JL, Rossi JS, Tsoh JY. Evaluating a population-based recruitment approach and a stage-based expert system intervention for smoking cessation. *Addict Behav*. 2001 Jul;26(4):583–602.
30. Tseng YH, Jaw SP, Lin TL, Ho CC. Exercise motivation and processes of change in community-dwelling older persons. *J Nurs Res*. 2003;11(4):269.
31. Velicer WF, DiClemente CC, Prochaska JO, Brandenburg N. Decisional balance measure for assessing and predicting smoking status. *J Pers Soc Psychol*. 1985 May;48(5):1279–89.
32. Williams DM, Papandonatos GD, Jennings EG, et al. Does tailoring on additional theoretical constructs enhance the efficacy of a print-based physical activity promotion intervention? *Health Psych*. 2011;30(4):432.
33. Woods C, Mutrie N, Scott M. Physical activity intervention: A Transtheoretical Model–based intervention designed to help sedentary young adults become active. *Health Ed Res*. 2002;17(4):451–60.

CHAPTER 5

Communication Skills to Elicit Physical Activity Behavior Change: How to Talk to the Client

Heather Patrick, Ken Resnicow, Pedro J. Teixeira, and Geoffrey C. Williams

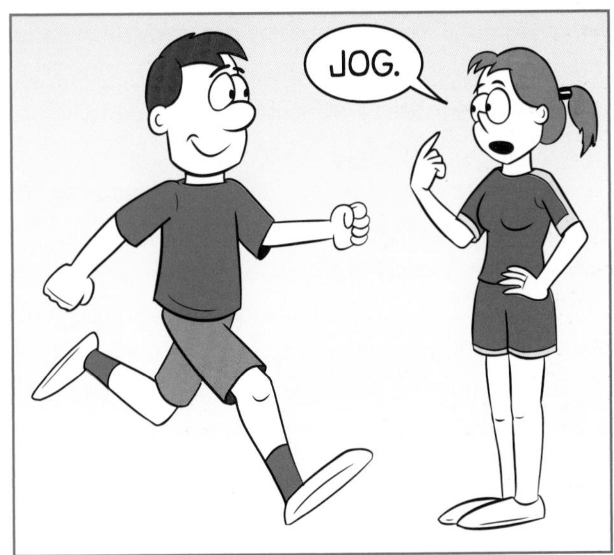

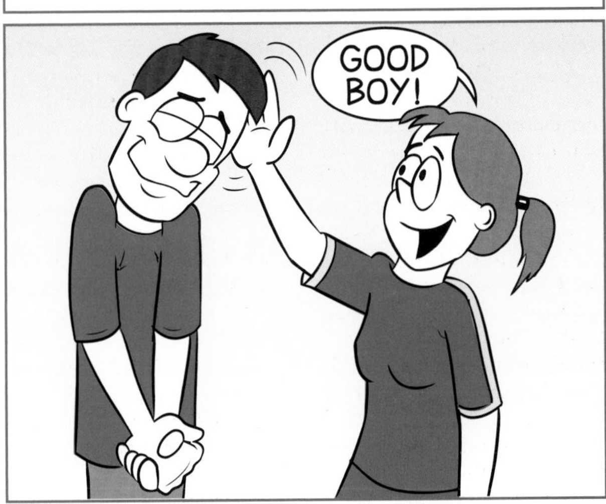

CONCEPT OVERVIEW

One of the biggest challenges facing practitioners is that physical activity (PA) counseling must take into account both individual motivational variables (*e.g.*, whether an individual wants to exercise or not, perceived barriers to being physically active) and the sociocultural context in which we live. A natural tendency for some practitioners is to attempt to motivate a client by showing clients the error of their ways; using fear messages or exhortation or by prescribing a ready-made exercise plan. However, these approaches often fail to yield the desired results. Indeed, in much the same way that most people in the developed world know that smoking tobacco is dangerous for their health, they also already know that being more physically active is something they "should do" to be healthier. Yet most are not doing enough of it. Information is not the key driver.

As a practitioner, you are uniquely positioned to energize and motivate your clients to be more physically active. Providing appropriate motivational support for your clients involves understanding the reasons they may not enjoy PA. This could include fears, discomfort, or other sources of resistance and ambivalence as well as the meaning of PA for their health and broader life values. Patient-centered counseling approaches offer a variety of techniques by which practitioners can support clients' optimal motivation, resulting in long-lasting health behavior change. This includes aligning their natural tendencies toward growth and health with their other life goals and values. Working with clients in this manner allows them to develop a plan for regular physical activity that is best suited to their specific needs, values, strengths, barriers, and life stage. Because clients play an active role in addressing barriers, exploring the meaning of PA, and developing their PA plan, a pattern of regular physical activity will more likely be maintained.

In this chapter, we take the perspectives of Motivational Interviewing (MI) (32) and Self-Determination Theory (SDT) (36,38) to identify client-centered ways in which practitioners can encourage increased physical activity. We have chosen to take these perspectives in particular for two primary reasons. First, MI and SDT have demonstrated efficacy in working with those who may be ambivalent about change, as well as those more ready to change (32,38). Second, an emerging body of evidence supports the efficacy of these approaches not only for the initiation of behavior change but also its maintenance. Although MI and SDT emerged in different ways—MI as a counseling style and SDT as a psychological theory—they are conceptually complementary in many ways (20,51), and both have been used to develop interventions that motivate long-term change of health behaviors, including tobacco cessation, reduction of alcohol intake, increases in fruit and vegetable intake, healthy weight management, and regular physical activity (19,38). More sophisticated discussions of the higher-level distinctions between MI and SDT have been provided elsewhere (29,50,51). For ease of presentation, we will discuss MI and SDT as distinct yet complementary approaches useful in a variety of contexts and settings. Thus, it is not the case that one is necessarily "better" than another in any given situation. We begin with a brief overview of MI and SDT to clarify their underlying assumptions about human motivation. Specific strategies used within MI and SDT are then described, along with the training necessary to successfully implement these techniques in clinical practice. Two specific client-centered counseling frameworks for physical activity (the 5 A's and MI's Explore, Guide, Choose) are presented, and an overview of the evidence for these approaches is provided. Examples and brief vignettes are included whenever possible to assist the reader in understanding how to put these techniques into practice.

A BRIEF OVERVIEW OF MOTIVATIONAL INTERVIEWING AND SELF-DETERMINATION THEORY

Motivational Interviewing

Motivational Interviewing (MI) is a set of general clinical techniques aimed at addressing clients' ambivalence toward change, overcoming resistance to change, and building autonomous motivation. Rather than using more directive or coercive approaches, MI works from the perspective of the client by aligning behavior change goals with the client's broader goals and values. Although it originally emerged out of addiction treatment, MI has since been used to modify a range of health behaviors relevant to chronic disease prevention and management, including healthy eating, physical activity, and weight management (19). MI is a "way of being" that uses strategies described later in this chapter such as reflective listening, shared decision making, and eliciting change talk.

Effective MI has been described as the strategic balance between "comforting the afflicted" and "afflicting the comfortable" (30). That is, MI techniques involve balancing the expression of empathy with the need to build sufficient discrepancy (*i.e.,* between the individual's current behavior and the behavioral goal and other personal values) to stimulate change. MI has been shown to be particularly effective with those who are ambivalent about change (3,15,24,28,31). This may be, in part, because of the nonjudgmental and encouraging tone that characterizes MI. Practitioners establish a nonconfrontational and supportive climate in which clients feel comfortable expressing both what they like and what they don't like about their current behavior. From the perspective of MI, it is often important to explore ambivalence prior to moving toward change (30).

Most practitioners learn to offer their professional advice based on their expertise and experience. They may do so in part to save time, and because they function from a paternalistic "I know what's best" approach for motivating their clients. However, an overly prescriptive approach often backfires, creating resistance from clients more than drive. Using an MI approach, clients do much of the psychological work themselves. Practitioners, therefore, serve as guides through the process, assisting clients in identifying their own pros and cons for their current behavior as well as the goal behavior, understanding what prevents them—both practically and perceptually—from reaching the goal behavior, and developing a plan of action once ambivalence has been explored and resolved. Within MI, practitioners typically do not directly attempt to dismantle denial or confront irrational or maladaptive beliefs. Instead, they may subtly help clients detect contradictions in their thoughts and actions, allowing them to experience discrepancy between their current actions and who they ideally want to be. MI practitioners rarely attempt to convince, cajole, or persuade. Instead, MI encourages clients to make fully informed and deeply contemplated choices, even if the decision is not to change. The counselor is careful to avoid pushing the client and creating further resistance.

Self-Determination Theory

MI emerged as a set of clinical techniques and thus is inherently practical in the clinical world. By comparison, Self-Determination Theory (SDT) evolved out of basic social science as a theoretical framework to understand the bases of human motivation (5,36). Much recent research in SDT has focused on applying its concepts clinically, including in the area of physical activity (13,39). There is a good deal of conceptual overlap between SDT and MI, though some differences remain. A sophisticated discussion of the complementarity and distinctions between MI and SDT is beyond the scope of this chapter. However, several recent publications have focused explicitly on this issue (20,26,29,47,50,51). Using the principles of SDT, Williams and others have developed and tested need-supportive therapy for health behavior change for physical activity, tobacco cessation, weight loss, and medication use (41,54,55). The SDT-based approach uses many MI-congruent techniques. Additionally, researchers and practitioners alike have begun to use SDT as the *de facto* theoretical perspective through which to understand how and why MI techniques work (30).

CONTINUUM OF MOTIVATION

SDT views motivation as having two central components: psychological energy, and the goal that the energy is directed toward. SDT has articulated a continuum of motivation which ranges from *amotivation* (*i.e.,* lacking psychological energy, or having no reason for engaging in a behavior, or seeking a particular health goal) to *extrinsic motivation* (engaging in behaviors for some separable outcome) to *intrinsic motivation* (engaging in behaviors for their own enjoyment or interest, and not for any other separable outcome). Figure 5.1 presents the motivation continuum, along with examples of each type of regulation, described in detail in the following text. Many health behaviors are extrinsically motivated; that is, they are engaged for some separable outcome (*e.g.,* to eliminate or reduce a symptom, to improve the quality or length of life, to minimize nagging from a well-intentioned spouse or clinician). Others, like physical activity or healthy cooking, can also be intrinsically motivating; that is, they can be interesting in their own right and strongly energized by the enjoyment they provide.

Within the motivation continuum there are several gradations varying in the degree to which extrinsic motivations are more or less internalized to the self (*i.e.,* how self-congruent these

		Extrinsic motivation				
Motivation	Amotivation	External regulation	Introjected regulation	Identified regulation	Integrated regulation	Intrinsic motivation
Definition	Lacking motivation or psychological energy.	Gaining rewards, avoiding negative consequences, including social sanctions.	Internal pressure resulting in feelings of shame or guilt.	Believing in the personal importance or value of the behavior.	The behavior is consistent with one's other goals and values.	The behavior is enjoyable and important in its own right.
Example	The client can't think of any reason for engaging in physical activity.	The client exercises to get a T-shirt. The client exercises so her trainer won't scold her for failing to meet exercise goals.	The client feels guilty about not exercising when he is spending a lot of money on a personal trainer.	The client exercises because she believes exercising is important for her health.	The client exercises because it is consistent with his goals for losing weight and getting healthier.	The client regularly attends an exercise class because it is fun.

FIGURE 5.1. The motivation continuum.

motivations are, and how closely they resemble intrinsic motivation) (5,35). The least internalized form of extrinsic motivation, *external* regulation, is characterized by engaging in behaviors to gain some reward, such as a financial incentive, or to avoid some negative consequence, including social sanctions like disapproval or disappointment from others. *Introjected* regulation is similar to external regulation in that behaviors are also enacted out of a sense of pressure or coercion—in this case, pressures that one puts on oneself to behave so as to avoid feelings of shame and guilt if one failed to perform a behavior as prescribed or up to one's standards.

Many clients may come into physical activity sessions with these "controlled" forms of motivation. And although these forms of motivation may be energizing for a time, this is often short-lived and frequently associated with poor psychological well-being when compared with more autonomous or internalized types of motivation. Importantly, although it may seem somewhat intuitive to offer extrinsic rewards to help to get people started with a regular exercise routine, the preponderance of evidence from basic social science research broadly, and from SDT in particular, suggests that such tactics are likely to interfere with the process of internalization (6,36,37). For instance, studies in tobacco cessation (4) and weight control (26) indicate that changes induced by financial incentives are generally not maintained in the long term. Thus, any short-term gains that may be achieved by using rewards, social punishments, or attempting to capitalize on the client's own propensity for feelings of guilt and shame, are outweighed by the long-term motivational consequences. Supporting clients to develop more autonomous, internalized forms of motivation is key, as internalized motivations have been shown to result in greater behavioral persistence (40).

Identified regulation is a relatively more autonomous form of extrinsic motivation. It is characterized by a belief that the target behavior is personally important and meaningful, and thus the behavior it energizes is maintained over time. For example, someone may pursue a specific physical activity goal—like training for and completing a marathon—because the individual believes it is an important goal to achieve. Finally, the most autonomous (*i.e.,* internalized) form of extrinsic motivation is *integrated regulation.* With integrated regulation, the individual believes that the behavior is important and meaningful and is also consistent with one's other goals and values. Thus, operating under integrated regulation a person may train for and complete a marathon because the activity is personally important and is also consistent with the person's broader goals and values for being healthy and active.

Importantly, SDT views motivation as dynamic. That is, even though people may have more external reasons for engaging in a behavior, they may develop more autonomous or internalized reasons over time. Practitioners are uniquely positioned to facilitate (or impede) this process. Also, it is important to keep in mind that different types of motivation can and do coexist relative to any behavior, including physical activity. For instance, some introjected motivation can be present even when someone exercises largely for autonomous reasons. From an SDT perspective, the important aspect for adherence and well-being is what type of motivation is predominant.

BASIC PSYCHOLOGICAL NEEDS

The supporting or thwarting of basic psychological needs is the primary mechanism through which motivation and self-regulation can be changed (6). SDT proposes three basic psychological needs: competence, relatedness, and autonomy. These needs are consistent with MI principles and techniques (20).

Competence

Competence refers to the need to feel capable of achieving desired outcomes. It is related to the concept of self-efficacy (*i.e.,* confidence), used in other health behavior theories (1) (also see Chapter 1 and 3). Discussing psychological and practical barriers to physical activity as well as goal setting and action planning can serve to meet the client's need for competence.

Identifying the level of physical activity your client is ready for (*i.e.*, reaching optimal challenge, not too much or too little) will also support his or her need for competence.

Relatedness

Relatedness refers to the need to feel connected to and understood by important others. Practitioners can support this need by being empathic, listening to the client's concerns and asking questions to seek clarification about what the client is expressing. Relatedness needs may also be supported through being physically active. For some, this may mean exercising with others or examining how physical activity can improve their social relationships.

Autonomy

Autonomy is the need to feel volitional, as the originator of one's actions. By serving as a guide to the client's own self-exploration and goal setting, practitioners can support this need and thus promote the development of more optimal, enduring forms of motivation and self-regulation for their clients. Clients' needs for autonomy are also supported by practitioners following the principles of client centeredness; providing choices or a menu of options for how to go about behavior change and by not pushing their own agenda, particularly when the client voices ambivalence or reasons against behavior change. For example, when talking with a client about types of exercise likely to promote health and cardiovascular fitness, some clients may automatically think of the experience of being told by a coach or gym teacher to run laps (often as punishment). As a practitioner, you can offer a list of possible activities the client may wish to try out that would achieve the same health benefits but be more enjoyable (*e.g.*, exercise classes such as Body Pump or Zumba, dancing, playing pick-up basketball games with friends).

Practitioners can guard against pushing their own agenda by using techniques such as reflective listening, as described later in this text. It is important for practitioners not to get attached to a particular outcome or agenda. Doing so interferes with clients' capacity to make an informed choice about the direction in which they want to go with prescribed behavior change, and to have ownership over the plan the client and practitioner develop together.

MI and SDT Techniques and Strategies

We now provide a general overview of MI and SDT techniques and strategies that can be used when working with clients around physical activity behavior change. Although we will be discussing a variety of techniques, it is not necessary to use all of these techniques with every client or in every session. Indeed, the amount of time one has to interact with the client in a given session, how long you have known the client, and the client's attitudes (regarding confidence and importance) toward PA behavior change will all determine which techniques are most appropriate in a given session. Think of these strategies as a clinical menu from which you can choose based on your available time and the client's particular needs. Because MI first began as a set of clinical techniques, we will use MI terminology but will draw analogies to SDT's need-supportive therapy for behavior change as well. Both MI and SDT are client-centered in their approach. Here, we delineate some specific techniques consistent with the tenets of these perspectives on client-centered counseling.

REFLECTIVE LISTENING

Reflective listening is a hallmark of client-centered counseling. It can be conceptualized as hypothesis testing or checking in with the client. In practice, this might take the form of, "If I heard you correctly, I think you're saying..." or more direct statements such as, "So, you are having trouble with...". The goal of reflective listening is to communicate to the client that you have heard and are trying to understand where they are coming from, affirm or validate their feelings and experiences, and further assist them in the process of self-discovery. This is, in part, a way to create a nonjudgmental environment from which the client can explore the positives and negatives of their current behavior and prescribed behavior change. From the perspective of SDT, which also uses reflective listening, this serves to support the client's needs for relatedness (*i.e.,* by conveying an interest in understanding where the client is coming from) and autonomy (*i.e.,* by withholding judgment about the client). Even if you "guess wrong" about what the client is trying to say, this can be beneficial as it helps the client to clarify his or her own thoughts, and the practitioner's openness to correction can further strengthen rapport.

Reflections range in complexity from the practitioner clarifying that he or she has understood the basic facts of the client's story to exploring meaning or feeling behind statements. At least seven types of reflections have been identified and defined and are described in the following text:

1. Content reflections
2. Feeling/meaning reflections
3. Amplified negative reflections
4. Double-sided reflections
5. Reflections on omission
6. Action reflections (including behavior suggestions, behavior exclusions, and cognitive suggestions)
7. Rolling with resistance

Content Reflections

Content reflections are perhaps the simplest form of reflection and involve reflecting the basic facts about the client's story. Although simple, content reflections are important for gathering background information and building rapport. This might take the form of a statement like, "You tried to exercise regularly before and were not able to stick with it."

Feeling/Meaning Reflections

Feeling/meaning reflections often take the form of direct statements about what the client seems to be feeling, why the person feels a certain way or how something is related to other important aspects of the person's life. Building on the content reflection cited earlier, a feeling/meaning reflection may go a step further: "Because you weren't able to stick with it before, you are afraid that you will fail again."

Amplified Negative Reflections

Amplified negative reflections involve exaggerating the negatives of behavior change and/or the positives of staying the same. Paradoxically, by arguing against change, the practitioner can exhaust the client's resistance. "So, for you it makes more sense not to exercise at all than to try to get into a regular routine and fail," or "You see no benefit in trying to exercise regularly." This technique may be particularly useful when clients get into a "Yes, but" resistance mindset.

Double-Sided Reflections

Double-sided reflections are particularly important because they convey to the client that the practitioner heard their reasons for and against behavior change. They also provide an opportunity for the practitioner to communicate to the client that they accept the client's ambivalence and are not going to push the client to change, thus supporting the client's need for autonomy. An example might be, "On the one hand, you see the benefits of being more physically active, but on the other hand you are concerned that exercising regularly would interfere with time you have with your family in the evenings."

Reflections on Omission

Through a *reflection on omission*, the practitioner can comment on what the client has *not* said. For example, if an otherwise happily married woman states that she has no one to exercise with, the counselor could reflect back, "So it sounds like your husband is not the answer." This can further build rapport and expresses to the client that the practitioner is not going to try to motivate with strategies that the client has already thought about, tried, and rejected (thus supporting autonomous motivation).

Action Reflections

Action reflections include potential solutions to the client's barriers or some element of a course of action. When possible, action reflections provide a menu of effective options from which the client can choose so as to support the client's need for autonomy. Because of their focus on actionable items, action reflections may also serve to support the client's competence needs. As reflections, these statements involve characterizing ideas the client has generated or contemplated. Thus, they do not involve giving unsolicited advice. There are three subtypes of action reflections: behavior suggestion, behavior exclusion, and cognitive suggestion (8).

Behavior Suggestions

Behavior suggestions can take several forms including:

1. Inverting the barrier (*e.g.,* "Starting with shorter, 10-minute bouts and building up to 30 consecutive minutes of moderate activity may feel less overwhelming and like a more attainable goal for you right now")
2. Nonspecific or umbrella strategies (*e.g.,* "So, finding a way to exercise around your house or during the work day may help.")
3. Specific strategies based on previous discussions with the client (*e.g.,* "Perhaps mapping out a walking route around your neighborhood would make it more reasonable for you to exercise regularly.")

Behavior Exclusions

Behavior exclusions involve reflecting back to the client that, given what they have said, there may be some options that would not work for them. The reflection on omission technique described previously is one way in which behavior exclusions can be included in action plans.

Cognitive Suggestions

Finally, *cognitive suggestions* are another way to express action reflections. These focus more on how a client may be thinking about physical activity rather than their behavior per se and often resemble the cognitive component of cognitive-behavioral therapy. (For example, "So, it sounds like when you miss an exercise session, you feel like you have failed. And when you start thinking that you have failed, you tend to abandon the effort altogether—which is what really interferes with your goals. Maybe not thinking of exercising regularly as all-or-none—you're either meeting the goal or not—would help to make it more doable for you to be more physically active and reach your exercise goals.")

Rolling with Resistance

Rolling with resistance is a unique kind of reflection. Confronting clients about their resistance can backfire, leading to defensiveness, rapport damage, and poor outcomes with respect to behavior change (23). Thus, instead of arguing with the client, MI suggests that practitioners "roll with resistance." By rolling with resistance, practitioners align with clients, essentially agreeing with them even in circumstances where the client is making factually incorrect statements. An example of a reflection characteristic of rolling with resistance might be, "You have a very busy life and you work a lot. So, coming home and sitting on the couch to watch TV is how you unwind at the end of the day." This approach is the opposite of amplified negative reflections, described previously.

Rolling with resistance reflections acknowledge the client's reasons for not changing. They also contribute to creating a social environment in which the client feels free to express resistance without feeling pressure to change or worrying about being judged. Rolling with resistance avoids thwarting clients' autonomy and relatedness needs by not forcing them to make changes in any particular way, and by providing an opportunity for them to explore the change at their pace so they can identify their own reasons for becoming physically active (autonomy). Rolling with resistance also avoids leaving clients feeling that you are judging them as weak-willed, or that you don't like them because they are not doing what you want them to do (*i.e.*, unconditional positive regard or relatedness). It further communicates you are not going to push them to change, but empathize with their struggles.

ELICITING CHANGE TALK

Eliciting change talk is another important component of client-centered counseling. Both MI and SDT start with the same basic assumption: that humans are naturally oriented toward growth, health, and well-being. Practically, this means practitioners do not need to tell people to be healthy; clients naturally want to do this, except in rare circumstance such as clinical depression or complete amotivation. Thus, the practitioner's role is to work with clients to identify and voice their personal sources of motivation, since clients are more likely to accept and act upon goals and plans that they articulate for themselves. The process by which counselors encourage clients to express their own reasons and plans for change is called *eliciting change talk*.

Measure Importance and Confidence

Importance and confidence "rulers" are one way to elicit change talk, and this approach has been used in both MI and SDT interventions. In the context of physical activity, this strategy uses two questions:

1. "On a scale from 0 to 10, with 10 being the highest, how important is it to you to be more physically active?"
2. "On a scale from 0 to 10, with 10 being the highest (and assuming you want to change this behavior), how confident are you that you could be more physically active?"

Practitioners then follow up each question with two probes. For example, if the client answered "7," the practitioner would first probe with, "You said on a scale of 0 to 10, you would rate the importance of being more physically active as a 7. Why didn't you choose a lower number, like a 4 or 5?" This would be followed by, "What might it take for you to get to a higher number, like an 8 or a 9?" These probes elicit change talk by providing an opportunity for the client to explore his or her reasons for behavior change as well as where there may be barriers and potential solutions. Assessing importance is one way to tap into the nature of the client's motivations as well as their broader values system.

SDT applications have sometimes modified this question slightly to ask clients how much they want to engage in behavior change (*e.g.*, being more physically active). Assessing confidence approximates the client's perceived competence and can also provide an opportunity to identify potential barriers.

Develop Discrepancy

Another technique for eliciting change talk and energizing motivation is to *develop discrepancy* between the client's current behavior and other life goals and values. Clients may choose from a list of values (*e.g.*, good spouse/partner, attractive, athletic, on top of things, energetic (30)) or they may generate three to five personal goals or values on their own. Self-generation of goals or values may be approached in the following way: "Now I'd like to get to know a little bit more about other aspects of your life and things that are important to you. If you were to think about the things that are most important to you, or perhaps some things you'd like to accomplish—either in the short term like the next 5 years or over the course of your life—what would those things be?"

The practitioner then explores with the client how becoming more physically active or starting a more regular exercise routine would support or interfere with the pursuit and achievement of those goals. For example, the client may acknowledge "spending time with family" as something that is important to them. The client may note that being more physically active may mean spending less time with family, which is less appealing. The client may also note, however, that by being more physically active they are pursuing a healthier lifestyle that is likely to contribute to longer length and quality of life, which would provide more time with family in the long run. Thus, rather than the practitioner telling the client what he or she should do and why it is important, the client is able to explore this territory on his or her own and align behavior change with broader life goals and values. The client's self-exploration supports autonomy needs and also promotes internalization of motivation for physical activity by bringing physical activity goals in congruity with other goals and values.

TRAINING: USING MI AND SDT TECHNIQUES SUCCESSFULLY

There is a considerable literature on MI training techniques, and SDT has used MI training protocols in teaching SDT practitioners how to utilize SDT and MI techniques in health promotion contexts. Thus, here we describe training as outlined for MI practitioners, though training for SDT practitioners is quite similar.

Introductory Training

Many practitioners are initially exposed to MI techniques in brief, generally didactic-only sessions like "grand rounds." More formal introductory training may begin with studying print materials and training videos. It may also involve attending an introductory training session lasting up to 1 to 3 days that covers the basic tenets of MI and the foundation for using MI techniques in practice.

Introductory workshops typically involve a mix of didactic instruction, demonstrations, and hands-on experience. The purpose of these sessions is to provide training participants with a general understanding of the spirit and method of MI and to provide practical experience in trying out the approach. Practitioners who have learned the basics of MI and had the opportunity to use MI techniques in their practice over time may wish to achieve additional proficiency.

Intermediate/Advanced Training

Intermediate/advanced clinical training often involves having audio or video recordings of sessions of the practitioner coded by a trainer, who provides feedback about how to further hone MI skills. Intermediate/advanced training is typically done over the course of a 2- or 3-day workshop and focuses primarily on demonstrations, opportunities for practice and review of audio- or video-recorded sessions that training participants have brought in from their clinical practice. Some studies have recently emerged to evaluate the efficacy of online and other autodidactic methods for MI training. These approaches show great promise and are critical for MI to be used on a broad scale. Additional information about MI Manuals and Training along with train-the-trainer materials can be found at http://www.motivationalinterview.org.

CLIENT-CENTERED APPROACHES FOR ELICITING PHYSICAL ACTIVITY BEHAVIOR CHANGE

The Traditional Approach: The 5 A's

Originally developed by the National Cancer Institute as an approach to addressing tobacco cessation in primary care, the 4 A's model (ask, advise, assist, arrange) has since been expanded to include a fifth step: agree, or "assess willingness to change." The 5 A's model (ask, advise, agree, assist, arrange), as described by the U.S. Preventive Services Taskforce, has been used to conceptualize brief interventions across a variety of behaviors implemented by a variety of health practitioners (*e.g.*, wearing seatbelts, alcohol use, etc.) (12).

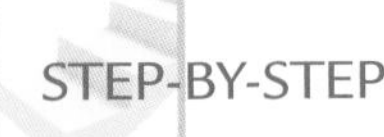

STEP-BY-STEP

Ask

Ask involves asking the client about health behaviors and risks and the factors that impact their decision to change as well as the goals and methods applied to such changes.

Advise

Advise involves giving the client clear, specific behavior change advice, including information about the health risks of not changing and benefits of implementing change. Within the 5 A's model, advice has been shown to be most effective when it is linked directly to the reason for which the person has sought care. For example, if a client came to a practitioner because they were concerned about their risk for cardiovascular disease, the practitioner may recommend the kinds of exercise that have been shown to lower cardiovascular risk (*e.g.*, moderate and vigorous physical activity).

Agree

Agree or *assess willingness to change* refers to the collaborative process by which the practitioner and client work together to determine whether the client wants to change and, if so, identify behavior change goals and strategies based on the client's interest and willingness to change the target behavior. By including the fifth "A" for "agree," this model directly supports autonomy because it is naturally aligned with engaging the client in the development of a plan and exploring and acknowledging client ambivalence.

Assist

Assist is the process by which the practitioner helps the patient to achieve the agreed-upon behavior change goals by obtaining the needed skills, confidence, and social or environmental supports. Assist directly supports clients' needs for competence.

Arrange

Arrange involves the practitioner working with the client to establish a schedule for follow-up contacts to provide ongoing support and adjust the treatment plan as needed. Multiple visits and unconditional support over time can be useful to motivating long-term change such as establishing a healthy pattern of physical activity. However, there is also the risk that the client perceives these visits (which ultimately will end) as an external source of reinforcement and motivation ("I have to show my personal trainer/doctor/etc. how well I'm doing"), which could undermine the development of more internal (and lasting) reasons to sustain new behaviors.

RELATIONSHIP AMONG MI, SDT, AND THE 5 A'S

It is important to note that although MI, SDT, and the 5 A's developed independently, because MI and SDT are primarily about the way in which the practitioner interacts with the client rather than nuts and bolts of specific clinical behaviors, it is possible to use a 5 A's, brief-encounter approach in a way that is MI- and SDT-congruent. For example, one may view MI and SDT as a more comprehensive approach to the first A: *Ask*. Additionally, one may use "Agree (willingness to change)," to elicit client autonomy and to explore and acknowledge client ambivalence, and move forward with "assist" only when the client has expressed a desire to change.

The one arena in which the 5 A's, MI, and SDT may be less complementary is *Advise.* In the context of PA counseling, advice may come in the form of providing information about current recommendations for levels and types of physical activity required to achieve certain health goals (*e.g.*, health benefits, reduced cardiovascular risk, weight loss, etc.). It may also come in the form of providing an exercise prescription or plan. MI and SDT would suggest that, to support clients' optimal motivation, it is important to develop an exercise plan in a collaborative, client-centered way rather than a more paternalistic or prescribing way. As described earlier, MI recommends against direct advice-giving and maintains that attempts to directly persuade a client may backfire because such persuasive attempts inherently "take sides" in the ambivalence. In turn, SDT maintains that one of the keys to supporting patient autonomy—providing structure—is achieved, in part, by explicitly guiding the client or patient through the various choices they have to best maintain or improve health and well-being.

For example, to the degree the client feels unsure about the most effective dose or type of exercise to achieve a certain fitness/health outcome, an explicit recommendation might be offered. However, even in SDT, advice is not intended to control the client, but rather to provide information about effective options of treatment. Further, in medical and health contexts in particular, explicit recommendations may be an expected component of interactions between practitioners and clients. Thus, a practitioners' refusal to provide such direction could thwart all three of the patient's psychological needs and may be experienced by the client as abandonment. However, SDT cautions that recommendations be given noncoercively, so as to provide information to the patient while still supporting the patient in making the decision himself or herself (*e.g.*, "Research has shown that incorporating regular exercise into your life is important for achieving the weight loss goals you have identified, but the choice is ultimately yours, and I will be here to support you in whatever decision you make.").

Indeed, more recent formulations of MI have allowed for practitioners to make recommendations when patients specifically ask for advice as discussed later in the three-phase model (Explore, Guide, Choose), and through action reflections described previously. From the perspectives of both MI and SDT, providing direct recommendations may occur at any point in the 5 A's model, depending on the client's expressed needs and goals. For example, in the context of Ask, the client may indicate being uncertain about what types of exercise they need to be engaging in to achieve a weight loss goal. This may be a circumstance in which the practitioner can provide information about current recommendations or provide options for the client to consider about the types of exercise he or she would like to engage in. Likewise, in the context of Agree, during which client and practitioner are working together to establish an exercise plan, the client may ask for suggestions on how to proceed toward a particular exercise goal. Regardless of when opportunities for direct advice-giving may present themselves, from the perspective of MI and SDT, it is critical for the practitioner to check in with the client to ensure that the practitioner is being responsive to the client's needs and is aligned with the client's goals rather than the practitioner's own agenda.

Both MI and SDT have used the *elicit-provide-elicit* framework for providing direct advice (29). That is, practitioners *elicit* from the client information about their knowledge and attitudes toward behavior change, where there may be knowledge gaps, etc., and then *provide* information and recommendations based on what the client has indicated or requested. Practitioners then *elicit* again, asking clients how they interpret the information that was provided and what the information means to them in the context of their current behavior. Case Scenario 5.1 provides a vignette that illustrates how the 5 A's approach might be used in a way that is consistent with the motivational perspectives highlighted in this chapter. Although we will discuss these techniques in a linear fashion, it is important to note that not all clients proceed through these phases in the order specified.

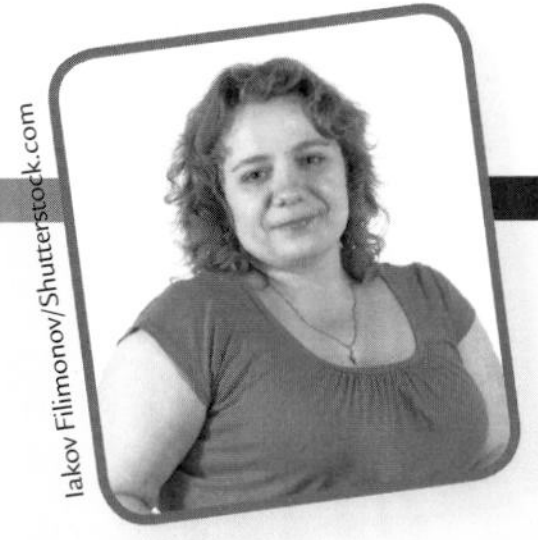
Iakov Filimonov/Shutterstock.com

Case Scenario 5.1

THE 5 A'S IN THE CONTEXT OF MI AND SDT

Your client is a 45-year-old married woman with two children; she is a computer programmer. She was a college athlete and was physically active during young adulthood but hasn't been active over the past 10 years. She has gained some weight (current BMI = 28), and she is struggling with negative body image. She is also worried about becoming obese. She has come to your fitness facility to get a plan for being more active and losing weight. In the following exchange, P is the Practitioner, and she is C, the Client.

Ask

P: Hi Mrs. Jones. How are you today?

C: I'm doing okay. I'm ready to start exercising again. I hate my body right now, and I'm worried about my weight. I used to be active, and I want to get back there.

P: So it sounds like you've been thinking about being more physically active. I'd like to learn a little more about what your daily life is like.

C: Well, my work keeps me in front of a computer all the time, and they always have food around the office that tastes so good—donuts, muffins, candy. I eat to take a break from my work. And I sit most of the day.

P: When do you like to exercise?

C: Well, in theory, I could exercise in the morning.

P: But it sounds like maybe that's not working for you?

C: Not really. Mornings are just so busy with the kids.

P: So, if mornings don't work for you, what might work–or what might you be willing to try?

C: I think I might be more of an evening exercise person. That's what I used to do when I was working out all the time. And since the gym is between work and home, evenings might work.

P: Okay. Let's see if I have this right. You are unhappy with your current weight and also concerned about becoming obese. You used to be active, but not recently–mostly because you've been busy. It also sounds like you tried to exercise in the mornings, but that didn't really fit in with your schedule that well. Do I have that right?

C: Exactly. And now that we're talking about this, I have to admit that, even though I know that being active is good for me, I really want to lose weight. I'm really unhappy with how I look right now, and I miss how good I used to feel when I was exercising regularly.

Comment: The summary at the end of this dialogue is important for enhancing motivation because it lets the client know you have heard her, and makes it more likely she will be able to hear your advice without feeling controlled. Acknowledging her weight and body image concerns is also key to understanding central motives around exercise, which may be addressed later.

continued

Case Scenario 5.1 *continued*

Advise

P: Now that I have a better sense of where you're coming from, let's talk about some recommendations for physical activity. Is that okay?

C: Yes, I think I have a general idea, but I'd like to know what I need to do–especially to lose weight.

P: It might help to think about exercise less as what you need to do and more as finding a routine that works for you. You might have heard that you need to get 150 minutes of moderate-intensity physical activity a week–or 30 minutes of activity on most days. These are activities like: brisk walking, bike riding, or water aerobics. But it might take more activity to lose weight. How does that seem to you?

C: Wow! 150 minutes seems like a lot. And I have to do more to lose weight? I definitely have my work cut out for me.

Agree/Assess (willingness to change)

P: 150 minutes sounds like a lot–and the thought of doing more can feel daunting. You might try thinking about it as something to work toward, with a smaller goal to start–like 10-15 minutes a day. How does that sound?

C: It definitely feels less overwhelming. But I don't want to set goals that are so small that I never get to where I need to be to lose weight.

P: It can be hard to find the balance between "do-able goals" and goals that are not challenging enough. Let's talk about some specifics and see how you feel then.

Assist

P: You might start with activities you like to do and build up from there.

C: I really like lifting weights, and I used to run, but at my current weight, it's really uncomfortable. Maybe I could use a stationary bike?

P: It sounds like you have some ideas about the kinds of exercise you like. Great! How many times a week could you get to the gym or exercise from home?

C: I would like to say every day, but I don't think that's realistic. Maybe 2 days at the gym?

P: That's a great start. What days of the week would you like to come?

C: I wasn't expecting to have to name days. Maybe one time during the week and one time on the weekend?

P: That sounds reasonable. Can you work out at home at all?

C: My kids love to ride their bikes. Maybe I can go out with them 1 or 2 nights a week.

P: That sounds like a great start! Just to summarize, what I have heard you say is that you are willing to start with some smaller goals, but ultimately you want to lose weight. For now your plan is:

- Come to the gym 1 weekday and 1 weekend day to lift weights and ride the stationary bike.
- Go out with your kids to ride bikes 1 or 2 nights a week.

How does that seem to you?

C: I'll give it a shot.

Case Scenario 5.1 *continued*

Arrange

P: I'd like to follow up with you, just to see how things are going and to give you an opportunity to talk about how this plan is working for you (or where w might need to make some changes). Could we plan to meet again in 2 weeks?

C: Sure. And maybe I'll see you when I'm here between now and then?

P: Absolutely. And if you're having trouble with anything in the mean time and want to touch base, just send me an email and we can set up a time to talk–on the phone or here at the gym. Or if I'm not working with another client and we're both here, you can just come talk to me then.

C: Great. That sounds like a plan that will work for me.

P: Sounds good. Remember, there are lots of ways to become more active. Sometimes it just takes a few tries before we find the right mix and scheduling that works best for you. And we can talk more about your weight loss goals–and how to achieve them–when we meet next.

An Alternative Approach: Explore, Guide, Choose

Based on Motivational Interviewing (MI), a three-phase model (Explore, Guide and Choose) delineated by Resnicow and Rollnick (30) represents another framework for working with clients toward behavior change. Like the 5 A's, this approach can be used in brief encounters.

STEP-BY-STEP

As with the 5As model described above, although we will discuss these processes in a linear fashion, it is important to note that not all clients or clinical encounters proceed through these phases in the order specified. Indeed, some clients will come into the interaction without much ambivalence, and thus, less time will need to be devoted to "exploring." Additionally, quality (*i.e.,* sources) and quantity of motivation are likely to fluctuate throughout the process of behavior change. As clients experience failures, reemergence of ambivalence and other motivational slumps, "exploring" and "guiding" may need to be covered again within the context of these new experiences.

Explore

Similar to the 5 A's *Ask*, the primary objective during the explore phase is to obtain a behavioral history, including prior attempts at behavior change. MI and SDT take this a bit further and view this phase as an opportunity for the practitioner to "comfort the afflicted," build rapport, and better understand the client's story. Key skills and techniques used in the explore phase include reflective listening, shared decision making (particularly with respect to agenda-setting), and open-ended questions. Because rapport building is an important component of this phase, the practitioner conveys empathy and demonstrates for the client that the practitioner will support autonomy and not push a change agenda. The explore phase includes very little action planning, although when action ideas come up in conversation, the practitioner may wish to provide a verbal acknowledgement of plans to revisit them later in the session.

Guide

Once the practitioner has heard and understood the client's story, and some rapport has been established, the discussion can proceed to guiding. This phase is characterized by "afflicting the comfortable" as it involves moving the conversation toward building motivation and therefore the possibility of change. The primary technique used in this phase is eliciting change talk, including building discrepancy between the client's current behavior (*e.g.*, not exercising) and the client's broader goals and values (*e.g.*, being healthy, spending time with family) and using the 0-to-10 importance/confidence rulers. The guiding phase concludes with the practitioner summarizing the discussion, highlighting the client's potential reasons for making a change, and checking in with the client about where that leaves the client with respect to pursuing change. If the client expresses a commitment to making a change, even a small one, the session can then move to a more practical discussion of how to implement the said change.

Choose

This is the action phase of the discussion and covers much of the territory covered by the last 4 of the 5 A's. Key objectives include helping clients identify a goal, building an action plan, anticipating barriers, and agreeing on a plan for checking in on progress. Skills and techniques used in the choose phase involve action reflections and include developing a menu of options for change and setting goals (including mini-goals or short-term objectives). It is important to keep in mind that, just like other reflections, action reflections are the practitioner's "best guess" for what the client has said or where the story is going. Thus, the client may refute suggestions or get into a "yes-but" mindset. This may result from underlying resistance or ambivalence that has not been resolved or from previous experiences the client has had with attempted behavior change and failure.

Even when clients refute suggestions, this provides important information about what does and does not work and what the client does or does not want to pursue. One technique that may help to minimize outright rejection and support autonomy is to provide multiple options within a reflection. For example, "Trying to get in a walk during your lunch hour or inviting the kids to come out with you on your neighborhood walk might be ways that you can be physically active without losing out on important family time." Because the provision of choice supports needs for autonomy, resistance is reduced. Case Scenario 5.2 provides a vignette illustrating the Explore, Guide, Choose approach.

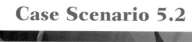

Warren Goldswain/Shutterstock.com

Case Scenario 5.2

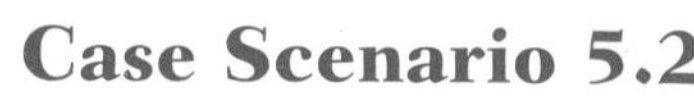

EXPLORE, GUIDE, CHOOSE

Your client is a 58-year-old married man who is a long-haul truck driver. He recently had a heart attack, and becoming more physically active is part of his cardiac rehabilitation. Although he was active in sports throughout high school, he has not been physically active much at all as an adult. His recent heart attack seems to have gotten his attention, though. In the following exchange, P is the Practitioner, and he is C, the Client.

Case Scenario 5.2 *continued*

Explore

P: I understand that your doctor has recommended that you become more physically active. How are you feeling about being more active in your daily life?

C: Well, my heart attack sure got my attention. And I've known for a while that I should be more active than I am. I sit a lot with my job. I used to really like sports when I was a kid, but that seems like forever ago.

P: So it sounds like you were jolted by your heart attack. You're concerned about how much time you spend sitting at work. You're also a little unsure about what it will be like to be more active at this point in your life—that maybe you won't be the star athlete you once were.

C: Yeah, I huff and puff just walking up stairs so I can't imagine doing... what did my doctor call it? Moderate to vigorous activity? For 30 minutes a day?!

P: Exercise may not seem like much fun, and getting to 30 minutes must seem daunting.

C: Yeah, but I know I need to do it. I don't want to have another heart attack or, worse, have to have bypass surgery.

Guide

P: So on a scale from 0 to 10, with 10 being the highest, how important is it to you to be more physically active?

C: Oh, it's real important. I'd say probably a 6 or 7.

P: So you would rate the importance of being more physically active as a 7. Why didn't you choose a lower number, like a 4 or 5?

C: Well, like I said, I definitely don't want to have another heart attack. And I know it's good for my health to exercise more.

P: And what might it take for you to get to a higher number, like an 8 or a 9?

C: Oh, I don't know. I mean, I think it's important to be active. I just don't know how realistic it is for me to fit it into my daily life. I'm out on the road a lot. So it's not like I can go to the gym whenever I want. And my job's not going to change, so I'm still going to be sitting all that time.

P: On the one hand, you see the benefits of being more physically active, but on the other hand you feel like the sedentary nature of your job might cancel out those benefits.

C: Yeah, and I just don't know how I'm going to do it. But I want to be healthy and active with my kids and to see them grow up.

P: This feels like a big change to undertake, but there are important parts of your life—like being healthy and being able to see your kids grow up—that would benefit from you taking better care of yourself by being more physically active.

continued

Case Scenario 5.2 *continued*

Choose

P: From what you've said so far, there are two barriers that you see to being physically active on a regular basis: (1) you are concerned about fitting physical activity into your busy work life, and (2) because your job will still require you to sit just as much you feel like maybe this undermines the benefits you might get from exercising regularly.

C: Well, I think it's important for me to know whether my effort is worth it. If I'm sitting like 10 hours a day, does it really matter if I get in that moderate to vigorous activity for only 30 minutes?

P: So you are wondering if exercise still pays even if you are sitting a lot the rest of the day. I would like to share with you what we know about that. It does, actually. We know from research that being active at a moderate level of intensity—so your heart rate is elevated a bit but you're not completely winded—for 30 minutes a day goes a long way toward improving your health. Of course, if you could be active for more than that, that's good too. What do you make of that?

C: OK. But I still don't know how I'm going to do it. I can't get to the gym.

P: You are looking for a way, other than going to the gym, to be active in a way that fits with your job.

C: I guess I could take little walk breaks when I stop to fill up the truck.

P: So what might that look like?

C: I don't know. Probably only 10 minutes or so. Not the full 30. Does that even count?

P: Absolutely. How might you make these walk breaks happen?

C: I could bring my sneakers and comfortable clothes with me...

P: So you can commit to getting in at least three 10-minute walk breaks each day when you're stopped to fill up your truck. Let's touch base again in about a month to see how that plan is working for you. You might find that this works out just fine, or that maybe we need to make some adjustments. Either way, let's plan to talk about what's working for you and what's not so that you can get closer to achieving your physical activity and health goals.

THE EVIDENCE FOR CLIENT-CENTERED APPROACHES

There is a solid evidence base for both MI and SDT in health behavior change settings. Early studies of MI and SDT focused on substance abuse and tobacco cessation, as well as engagement in sports and physical education (18,42,49). Here we limit our overview to the evidence for MI and SDT in leisure-time physical activity. In addition, there is considerable support for the 5 A's model, particularly for use as a brief treatment (3–10 minutes, for two to four visits) for tobacco and alcohol abuse and dependence, though a more detailed description of this evidence base is beyond the scope of this chapter (10,53).

Motivational Interviewing and Physical Activity

Several systematic reviews and meta-analyses of MI applied to behaviors relevant to chronic disease prevention and management have been published in recent years. In a review of brief MI interventions by Dunn and colleagues, MI was found to be more effective for facilitating exercise (and diet) change than change in other health behaviors (8). In a meta-analysis of 30 randomized controlled clinical trials examining the effectiveness of adaptations of MI (*e.g.*, MI interventions that also include non-MI components such as norm-based feedback), Burke, Arkowitz, and Dunn (2) reported that adaptations of MI were as effective as other active treatments and more effective than no treatment and placebo controls for improvements in exercise adoption and maintenance (follow-ups ranged from 4 weeks to 1 year), as well as several other health behaviors. In their meta-analysis of 72 randomized, controlled trials involving diet, exercise, diabetes, and substance abuse, Rubak, Sandbaek, Lauritzen, and Christensen (34) found that, overall, MI outperformed traditional advice-giving in 75% of the studies reviewed. Resnicow, Davis, and Rollnick (27) reviewed youth studies that used MI to modify diet or physical activity, diabetes, and other behaviors such as smoking and found some evidence for the feasibility and utility of MI with children and adolescents. Their review also included some adult studies that used MI to promote change in diet or physical activity (27). Van Dorsten (48) reported that MI substantially improved diet and exercise behaviors, treatment adherence, and weight loss in 10 studies targeting weight loss and/or exercise.

In another review, 24 published empirical studies were identified that used MI as an intervention for diet and/or exercise behaviors (21). Across these studies, MI was shown to be effective for diet and exercise behavior change both alone and in combination with other interventions. With regard to exercise, clients receiving an MI intervention reported greater exercise self-efficacy and increased physical activity behavior. MI has also been shown to facilitate healthier eating (*i.e.*, reduced caloric intake, increased fruit and vegetable consumption) and improve weight loss outcomes (*e.g.*, decreased BMI) (21). Finally, Lundahl and colleagues (19) published a meta-analysis on 119 studies with outcomes including substance use, gambling, engagement in treatment, and—more germane to the present discussion—health-related behaviors such as diet and exercise. Across studies, MI produced statistically significant, though small (average $g = 0.28$) effects compared to weak comparison groups. When judged against specific treatments, MI yielded statistically nonsignificant results. Further analyses suggested that feedback (*e.g.*, via motivational enhancement therapy), delivery time, manualization, and delivery mode (group vs. individual) moderated outcomes. It is worth noting that previous reviews and meta-analyses, as described earlier, found that MI was more effective for physical activity and exercise than for substance use treatments. The Lundahl and colleagues (19) meta-analysis did not present results differentiated by behavioral outcome. Taken together, these reviews and the studies that comprise them provide strong evidence for the clinical utility of MI for physical activity behavior change and that additional research is needed to better elucidate the clinical utility of MI for pediatric physical activity promotion and obesity prevention.

Self-Determination Theory and Physical Activity

As a general theory of human motivation SDT has addressed both the characteristics of motivation toward prescribed behavior (*i.e.*, the extent to which motivations are more or less internal to the self) and the importance of psychological need support (*i.e.*, for one's inherent needs for autonomy, competence, and relatedness) from the social context in facilitating the emergence of more internal forms of motivation. Several studies applying SDT to physical activity demonstrated associations between internalized or autonomous forms of motivation (*i.e.*, intrinsic, integrated, identified) and greater exercise behavioral engagement, adherence to exercise recommendations over time, perceived competence, and psychological well-being. These were primarily observational studies (7,17). Additional evidence has demonstrated that the socioenvironmental context provided by the support of psychological needs for autonomy, competence, and relatedness facilitates internalization of motivation which is, in turn, related to exercise behavior (9,14).

Recently, investigators have begun testing SDT-based interventions for physical activity. For example, studies that experimentally prime more autonomous motivations, through the use of need-supportive techniques (described earlier), evidenced increased exercise intentions and behaviors (9,14). Interventions implemented in applied settings such as primary care and personal training have also been developed and are being tested (9,11,25). Given the role of physical activity behavior in various health outcomes, SDT-based interventions targeting cardiovascular health, diabetes, and overweight/obesity have also used SDT techniques to promote physical activity. Very recently, a systematic review of 66 empirical studies of SDT and exercise/PA (observational and experimental) found that autonomous forms of motivation, both extrinsic and intrinsic, consistently predicted increased PA participation, in some cases in the long term (46). In this review, higher levels of internal goals for exercising (*e.g.*, affiliation and social engagement, challenge, and skill development) were also clearly associated with exercise participation. Reviewers concluded that reporting high perceived competence for exercise positively predicts more adaptive exercise behavioral outcomes.

For example, in a study of patients in a community-based primary care practice, sedentary patients who worked with a SDT-trained physical activity counselor, compared to those who worked with a physical activity counselor using usual care practices, experienced greater need support in the health care climate. This predicted greater increases in autonomous self-regulation for physical activity and, in turn, increases in perceived competence for physical activity. Both autonomous self-regulation and perceived competence for physical activity predicted greater increases in physical activity behavior (*i.e.*, number of days in the past 6 weeks in which the participant engaged in light, moderate, or intense leisure-time activity for 20 minutes or more) (11).

In a one-year, SDT-based intensive behavioral intervention for weight loss among overweight and obese women, moderate and vigorous PA was significantly higher for women in the intervention compared to the control at the end of the intervention and at 1 and 2 years post-intervention (40,41). The intervention explicitly targeted increasing intrinsic motivation—namely enjoyment of physical activity—and autonomous regulation more generally. The effect of the intervention on autonomous regulation was notable because it was large, it was sustained over 2 years, and it mediated the effect of the intervention on physical activity 1 year after the intervention was over (40). Further evidence from this study has suggested a "motivational spill-over" whereby autonomous self-regulation for exercise predicted autonomous self-regulation for healthy eating over 1 year (22). Thus, facilitating autonomous self-regulation in one health domain may increase autonomous self-regulation in other, related domains. In sum, the studies summarized here represent a strong evidence base for using the tenets of SDT to promote physical activity behavior change.

Tailoring and Cultural Considerations

Although many patients report great satisfaction and improved outcomes from patient-centered approaches (33,44,52) such as MI or SDT, some individuals indicate that they prefer a more directive, educational style (45). In one recent study (43), where rural African American women viewed an MI training video showing both MI- and non-MI-consistent practices, many expressed concern that the MI consultation was too patient-centered. One participant commented, "He [provider] was asking the patient more about his decision, instead of him [provider] telling him." Another patient stated, "He [health care provider] [was] not giving the patient much information. He's supposed to know; he's a doctor." Many patients implied that a more practitioner-centered, directive approach, where the health care provider did most of the talking and offered unsolicited advice, was desired. As described earlier, SDT supports providing that advice when the client asks for it. Practitioners, therefore, need to tailor their intervention style to clients' preferences and cultural background.

Several issues are worth keeping in mind when working with diverse populations that may have different expectations about encounters with health professionals. MI and SDT, as client-centered approaches, are oriented toward tailoring the clinical approach based on the client's expressed preferences, concerns, and goals. Thus, it is possible to be clinically consistent with the tenants and techniques of MI and SDT while providing varying degrees of structure, advice, and so forth. Further, from the perspective of SDT, autonomy is not synonymous with independence. Rather, functioning in an autonomous way involves perceiving that one is the originator of one's actions, which may involve varying degrees of input from others.

This has been a critical issue of study in the area of cross-cultural research on basic psychological needs. Evidence has consistently demonstrated the universality of the need to be autonomous (5). However, the circumstances under which people experience autonomy may differ. For example, in more collectivist cultures, it is not uncommon for people to consult with family, friends, or other community leaders prior to making important decisions—including decisions about health and health behavior. They may seek input from others and experience this input in more or less autonomous ways. That is, they may volitionally choose to seek input from valued others or they may feel pressured or coerced to do so. Thus, it is not the seeking of input or direct advice-giving per se that is more or less autonomy supportive. Rather, it is the way in which the seeking of advice is approached and the way in which advice is delivered that is key.

TAKE-HOME MESSAGE

Working with clients who are ambivalent or amotivated about health behavior change can be challenging. Indeed, there is much in modern society that makes physical inactivity the default, and getting people to move from that default (psychologically and behaviorally) poses unique opportunities for practitioners. This chapter has provided some options for working with clients to promote physical activity, even in these difficult circumstances. First, consistent with MI and SDT, practitioners may wish to begin with the assumption that humans are naturally oriented toward growth, health, and well-being, while simultaneously acknowledging that many clients may be ambivalent about behavior change. By starting with these assumptions, practitioners are better equipped to show empathy for the challenges clients face and to attempt to understand where clients are coming from. Starting from the position that clients are able to enact change and providing empathy with their struggles enables practitioners to work with—rather than against—clients in their ambivalence and resistance to change by supporting their psychological needs. Thus, practitioners can help "plant the seeds" of lasting motivation and guide clients toward healthy levels of physical activity.

From the perspective of both SDT and MI, health professionals working in the exercise/PA arena would do well to not be excessively focused on producing immediate behavior change in their clients or patients, even if they themselves feel some internal or external pressure to produce results. Instead practitioners are encouraged to:

1. Explicitly focus on long-term behavioral outcomes (months, years) and share with clients the importance and value of lasting change (and what it may take to reach it);
2. Do their utmost to create the best counseling and experiential environment for clients' internal motivation to arise (when and if it does) instead of feeling that it is the role of the counselor to "motivate" the client;
3. Be confident in the client's natural desire to be healthy and vital, trusting that it is he or she, when and if adequately motivated, who will ultimately find the best solution to overcome what stands between him/her and a more physically active lifestyle.

REFERENCES

1. Bandura A. *Self efficacy: The exercise of control.* New York: Freeman; 1997.
2. Burke BL, Arkowitz H, Dunn C. The efficacy of motivational interviewing and its adaptations. In: Miller WR, Rollnick S, editors. *Motivational Interviewing: Preparing People for Change.* New York: Guilford Press; 2002. p. 217-50.
3. Butler C, Rollnick S, Cohen D, Bachman M, Russell I, Stott N. Motivational consulting versus brief advice for smokers in general practice: A randomized trial. *British J Gen Pract.* 1999;49:611–6.
4. Cahill K, Perera R. Competitions and incentives for smoking cessation. *Cochrane Database of Systematic Reviews*, 4. Art. No.: CD004307; 2011.
5. Chirkov VI, Ryan RM, Kim Y, Kaplan U. Differentiating autonomy from individualism and independence: A self-determination theory perspective on internalization of cultural orientations and well-being. *J Pers Soc Psychol.* 2003;84:97–110.
6. Deci EL, Ryan RM. The "what" and "why" of goal pursuits: Human needs and the self-determination of behavior. *Psychol Inq.* 2000;11:227–68.
7. Duncan LR, Hall CR, Wilson PM, O J. Exercise motivation: A cross-sectional analysis examining its relationships with frequency, intensity, and duration of exercise. *Int J Behav Nutr Phys Act.* 2010;7:1–9.
8. Dunn C, DeRoo L, Rivara FP. The use of brief interventions adapted from MI across behavioral domains: A systematic review. *Add.* 2001;96:1725-43.
9. Edmunds JK, Ntoumanis N, Duda JL. Perceived autonomy support and psychological need satisfaction in exercise. In: Hagger MA, Chatzisarantis NLD, editors. *Intrinsic Motivation and Self-Determination in Exercise and Sport.* Champaign (IL): Human Kinetics; 2007. p. 35–51.
10. Fiore MC, Jaen CR, Baker TB et al. Treating tobacco use and dependence: 2008 update. http://www.surgeongeneral.gov/tobacco/treating_tobacco_use08.pdf; 2008.
11. Fortier MS, Sweet SN, O'Sullivan TL, Williams GC. A self-determination process model of physical activity adoption in the context of a randomized controlled trial. *Psychol Sport Exer.* 2007;8:741–57.
12. *Guide to Clinical Preventive Services, 2012.* AHRQ Publication No. 12-05154, October 2012. Agency for Healthcare Research and Quality, Rockville (MD).
13. Hagger MS, Chatzisarantis NL. *Intrinsic Motivation and Self-Determination in Exercise and Sport.* Champaigne (IL): Human Kinetics; 2007.
14. Hagger MS, Chatzisarantis NLD, Barkoukis V, Wang CKJ, Baranowski T. Perceived autonomy support in physical education and leisure-time physical activity: A cross-cultural evaluation of the trans-contextual model. *J Educ Psychol.* 2005;97:376–90.
15. Heather N, Rollnick S, Bell A, Richmond R. Effects of brief counselling among male heavy drinkers identified on general hospital wards. *Drug Alc Rev.* 1996;15(1):29–38.
16. John LK, Lowenstein G, Troxel AB, Norton L, Fassbender JE, Volpe KG. Financial incentives for extended weight loss: A randomized-controlled trial. *J Gen Inter Med.*; 2011.
17. Kwan BM, Caldwell Hooper AE, Mangan RE, Bryan AD. A longitudinal diary study of the effects of causality orientations on exercise-related affect. *Self Ident.* 2011;10:363–74.
18. Lonsdale C, Sabiston CM, Raedeke TD, Ha ASC, Sum RKW. Self-determined motivation and students' physical activity during structured physical education lessons and free choice periods. *Prev Med.* 2009;48:69–73.
19. Lundahl BW, Kunz C, Brownell C, Tollefson D, Burke BL. A meta-analysis of motivational interviewing: Twenty-five years of empirical studies. *Res Soc Work Prac.* 2010;20:137–60.
20. Markland D, Ryan RM, Tobin VJ, Rollnick S. Motivational interviewing and self-determination theory. *J Soc Clin Psychol.* 2005;24:811–31.
21. Martins RK, McNeil DW. Review of motivational interviewing in promoting health behaviors. *Clin Psychol Rev.* 2009;29:283–93.
22. Mata J, Silva MN, Vieira PN, et al. Motivational "spill-over" during weight control: Increased self-determination and exercise intrinsic motivation predict eating self-regulation. *Health Psychol.* 2009;28:709–16.
23. Miller W. Motivational interviewing with problem drinkers. *Behav Psychotherapy.* 1983;11(2):147–72.
24. Miller W, Rollnick S. *Motivational interviewing: Preparing people to change addictive behavior.* New York: Guilford Press; 1991.
25. Patrick H, Canevello A. Methodological overview of a self-determination theory-based computerized intervention to promote leisure-time physical activity. *Psychol Sport Exer.* 2011;12:13–9.
26. Patrick H, Williams GC. Self-determination theory: Its application to health behavior and complementarity with motivational interviewing. *Int J Behav Nutr Phys Act.* 2012;9:18.
27. Resnicow K, Davis R, Rollnick S. Motivational interviewing for pediatric obesity: Conceptual issues and evidence review. *J Amer Diet Assoc.* 2006;206:2024-33.
28. Resnicow K, Jackson A, Wang T, De AK, McCarty F, Dudley WN, et al. A motivational interviewing intervention to increase fruit and vegetable intake through black churches: Results of the Eat for Life trial. *Am J Pub Health.* 2001;91(10):1686–93.
29. Resnicow K, McMaster F. Motivational interviewing: Moving from why to how with autonomy support. *Int J Behav Nutr Phys Act.* 2012; 9:1–15.
30. Resnicow K, Rollnick S. Motivational interviewing in health promotion and behavioral medicine. In: Cox WM, Klinger E, editors. *Handbook of Motivational Counseling: Goal-Based Approaches to Assessment and Intervention with Addiction and Other Problems.* 2nd ed. New York: John Wiley & Sons; 2011.
31. Rollnick S, Miller W. What is motivational interviewing? *Behav Cog Psychotherapy.* 1995;23(4):325–34.
32. Rollnick S, Miller W, Butler C. *Motivational Interviewing in Health Care: Helping Patients Change Behavior.* Rev. ed. New York: Guilford; 2008.

33. Roter DL, Hall JA. Physician gender and patient-centered communication: A critical review of empirical research. *Annual Rev Public Health*. 2004;25:497–519.
34. Rubak S, Sandbaek A, Lauritzen T, Christensen B. Motivational interviewing: A systematic review and meta-analysis. *British J Gen Prac.* 2005;55:305-12.
35. Ryan RM, Connell JP. Perceived locus of causality and internalization: Examining reasons for acting in two domains. *J Pers Soc Psychol.* 1989;57:749–61.
36. Ryan RM, Deci EL. Self-determination theory and the facilitation of intrinsic motivation, social development, and well-being. *Am Psychol.* 2000;55:68–78.
37. Ryan RM, Deci EL. When rewards compete with nature: The undermining of intrinsic motivation and self-regulation. In: Sansone C, Harackiewicz JM, editors. *Intrinsic and Extrinsic Motivation: The Search for Optimal Motivation and Performance*. New York: Academic Press; 2000. p. 13–54.
38. Ryan RM, Patrick H, Deci EL, Williams GC. Facilitating health behaviour change and its maintenance: Interventions based on self-determination theory. *Eur Health Psychol.* 2008;10:2–5.
39. Ryan RM, Williams GC, Patrick H, Deci EL. Self-determination theory and physical activity: The dynamics of motivation in development and wellness. *Hellenic J Psychol.* 2009;6:107–24.
40. Silva MN, Markland DA, Carraca EV, Vieira PN, Coutinho SR, Minderico CS et al. Exercise autonomous motivation predicts 3-yr weight loss in women. *Med Sci Sports Exer.* 2011;43:728–37.
41. Silva MN, Vieira PN, Coutinho SR, et al. Using self-determination theory to promote physical activity and weight control: A randomized controlled trial in women. *J Behav Med.* 2010;33:110–22.
42. Smith A, Ntoumanis N, Duda JL. An investigation of coach behaviors, goal motives, and implementation intentions as predictors of well-being in sport. *J App Sport Psychol.* 2010;22:17–33.
43. Stephania TM, Khensani NM, Bettina MB. Perceptions of physical activity and motivational interviewing among rural African-American women with type 2 diabetes. *Women's Health Iss.* 2009;1–7.
44. Stewart MA. Effective physician–patient communication and health outcomes: A review. *CMAJ Can Med Assoc J.* 1995;152(9):1423–33.
45. Swenson SL, Buell S, Zettler P, White M, Ruston DC, Lo B. Patient-centered communication: Do patients really prefer it? *J Gen Intern Med.* 2004;19(11):1069–79.
46. Teixeira PJ, Carraça EV, Markland D, Silva MN, Ryan RM. Exercise, physical activity, and self-determination theory: A systematic review. *Int J Behav Nutr Phys Act.* 2012; 9:78.
47. Teixeira PJ, Palmeira A, Vansteenkiste M. The role of self-determination theory and motivational interviewing in behavioral nutrition, physical activity, and health: An introduction to the IJBNPA special issue. *Int J Behav Nutr Phys Act.* 2012;9:17.
48. Van Dorsten B. The use of motivational interviewing in weight loss. *Curr Diabetes Rep.* 2007;7:386-90.
49. Vansteenkiste M, Mouratidis A, Lens W. Detaching reasons from aims: Fair play and well-being in soccer as a function of pursuing performance-approach goals for autonomous or controlling reasons. *J Sport Exer Psychol.* 2010;32:217–42.
50. Vansteenkiste M, Resnicow K, Williams GC. Self-determination theory and motivational interviewing as examples of development from a meta-theory (top-down) vs. from clinical experience up (bottom-up): Implications for theory development, research and clinical practice and interventions. *Int J Behav Nutr Phys Act.* 2012;9:23.
51. Vansteenkiste M, Sheldon KM. There's nothing more practical than a good theory: Integrating motivational interviewing and self-determination theory. *British J Clin Psychol.* 2006;45:63–82.
52. Wanzer MB, Booth-Butterfield M, Gruber K. Perceptions of health care providers' communication: Relationships between patient-centered communication and satisfaction. *Health Comm.* 2004;16(3):363–83.
53. Whitlock EP, Orleans CT, Pender N, Allan J. Evaluating primary care behavioral counseling interventions: An evidence-based approach. *Am J Prev Med.* 2002;22(4):267–84.
54. Williams GC, Minicucci DS, Kouides RW, et al. Self-determination, smoking, diet and health. *Health Educ Res.* 2002;17:512–21.
55. Williams GC, Niemiec CP, Patrick H, Ryan RM, Deci EL. The importance of supporting autonomy and perceived competence in facilitating long-term tobacco abstinence. *Ann Behav Med.* 2009;37:315–24.

CHAPTER 6

How to Deliver Physical Activity Messages

Gregory J. Norman, Julia K. Kolodziejczyk, Eric B. Hekler, and Ernesto R. Ramirez

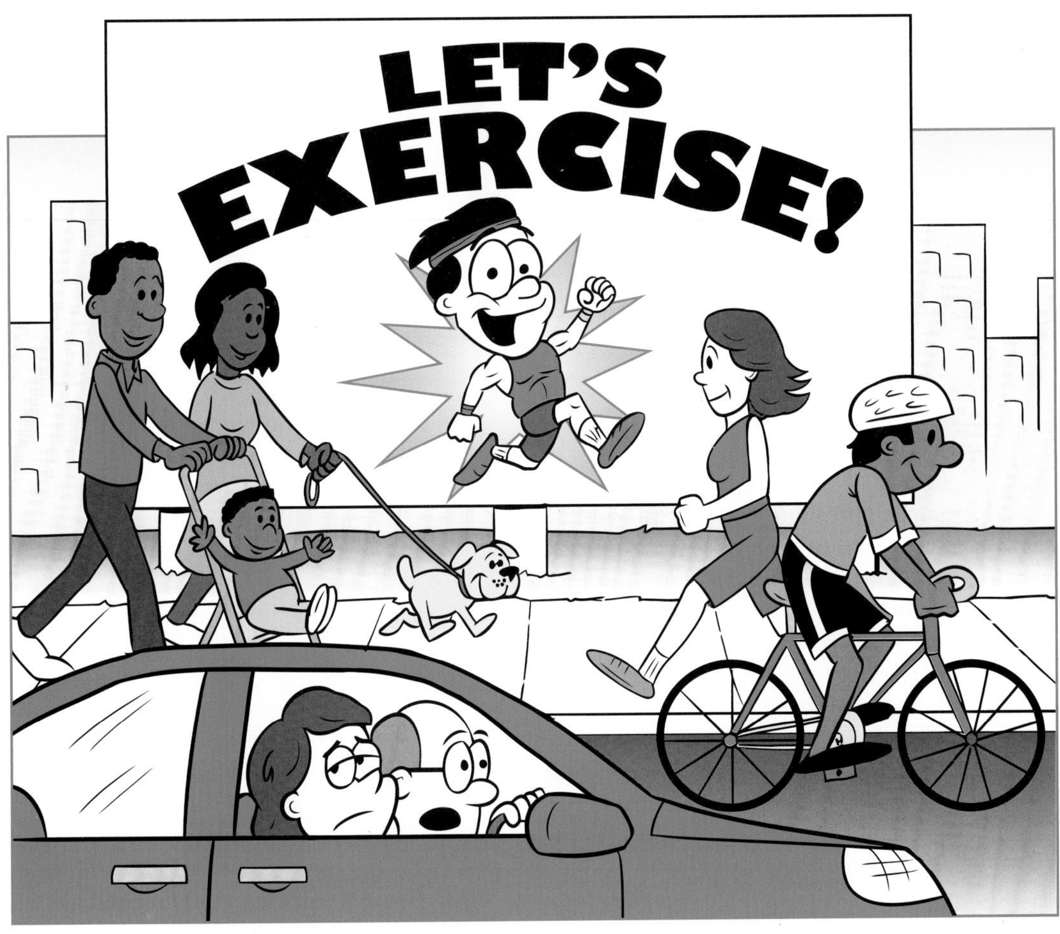

"I KNOW I SHOULD START EXERCISING, BUT I DON'T KNOW WHERE TO BEGIN!"

CONCEPT OVERVIEW

ELECTRONIC TECHNOLOGIES AS COMMUNICATION CHANNELS FOR PHYSICAL ACTIVITY MESSAGE DELIVERY

In this age of electronic media and wireless communication, there are multiple ways to deliver a physical activity program. The Internet, computers, and mobile phones can be harnessed to customize and automate physical activity intervention programs that can provide instruction, motivational messages, goal setting, and feedback in ways never before possible. In addition, there are new types of devices to use with these technologies for collecting information from individuals about their activity patterns. Devices such as pedometers, heart rate monitors, and GPS units—as well as technologies that have accelerometers, gyroscopes, and temperature sensors built into them—can provide monitoring and feedback to individuals, coaches, or health care providers about activity levels and other health indicators. This chapter sorts through and explains the barrage of electronic technologies and how they have been implemented and evaluated as channels for delivering physical activity programs. Before we delve into each type of technology and present step-by-step recommendations for their use, we will provide some background on ways of thinking about communication systems.

A COMMUNICATION MODEL APPLIED TO DELIVERING PHYSICAL ACTIVITY INTERVENTIONS

Berlo's (10) S-M-C-R model of communication defines communication as a process that works through a *Source* that delivers the *Message* through a *Channel* to a *Receiver*. When we apply the S-M-C-R model to deliver physical activity interventions, the *Source* is you and your intervention system, which includes the decision rules that determine the appropriate *Message* to send. The *Message* is the content of the intervention and is delivered through different *Channels,* such as printed materials, Web sites, text messages, or Twitter "tweets" that are *Received* by users interested in changing or maintaining their physical activity level. Velicer and colleagues (111) added the *Feedback* channel to the S-M-C-R model to explain how a behavior change intervention determines the specific elements on which to tailor the intervention for the *Receiver*. This information could come from survey responses to questions about motivation and barriers to being physically active and from sensor data collected from a pedometer, accelerometer, or other data capture device to determine levels and patterns of physical activity.

For the technologies presented in this chapter that serve as the Source—*Message* channels and *Feedback* channels (S-M-C-R-F)—we emphasize designing interventions to influence physical activity through human computer interaction (HCI) rather than computer mediated communication (CMC) (36). In HCI, the *Receiver* interacts with computerized message channels such as mobile phone texting or a Web site that delivers content determined by computer algorithms and *Feedback* channels such as a sensor device that captures physical activity levels. CMC, on the other hand, facilitates person-to-person communication through technologies such as instant messaging, Skype, or WebEx. The distinction between HCI and CMC is subtle but important. One important difference is that CMC allows for one-to-one communication and does not "scale up" to allow you to reach a large number of individuals in a timely and cost-effective manner. The automatic approach of HCI is designed to mimic the experience that occurs through CMC and face-to-face interactions.

HCI opens the range of possibilities for how physical activity interventions can be delivered. One-to-one, face-to-face interaction was the typical way people received a physical activity intervention through a trainer or health care provider. Similarly, one-to-many interactions to deliver an intervention were typically delivered through group sessions or classes. Now, HCI can simulate many of the aspects of one-to-one interactions but deliver "customized" programs to many people through interactive Web sites, mobile applications, and computer-tailored print materials. Thus, HCI allows scaling of one-to-one interactions so they can be delivered as one-to-many interactions. In addition, social media technologies such as Facebook allow for many-to-many delivery for physical activity promotion. Many-to-many delivery can happen, for example, when you post a physical activity tip on your Facebook page and many people see your post and repost your tip on their pages, linking you to people who you did not contact directly. This chapter presents multiple examples of types of HCI actions possible with different communication technologies.

Continuing with how the S-M-C-R-F model applies to technologies for delivering physical activity interventions, there are important aspects about the *Receiver* to consider. Ideally, you want to develop and direct your intervention program to those in different phases of physical activity "readiness" (97). For example, knowing a person is new to physical activity and is in the Adopter phase would lead you to develop a program different from one designed for someone who is already active and needs motivation to stay a Maintainer. Similarly, someone who was previously active but currently is not—for example, because of injury or pregnancy—would likely get a different kind of intervention geared toward the Relapse phase. Many other aspects of the *Receiver* may be important to determine, which can help customize the intervention *Message*, such as age, gender, and physical activity goals. The latter might be a key part of your intervention program, and you will need to determine whether someone is interested in intentional leisure types of physical activity (*e.g.,* running, swimming, team sports) or increasing activity through incidental-utilitarian types of activity such as taking the stairs instead of the elevator or walking to destinations instead of driving.

This brings us to the type of *Message* content you will need to develop that will be delivered in your physical activity intervention. Kreuter (61) conceptualized a spectrum of communication content types, from a completely generic content to a completely individualized tailored content. With generic content, there is the assumption that "one size fits all" and intervention content does not need to be altered based on characteristics of the individual. "Tailored" intervention content is designed for one particular individual based on his or her specific characteristics (*e.g.,* motivation level for physical activity, perceived barriers to being active). In between generic and tailored communication is content "targeted" to a subgroup of people, usually based on one or more demographic characteristics (*e.g.,* age and sex). The type of *Message* content you use in your intervention may be determined by factors such as the nature and size of the target population, the budget, and HCI technologies that will be used in the *Message* and *Feedback* channels of your intervention. In this chapter, we will mainly focus on developing tailored interventions and how different technologies facilitate delivering tailored message content.

The sections of this chapter focus on the communication *Channels*, both for content and for feedback to the *Source*. We begin with computer-generated print materials, and then turn to electronic media such as Internet, video, and interactive voice recognition (IVR). Next, we present two newer technologies for intervention delivery: Short Message Service (SMS) text messaging and social networking platforms. From there, we switch to the feedback devices such as pedometers, accelerometers, heart rate monitors, and GPS units. The chapter concludes with ways that *Message* and *Feedback* channels can be integrated into smart mobile applications and other technology platforms. This chapter is geared to those interested in creating their own physical activity intervention program either through developing a "custom" system or by using "off the shelf" commercial products.

COMPUTER-GENERATED PRINT MEDIA

The "gold standard" for delivering physical activity programs is face-to-face contact with a health professional or a certified personal trainer (79). However, the time and cost of these programs often makes them inaccessible to many people. There is a long history of physical activity instructions and self-help materials delivered through books, pamphlets, and newsletters. Print materials can be used to provide a structured self-help program or to supplement face-to-face training sessions. Print materials can be handed out at the point of service, such as athletic clubs, gyms, health care clinics, and work-sites, or they can be mailed directly to patients, employees, club members, and clients. Electronic print materials can also be e-mailed to individuals or made accessible on Web sites. Providing print materials is a way for health professionals to deliver information to their patients that they do not have time to cover during a clinic visit or as a means to reinforce messages they give at a counseling session. The printed materials serve as a reminder to the individual and information that the client can refer to between clinic visits or sessions.

Since the early 2000s, considerable information about physical activity has become available on the Internet, and 8 in 10 U.S. Internet users have searched for health information on the Web (http://pewinternet.org). Thus, Internet sources have a wide reach for interested consumers, yet the quality of information and appropriateness to the individual may vary considerably. Electronic print materials can consist of existing generic print materials simply provided directly on the Web. Organizations such as the *American Heart Association, American College of Sports Medicine, the American Academy of Family Physicians*, and *American Council on Exercise* (*ACE*) have online materials available. However, a major advantage of electronic print media is the potential to customize materials either for groups or to individuals. Customizing information to a group is often called "market segmentation" or "targeting." For example, developing a monthly physical activity newsletter just for seniors would provide specific information about types of physical activity that would appeal to this population age segment.

On the other hand, tailored materials are designed to mimic the strengths of individual counseling such as interpersonal contact, interactivity, and immediacy of feedback. Tailored information can range from superficially "personalized" materials that use a person's name to generate interest but deliver generic information, to highly individualized tailoring that provides feedback based on assessed knowledge, attitudes, and behavior history.

Tailored electronic print materials require information to be collected to tailor the messages and feedback. Information can be collected by mail, at a kiosk, or online. How data are collected and the information is delivered determine the immediacy of the information. There will be a significant delay if a person must mail a survey and the survey information has to be entered into a computer system to generate a tailored feedback report. In comparison, a computer kiosk or online assessment can be completed and immediately tailored for the individual, and delivered to them.

Evidence

Multiple reviews of tailored health behavior studies generally have concluded that tailoring "works" (84). For example, when reviewing eight studies that specifically compared tailored to nontailored print materials, Skinner and colleagues (102) found tailored information enhances the impact of the printed intervention materials (in terms of being better remembered, read, and perceived as relevant) compared to nontailored materials. Skinner et al. also found tailored print materials to be more effective than nontailored for changing health behaviors (*e.g.*, diet, physical activity, smoking, mammography screening).

However, only one of the eight studies focused on physical activity. Similarly, from a review of 30 studies on physical activity and diet behavior change, Kroeze (63) concluded that the evidence in support of computer-tailored interventions for diet was strong. However, from the 10 physical activity–tailored intervention studies, the evidence was not sufficient to conclude in favor of computer-tailored interventions.

Several studies have demonstrated that tailored print material interventions work for promoting physical activity. For example, Marcus and colleagues (72) demonstrated that stage-targeted materials outperformed standard *American Heart Association* generic print materials. Marcus (73) compared tailored print materials to tailored Internet delivery, and to standard Internet delivery, which consisted of links to six publicly available physical activity Web sites. The tailored print and Internet groups received the same information and groups were instructed to complete physical activity logs. Participants in all three groups (N = 249) increased activity from being sedentary to between 80 to 90 minutes of physical activity a week over 12 months. The findings suggest that all three types of programs were effective likely because they included prompted self-monitoring with physical activity logs, which is known as an important behavior change strategy.

A similarly designed study randomized sedentary adults to print and telephone-delivered tailored interventions, or to a control group condition (74). A total of 14 contacts were made over 12 months with materials either mailed or delivered by telephone health counselors in the print and telephone groups, respectively. Although both intervention programs increased physical activity by an additional 40 minutes/week compared to the control condition at 6 months, by 12 months only the print materials condition was significantly more active than the telephone and control groups. These findings suggest that both intervention modes may be effective for helping people in the adoption of physical activity, but the print materials may be more effective than telephone counseling for maintaining physical activity. It may be that having the printed tailored intervention materials available to review at any time is helpful in keeping a person motivated to be physically active.

Some studies have examined the effect of tailored print materials targeting both physical activity and diet behaviors. Van Keulen (55) randomized individuals to receive either four computer-tailored letters, four motivational interview telephone calls, a combined intervention (two letters and two calls), or a control group. Interventions were delivered within 12 months and all three interventions improved physical activity and diet compared to the control group. Another study randomized breast and prostate cancer survivors to receive a 10-month program of either tailored or nontailored mailed print materials for improving physical activity and diet behaviors (29). Although cancer survivors in both programs improved health behaviors, the tailored program was found to be more effective.

Unfortunately, there is no definitive evidence on how much printed materials need to be tailored to be effective, or exactly what factors need to be tailored. For example, demographic characteristics, level of motivation, perceived barriers, and use of behavior change constructs are just some of the factors that could be the basis for tailoring intervention materials. It is also not known how often tailored interventions need to be delivered. For example, counter to intuition, a single mailing of print materials was more effective at promoting physical activity than multiple mailings (75).

Step-by-Step

Kreuter (61) outlined a five-step process for developing tailored intervention materials. The steps presented in Table 6.1 incorporate Kreuter's steps, with additional decisions that need to be made when developing a print-based tailored intervention program.

TABLE 6.1 Steps in the Process of Developing a Print-Based Tailored Intervention

Step	Key Questions and Tasks
1. Preliminary Steps	What is the purpose of program? Is it to supplement or enhance a "face-to-face" program, or will this be a "stand-alone" self-help program? Who is your target audience? Will the program target multiple phases of physical activity, such as adoption, maintenance, and relapse? In what setting will the printed materials be distributed? Possibilities include an individual's home, gym, worksite, or health care clinic. The setting may influence the look, content and "branding" of the print materials.
2. Intervention Content	Will the structure of the intervention be a newsletter, a report, or a pamphlet? Will the content be based on a scientific theory and evidence? Theories and models of persuasion and behavior change can be drawn from fields of communication, psychology, and sociology (Neuhauser 2003). On which determinants of physical activity do you want to focus? How extensively will the content be tailored?
3. Partnering with Experts	The decisions in steps 1 and 2 will lead you to determine who to partner with to develop the printed materials. Do you need a graphic designer, computer programmers, a printing company, copyeditor, or health care professionals?
4. Gathering and Storing Information	How will the determinants of physical activity be measured? Do validated survey measures exist? How will collected information be stored in a database?
5. Creating the Intervention System	Create tailored messages that vary by levels of the measured determinants. Develop algorithms and a computer program for determining how survey responses about determinants are linked to specific tailored messages. The algorithms are rules or decisions that the computer follows to "act" like the human expert (*e.g.*, coach, counselor, health care provider).
6. Other Considerations	Consider what the appropriate reading level should be for your printed materials. It is recommended that health literature be written at a 6th-grade reading level so it is accessible to lower literacy individuals. What is the time frame for the delivery of the intervention materials? For example, will it be weekly, monthly, or semiannually? The time frame is an important consideration and relates to the overall structure of the printed materials and how much content will need to be developed.

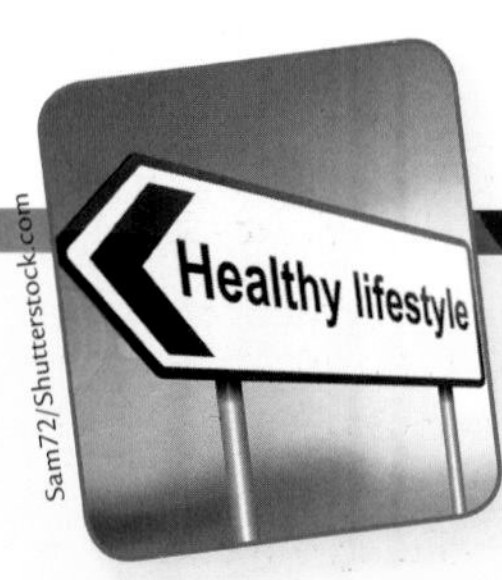

Sam72/Shutterstock.com

Case Scenario 6.1

You are hired by a large business to assist with a yearlong "Workplace Wellness" initiative for their employees. Your job is to create print materials to help employees increase their physical activity levels.

Worksite: Customer service center
Number of employees: 500
Age range: 18–60

Case Scenario 6.1 *continued*

Gender: 65% women

Education: 25% high school graduate, 65% college degree, 10% graduate degree

Main physical activity barrier: Most of the employees sit at a computer for 8 hours a day, 5 days a week.

Because you will not be providing any other counseling to these individuals, the materials must stand-alone and be self-explanatory. The materials need to target multiple phases of physical activity (*i.e.*, adoption, maintenance, and relapse) as this is a yearlong program and the employees will likely start at different physical activity levels. You determine that the best way to deliver these materials is via e-mail, as this method is efficient and inexpensive. In addition, the employees may be more likely to read the materials if the e-mail comes from a reliable source like the Human Resources or Health Services department. The materials will be in a newsletter that employees can easily print out or that can be read on the computer. The content will be based on Social Cognitive Theory. Because the employees are sedentary for most of the week, the focus of the materials will be on environmental determinants of physical activity such as access and time barriers. About 40% of the content will be generic, but given the demographics of the company, you decide it is best to tailor the remaining 60% of the content on age, gender, and the current phase of physical activity. You hire a behavioral health consultant to help base the content on evidence-based behavior change theories and a computer software engineer to help you create computer algorithms for tailoring the content. You also plan to hire a copyeditor and a graphic designer so the product has a professional look and is attention grabbing. The determinants of physical activity will be measured quarterly with a validated, electronic questionnaire distributed to the employees via e-mail. Information will be collected on a secure database. Finally, the computer algorithms will link the information collected from these questionnaires to specific tailored messages to create the tailored print materials.

ELECTRONIC MEDIA: INTERNET AND INTERACTIVE VOICE RESPONSE

Electronic media such as Internet-based and automated telephone systems have the potential for reaching many individuals at a low cost. For example, the Internet has global reach, with widespread adoption in the U.S. (*e.g.*, 79% of adults use the Internet: pewinternet.org, August 23, 2011) and about 30.2% (approximately 2.1 billion people) of the global population, with rapid growth observed in developing areas such as Africa (2527% growth since 2000) and the Middle East (1987% growth since 2000: Internet World Stats, 2011). There are many advantages of computer/Web-based interventions for health behavior change, such as ease of dissemination, access, anonymity, interactivity, and graphical interfaces. Further, after initial setup costs, maintenance of these Web sites is relatively low-cost (8). Interactive voice response (IVR) systems are computer-directed interactions via the telephone (*e.g.*, when you call a company, your initial interactions are often with a computer-automated voice, which is an IVR system). These technologies have gained popularity, not only for call service centers but also for health promotion because they can be automated to provide a variety of health services ranging from automated appointment reminders to data gathering and physical activity coaching.

Evidence for Internet Interventions

Several scientific reviews have explored the value of Internet-based interventions (16,28,82, 114). In general, most reviews have suggested insufficient evidence for Internet-based interventions as an effective strategy for physical activity interventions. Despite this, a more meta-analysis exploring the efficacy of Internet-based interventions as social marketing for behavior change more generally, not just for physical activity promotion, showed "small but statistically significant effects" across 30 studies (28). Almost all of these previous reviews highlight the early nature of Internet-based programs, along with the need for additional research.

When interventions did show evidence of working, it tended to be when they were compared to no-treatment control groups (12,49,50,78,103). There was less supportive evidence of Internet-based interventions relative to other active forms of intervention, such as tailored print-based media (73). A study comparing two Web sites showed that a neighborhood-focused Web site that was updated often resulted in significantly improved physical activity participation over a 26-week period relative to a nontailored motivationally focused Web site (34).

Short-term intervention programs seem to be more effective than longer-term programs (28). A major problem of most Internet-based interventions is that people stop using the program regularly with many showing low return visit rates to the Web sites (32). Internet-based interventions had attrition rates greater than 20%, suggesting the continued need to explore methods for improving adherence.

When designing a Web-based intervention, there are two major types of design features to consider: those features that improve the return/retention rate of the use of the Web site and those features that promote physical activity. Each of these types of features will be discussed in turn based on previous literature and specific recommendations will be given.

Previous research has explored differences in attrition rates that occur based on recruitment strategies (*e.g.*, clinical trials vs. commercially available Web sites). Research from clinical trials suggests the value of including multiple methods of communicating (*i.e.*, e-mail , text message) along with peer interaction / social support to improve adherence to Web-based interventions (16,18,114). A few studies have explored program adherence using a Web-based intervention among individuals not part of a clinical trial (81,112). Results from one study suggest that only 4.8% of the individuals who visited the open-access Web site registered to use it, and even among registered users, the vast majority (*i.e.*, approximately 92%) stopped using the Web site after one month and did not return despite e-mail reminders. This dropout rate was markedly higher compared to participants in the clinical trial (*i.e.*, 40% drop out by month one) who were instructed to access the same Web site.

Another study explored dropout and retention rates for a commercially available weight-loss Web site, *The Biggest Loser, Australia* (81). This Web site was advertised on *The Biggest Loser, Australia* TV show and included a paid subscription plan ranging from 12 weeks to 52 weeks. When looking at data from those who paid for the subscription, the number of participants returning after the first month to use the Web site dropped to fewer than 50% of the eligible participants by weeks 9–12 of the program among those who signed up for a 12-week subscription. Among participants who signed up for a 52-week subscription, nonuse rates increased the most during the first 16 weeks of the program, with a relatively steady rate of nonuse of approximately 60% occurring from week 21 onward.

Web sites need to be designed with content easily accessible at all page levels of the site. One study explored what factors (*e.g.*, demographics, self-determination beliefs) predicted surfing depth in a physical activity and nutrition behavior change Web site (51). This study highlighted a variety of good practices for the development of a Web site. From a design standpoint, the researchers did a small prototyping phase with a small sample of the target population. In addition, participants determined how difficult (*i.e.*, how many clicks) it was to get to various information within a Web site, thus aiding in understanding how the structure of the information impacts use. As a result, the researchers gathered a great deal of valuable metrics for understanding user behavior (*e.g.*, number of clicks, time spent on each page—information that can be gleaned using tools like Google Analytics). Findings from this study suggested that the Web site had an average penetration of only two layers (*i.e.*, two additional clicks to content areas beyond the home page), which is lower than the four to eight clicks more commonly observed in other successful Web sites. Although e-mail reminders were shown to help increase the depth of exploration, the results were considered largely inconclusive based on the relatively small depth that participants entered into the Web page.

The aforementioned studies highlighted that use of these Web site interventions was higher among the highly educated, the overweight, and women (19,80,112). An interesting opportunity for practitioners is the development of intervention Web sites that work more effectively among other population segments, particularly men—which has been highlighted more generally within physical activity promotion research (87,113).

With regard to promoting behavior change, a variety of theories have been used when developing Web-based interventions, with the most effective Web-based interventions using Social Cognitive Theory, the Transtheoretical Model (see Chapters 1 and 4), and/or the Theory of Planned Behavior (16,115). In addition, although results are inconclusive, physical activity interventions that frame information based on tailored messages, gain-framed messages, and to improvements self-efficacy appear to hold the most promise for improving physical activity (67). Two qualitative reviews have each identified five key components to effective weight-loss intervention Web sites. One suggested self-monitoring, counselor feedback and communication, social support, use of a structured program, and use of an individually tailored program as key components (56). The other review concluded that intervention developers should aim to re-create the human experience, personalize it to the individual, create a dynamic experience, provide a supportive environment, and build upon sound behavior change theory (9) (see Chapter 3). As can be seen, common parallels between these two studies are a focus on personalizing/tailoring, social support, solid communication techniques, and structured/evidence-informed/theoretically based programs.

Evidence for Interactive Voice Response (IVR) Systems

Several studies suggest that telephone-based interventions delivered by humans can be widely disseminated and result in improved physical activity (30,117). Researchers have also explored the use of interactive voice response (IVR) systems (also known as automated telephone-linked computer systems) as a health care tool (85). These systems have high potential value because they can be used for simple tasks such as appointment reminders and for complicated tasks such as delivering fully automated advice and feedback about physical activity as well as other health behaviors. A meta-analysis of IVR telephone systems showed that automated calls were effective at promoting improved processes of care (*e.g.*, coming to appointments) and disease states (*e.g.*, improved glycemic control) (69).

Although there is limited research on IVR systems for promoting physical activity, several results have been promising (59). For example, the most rigorous study to date examining the utility of IVR telephone systems showed that an automated phone system was more effective than an attention control condition at promoting physical activity for 12 months and was equally as effective as a human-delivered telephone counseling program (59).

Some studies have identified characteristics that improve IVR user acceptance. Specifically, IVR systems are less accepted when: (a) similar content is repeatedly given, (b) interactions are inflexible and feel driven by the needs of the computer rather than the user, (c) users feel like the system is condescending, (d) the IVR system makes the users feel guilty, (e) little introduction leads to poor perceptions of the system, including the perception that the system is a telemarketer, and (f) intervention content was not delivered quickly enough (3,33,42). Several studies have also identified ways to improve IVR systems. For example, IVR systems that were generally accepted included a detailed description of the IVR system prior to its use, and a chance to contact a human if problems arose with the program (42,59). Interestingly, some participants expressed a strong affinity for the automated voice akin to that of a mentor or close friend (54).

As with other technology systems, there are several companies who have already developed the basic architecture for IVR systems. Development of an IVR system often involves contacting these companies and working on developing appropriate content, including a specific set of decisions and rules about the appropriate times to call.

Step-by-Step

Table 6.2 summarizes key steps to take when developing an electronic media intervention. Although Table 6.2 begins with similar preliminary steps identified in Table 6.1, Table 6.2

TABLE 6.2 Steps in Developing an Electronic Media Intervention

Step	Key Questions and Tasks
1. Identify the user group.	Who will use the system? What behaviors will be promoted? What are the known constraints? Be as specific as possible.
2. Observe.	What is the potential user currently doing related to the behavior? Why? Among those doing well, why are they doing well? Among those doing poorly, why?
3. Identify theory(ies).	Which theories of behavior change fit best with the issues observed with the group? Which theory has the most empirical support? What does current theory not include that was observed?
4a. Develop prototypes.	Develop potential ideas. Highlight differences and come up with competing hypotheses.
4b. Test users.	Concept phase: Goal is to see if how you defined your concept is how potential users see it. Show prototypes and observe if they are "getting it" as expected. User experience: Goal is to identify the simplest, most intuitive means of moving through the system. Observe how a participant moves through a system focused on trying to understand expectations of the user. Note the full system does not need to be functional (*e.g.*, the backend storage and data processing) to get a sense of user experience. Functional Prototype: Put it altogether, including the back-end and see if it works as planned. Previous steps will help to minimize painful lessons.
4c. Iterate	Aggregate lessons learned from user testing and go back as far as step 1 but likely 4a, depending on the results. During iteration, the goal is to move from concept prototypes to user-experience prototypes to fully functional prototypes.
5. Test system among "experts."	When the fully functional prototype is up and running, have several folks, including individuals who may not be your user testers but may be knowledgeable and around (*e.g.*, colleagues) to use it to help identify obvious bugs in the system. Iterate based on lessons learned.
6. Test within a small sample group.	Goal is to identify other glaring problems with the system.
7. Launch the system (but remember to monitor and update).	Be prepared to monitor the system while it is going and to fix/iterate problems that arise, particularly by monitoring system use via tools such as Google Analytics.

includes additional development steps such as developing prototypes, iterative development cycles, and user testing that are critical for building interactive electronic media programs.

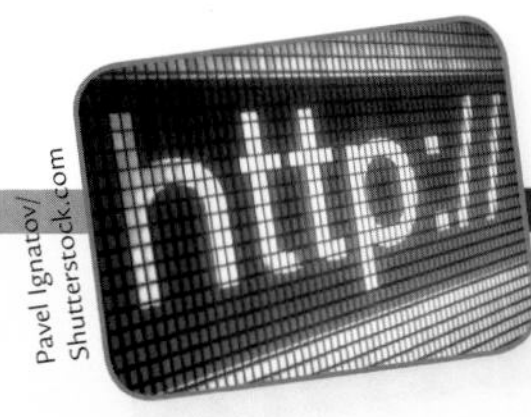

Pavel Ignatov/ Shutterstock.com

Case Scenario 6.2

You are developing an intervention to increase walking and strength training for older adults who are caregivers of frail spouses.

Gender: Mostly women

Age: 65 and over

You begin by observing older adults using Web pages in their homes and conduct interviews with them about opportunities for being active. This lets you "walk a mile in their shoes." Next, you decide that you want to include theory-based behavior change strategies such as self-monitoring, goal setting, and framing information in a gain-focused manner. Afterward, you begin the process of developing prototypes and user testing. In the concept phase, you mock-up several drawings and text descriptions of different goal setting formats. When you show participants the different goal framings, you find out the wording does not elicit the concept you intended and you have to go back and create new paper prototypes for goal setting. In the user experience phase, you test different self-monitoring formats by exploring ease of use and observing how users enter their information into the system. When a fully functional prototype is built, you have new users test the systems for longer lengths of time. In addition, you invite several colleagues to try the system for a few days, and they find several instances of system crashes, incomplete links, and poorly worded content. These errors are corrected and another group of users test the system. These users respond with general interest to the Web site but feel some parts are cumbersome. You revise the user interface to conform better to the users' needs. At this stage, your system has been well vetted, and your IT team can continue to monitor and resolve minor problems to maintain your Web site.

TEXT MESSAGING

Short-messaging services (SMS; also known as text messaging) is an inexpensive, instantaneous form of two-way communication that transmits brief written messages via a mobile phone. It is the most widely available and frequently used mobile data service (66,104). Almost everyone in the U.S. has a cell phone, with 302.9 million wireless subscribers as of Dec 2010 (*i.e.*, 96% of the total U.S. population, with over 26.6% in wireless-only households; www.ctia.org). In addition, 98% of cell phones worldwide have SMS capabilities with 187.7 billion monthly text messages sent in the U.S. The popularity of texting may even increase as cell phone companies are increasingly including unlimited texting in calling plans. What makes mobile phone technology unique compared to other forms of communication, such as landlines or the Internet, is that mobile phone ownership and the use of cell phones is as prevalent among those from lower socioeconomic groups as among those from the general population (60,121). SMS is often used for "push" technology, where information is transmitted to a user without the user having to initiate the request. Push technology contrasts with other mobile technology that may require a "pull" from a user, such as calling a telephone number or accessing an Internet Web site. Pull technology is also used in SMS when messages ask the user to respond or when the user initiates dialogue to receive information. Push and pull technology and other features of SMS may be particularly useful to help individuals make healthful lifestyle decisions made continuously throughout the day, such as reducing screen time or engaging in a daily workout.

Using SMS for promoting health behavior is a rapidly growing area (35,62) as mobile phones have many capabilities that can be used for health promotion (88). SMS technology can collect and deliver time- and context-sensitive information in succinct messages that can be read discreetly. These messages are asynchronous—that is, they can be accessed any time or place convenient for the user. The messages will also be stored on the phone even if the phone has been turned off, and messages will be delivered when the phone is turned back on. SMS technology can reach rural areas or places with limited cellular service because it requires a lower bandwidth compared to phone calls made with mobile phones. These SMS features can be useful for a wide variety of health behaviors and conditions, such as simple appointment reminders or complicated tasks like weight loss counseling (88,89).

One of the reasons SMS is effective at promoting health behavior is that many SMS features relate to important constructs in behavior change theories such as cues to action, reinforcement, goal setting, goal reminders, and feedback. In addition, research has shown that SMS programs improve social support (40), self-monitoring (99,100), perceived control (49), anxiety (93), and self-efficacy (40) (also See Chapter 3).

Evidence

SMS has shown to be effective at improving many health-related behaviors such as diabetes management (39,40) and smoking cessation (15,94). To date, two studies focused on physical activity have shown positive results. In a nine-week trial conducted by Hurling and colleagues (49), 77 healthy adults received access to an interactive Web site with a feedback facility, wrist accelerometers for self-monitoring, and tailored supplemental messages. Participants choose to receive the messages by either e-mail or SMS. These messages offered participants solutions for perceived barriers and included scheduled reminders for weekly physical activity. This text message program helped increase moderate-intensity physical activity by approximately 2.25 hours per week. In another study conducted by Shapiro and colleagues (100), 58 children and their parents used SMS to self-monitor physical activity levels for 8 weeks. After three 90-minute educational group sessions, the children and parents were instructed to send two messages a day denoting their physical activity, and for each message they received automated SMS feedback. The results showed that using SMS improved adherence to self-monitoring physical activity. However, a third study by Newton (83) did not find that SMS was effective at increasing physical activity. In this 12-week trial, 78 adolescents received a pedometer and generic motivational messages to increase step count. The results showed that sending text messages to adolescents decreased step count and did not change BMI. The null results found in this SMS trial may be because of to the use of generic messages rather than tailored messages.

Other SMS research has been conducted where physical activity was not the primary aim in the trial, but it was incorporated into the program. Four of these studies, which focused on weight loss as the primary aim, sent diet and physical activity messages to participants. In a study conducted by Joo and Kim (52), a weight reduction program that included access to a public health center and pedometers, printed materials, an initial nutritional assessment by a registered dietician, and SMS, helped participants lose 1.6 kg of weight in 12 weeks. Patrick and colleagues (89) found that their SMS program, which was supplemented with brief monthly counseling calls and printed materials, helped decrease participants' weight by 2.88 kg in 4 months. Haapala and colleagues (44) found that their SMS program, which did not include supplemental intervention strategies, decreased participant weight by 4.5 kg in 12 months. Gerber and colleagues (41) also conducted an SMS-only weight management program that focused on perceptions of use and found that women receiving text messages about weight loss had positive attitudes toward the incoming messages. Two studies focused on Type 2 diabetes control and incorporated physical activity messages into the program. Both of these studies were primarily SMS-based and were supplemented with a Web site. At 12 months, both studies (57,120) showed that SMS improved HbA1C among other measures related to diabetes control. With the exception of only one study, all of the aforementioned SMS research conducted has shown that SMS is effective at either improving physical activity levels or assisting in health promotion related to physical activity.

Frequency of text message transmission and duration of the program are important program characteristics. In general, frequency of messages usually reflects the expected frequency of the target behavior (35). For physical activity SMS studies, frequency varied greatly among the different programs. One study with a physical activity component showed success with sending up to five messages a day (89) and others found success with weekly messages (41,49,52,57,120). Another study left it up to the participants to decide on the number of text messages they wanted to receive (44). As for the duration of the program, most of the successful physical activity or health promotion studies were between 6 to 12 months.

It is important to note that SMS programs are often combined with other intervention strategies or materials, such as interactive Web sites, a paper diary for self-monitoring, consultations with health professionals, or printed materials. All of the physical activity SMS studies have included supplementation in their programs. Most common was use of Web sites (44,49,57,120), counseling calls (41,89), or interaction with health professionals (57,120).

Step-by-Step

There are many companies that offer SMS services available to individuals or businesses. One of the most popular health SMS-based programs available to individual consumers is "text4baby" that offers women support through pregnancy. To date, there are no SMS programs for physical activity commercially available to individuals, but some companies offer these programs to businesses. For instance, Santech Inc. (www.santechhealth.com) is one company that offers tailored mobile phone diet and physical activity-based programs, such as "Text4Diet" that is a program geared toward weight loss in the general adult or teen populations.

There are also ways to create your own SMS programs for clients. After deciding on what SMS program characteristics are a good fit for you and your client (*e.g.*, personalization, interactivity), you can search online for companies that offer bulk-messaging services. Many of these programs are free (*e.g.*, Google Voice) or have a small fee per message sent (*e.g.*, www.bulksms.com; callfire.com). These Web sites offer many advanced features that make sending general nontailored messages simple and effortless because you can easily create address books, automatically schedule messages, track message delivery, and much more. See Table 6.3 for tips on how to write an effective text message. See Table 6.4 for sample physical activity messages.

TABLE 6.3 How to Write an Effective Text Message

What to Include	Why	Example
Positive affect	• Attention grabbing • Message becomes more salient • Increases feedback	• Using words like "happy," "sweet," or "nice"
Gain-framed	• Persuasive	• Framing message in terms of benefits rather than costs of physical activity
Nonverbal cues	• Readers better interpret the message • Increases socio-emotional appeal • Using playful language creates a friendly, informal, conversational tone and in turn fosters relationships • Manipulation of grammatical markers: indicate pauses (....), express exclamation (!), or signal tone of voice (SHOUT) • Minus features: an absence of certain language standards present in normal writing, such as a lack of capitalization at the beginning of a sentence	• Vocal spelling: "weeeeellll" • Lexical surrogates: "mhmm" • Spatial arrays (emoticons)
Powerful language	• Attention grabbing • Message becomes more salient	• Powerful: "always" or "never" • Powerless: "sort of," "maybe," tag questions ("isn't it?"), hesitations ("um"), intensifiers ("really"), or fragmented sentences
Clarity	• Less mental processing effort • Less distraction	• Regular text supplementation (only when completely necessary) • Pictures • Animation • Audio • When using shortcuts, shortening words (e.g., "wk" for "week") is clearer than respelling (e.g., "c u" for "see you")

TABLE 6.4 Physical Activity Text Message Samples

Education
By exercising as little as 30 min a day, you can improve your health and live longer!
Physical activity boosts mental wellness—It can increase relaxation, concentration, and happiness
Strategies
Start with a small physical activity goal and commit regularly
Use variety to keep your interest up. Walk one day, swim the next, go for a bike ride on the weekend
Tips
The simplest change you can make to improve your heart health effectively is to start walking. It's enjoyable, free, easy, and great exercise
Look for chances to be more active during the day. Walk the mall before shopping or take the stairs instead of the escalator
Reminders
Remember to put on your pedometer today!
Grab a friend and go for a 30 min walk before the day is over
Motivational
The time to get moving is NOW!
Stick to your goal of getting 12,000 steps on your pedometer today. You can do it!

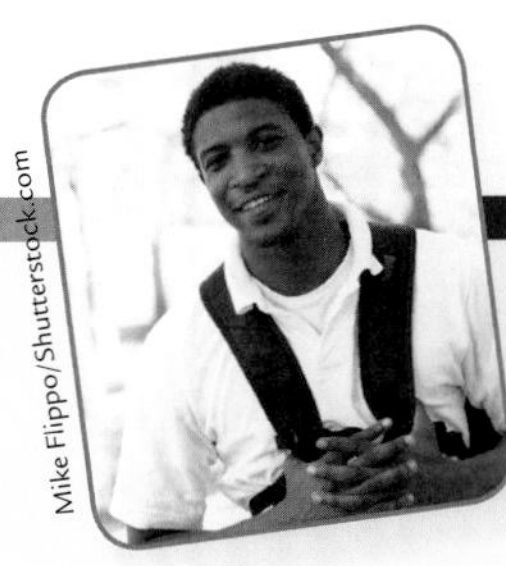
Mike Flippo/Shutterstock.com

Case Scenario 6.3

This case scenario presents the use of tailored, one-way messages to serve as prompts and cues to action.

Client: Brian

Client information:

- 18-year-old male
- A high school cross-country runner

Brian has asked you to help him prepare for cross-country team tryouts in the fall.

After designing a workout for him, you want to send it via SMS daily reminders so he can easily stay on track throughout the summer. One tailored, one-way pushed message each day will serve Brian's needs. See Table 6.5 for sample text messages that could be sent to Brian to help him prepare for the upcoming cross-country season.

continued

Case Scenario 6.3 *continued*

TABLE 6.5 Sample Text Messages for Brian's Cross-Country Running Training

Day	Text Message
Monday	Hi Brian- today's workout: 45 min tempo run. It's hot outside today- remember to hydrate
Tuesday	Brian, today's workout is 60 min interval training (10 x 400m)
Wednesday	Today's workout: 30 min easy with 15 min extra stretching. Keep up the good work, Brian!
Thursday	Hi Brian- today's workout 45 min Fartlek; incorporate at least 3 hills
Friday	Today's workout is 45 min interval training (5 x 1000). Brian, get to the track before 4pm, it closes at 6pm today
Saturday	Brian, here is today's workout: 10k long run. Remember to run at a conversational pace
Sunday	Good job this week, Brian!

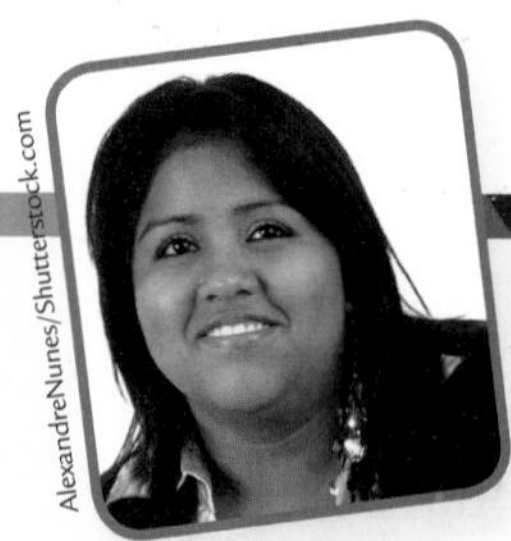
AlexandreNunes/Shutterstock.com

Case Scenario 6.4

This case scenario presents the use of tailored, two-way messages that serve as personalized feedback, social support, and goal setting.

Client: Megan

Client information:

- 35-year-old female
- Employed full-time, married, two children
- Overweight (BMI = 29)

Megan's doctor recommends that she exercise at least 30 minutes a day to lose weight. She has come to you for help, and she does not have time to come in for counseling because of her busy schedule. Two tailored, pushed messages each day will serve Megan's needs. Some messages will also need to be interactive to uncover Megan's personal barriers to meeting her exercise goal. See Table 6.6 for sample text messages that could help Megan exercise at least 30 minutes a day.

Case Scenario 6.4 *continued*

TABLE 6.6 Sample Text Messages to Help Megan Exercise 30 Minutes a Day

Day	Text Message
Mon AM	Megan, what is preventing you from exercising 30 min a day? A) I forget B) I don't have time C) It's too hard D) Something else (*Megan answers B*)
Mon PM	Breaking up your physical activity into 3 ten-min sessions throughout the day will give you the same benefit as doing 30 min at one time
Tues AM	You can do little things throughout the day to increase your physical activity-like taking the stairs instead of the elevator
Tues PM	Combo physical activity with time spent with your friends/family. Take walks together or just play at the park
Weds AM	Hi Megan- How much physical activity did you do yesterday? A) <30 min B) 30 min C) >30 min (*Megan answers A*) Megan, you should aim for at least 30 min of physical activity per day. Try again tomorrow :)
Weds PM	To increase your daily physical activity, try incorporating walking meetings outdoors with coworkers
Thurs AM	Need more time in your day to get a workout in? Put your gym clothes in your car in the morning—you'll be ready to go after work
Thurs PM	Try wearing wrist weights as you do chores around the house—this is a great way to combine exercise and chores.
Fri AM	Hi Megan- How much physical activity did you do yesterday? A) <30 min B) 30 min C) >30 min (*Megan answers B*) Good job, Megan! Keep up the good work. Try increasing your workouts by 5 min tomorrow
Fri PM	Increasing your physical activity is easier if you can distract yourself. Try chatting with friends while you walk or put on your favorite music

Limitations

Although SMS offers many valuable features that can be used for promoting physical activity, there are limitations with this technology. First, the main limitation is that information sent via SMS must be brief because each message must be 160 characters or less. Senders may send multiple messages at once, but because of the small screens on cell phones, lengthly messages are difficult to read (e.g., surveys). Second, there is usually a time commitment to set up an SMS program (*e.g.,* writing messages, importing mobile phone numbers). Third, some messages may not be received because of disconnected mobile phone or full in-boxes, but messages are usually received when the phone is in service again. The SMS program also can be disrupted if the cell phone is lost or stolen. However, the same limitations exist with other forms of communication such as the postal system. Fourth, using SMS technology may marginalize certain populations, such as those who are illiterate or do not have access to a mobile phone for financial reasons; however, these limitations will be reduced as mobile technology advances (incorporating voice response systems or sending pictures instead of texts) and the total cost of cell phone ownership decreases. Finally, using SMS for health promotion is in an early stage of research, and there are still many open questions on best practices for effective behavior change.

SOCIAL MEDIA

Social networking sites (*e.g.*, Facebook, My Space) are a type of social media comprised of personal Web pages that facilitate communication with other users. On these Web pages, users build online profiles, and share updates about themselves, including photos and links to their favorite groups or events, and comment on others' updates. A key feature of these sites is that users can link to others' profiles, which is how the social network develops (31). Users can choose from thousands of different health-related groups and applications that interest them (*e.g.*, *Diabetes Daily*, *Ultra Running*, and *National Health and Wellness* from Facebook). These sites can educate, engage, and empower clients and health professionals because they offer a source to learn about health issues and interact with a community of individuals with similar interests. Social networking sites are one of the most popular forms of social media (98) and, as such, they have great potential to advance health promotion.

Over the last 5 to 10 years, social networking sites have become one of the most popular sites to visit on the Internet. As of November 2010, 93% of teens (12 to 17 years old) were online, and of these users, 73% used a social networking site. Adults (>18 years old) were not far behind with 77% online, and of these users, 61% used social networking sites. Furthermore, 80% of all daily Internet users visit social network sites (http://pewinternet.org). Although young adults are still more likely to access social networks sites, the fastest growing demographic of Facebook users is older adults (>65 years old)—three times as many older adults signed up for Facebook in May 2010 than in May 2009 (119). Also, social media use in the United States is independent of education, race/ethnicity, or health care access (21). As social network technology advances and access increases, it is anticipated that the popularity of online social networking will continue to grow worldwide (48).

The popularity of social networking sites can be attributed to their many unique features. Not only are these sites easy to use and cost effective (*i.e.*, most are free), but they are also user-controlled and generated. In other words, social media sites are not static: They are interactive or users publish their own content and comment on other peoples' content. These sites are also easily accessed because they can be adopted on a variety of devices (*e.g.*, computer, mobile phone, electronic tablet). Social network sites differ from other online communities because of their ability to enable users to display their social networks. This unique feature of visually displaying a list of friends accessible to others is hypothesized to result in connections among individuals that would not have otherwise been made (13). Overall, online social networks allow users to connect and communicate to other users more quickly and easily than other forms of social media.

The connections made through online social networks have great potential for positively influencing health because an individual's social environment plays an important role in many different types of health behavior (86,116), including physical activity (6). One reason is because social networks can affect the perception of social norms, or customary rules that govern behavior in groups of people, which is a dominant force that shapes behavior (22). Perception of social support is another factor within an individual's social environment associated with more positive health behavior and health outcomes in general (110). In addition to affecting an individual's social environment, online social network sites also allow access to information and resources (91), which has been shown to increase empowerment (38,70). Empowerment plays an important role in supporting behavior as individuals seek positive health behavior and lifestyle changes (4,5). Taken together, these psychological constructs can have a powerful impact on individuals' health behavior and outcomes.

Evidence

Research on the use of social networks for health promotion is limited, but evidence is growing especially in the area of health communication. In a Facebook study regarding diabetes, researchers found that about 65% of posts included unsolicited sharing of diabetes management strategies, more than 13% of posts provided specific feedback to information requested by other users, and almost 29% featured an effort by the poster to provide emotional support to other members of the community (43). In another study that focused on breast cancer survivor groups on Facebook, researchers found that this social network site had over one million members and 620 groups. Within these groups, 44.7% were created for fundraising, 38.1% for awareness (about 900K members), 9% for product or service promotion related to fundraising or awareness, and 7% for patient/caregiver support (65). These studies demonstrate that Facebook provides a forum for many different types of health communication, from reporting personal experiences and receiving feedback to reaching mass groups of people for awareness of important public health issues.

To date, one health behavior change intervention has used online social networks. In this physical activity-based Facebook intervention, researchers evaluated StepMatron—a Facebook application designed to provide a social and competitive context for daily pedometer readings to motivate physical activity (37). Researchers found that participants who used the Facebook application to record steps had logged more steps than simply recording steps without the social context. Although more research needs to be conducted in the area of behavior change and social networking sites, the findings from the StepMatron study offer encouraging results that demonstrate the potential of online social networks to motivate behavior change (37).

Step-by-Step

Table 6.7 is a list of some popular social networking sites. Peruse these sites and see which ones have the features and functionality that meet your needs. From the Practical Toolbox 6.1 recommends other resources to consult for more in-depth step-by-step information.

TABLE 6.7 Some Popular Social Networking Sites

Social Network Site	Description
Facebook: http://www.facebook.com	The largest general social networking site worldwide
My Space: http://www.myspace.com	Entertainment (music, movies, celebrities, TV, and games) social networking site
Linked In: http://www.linkedin.com	Business and professional social networking site
Hello Health: http://www.hellohealth.com	Social networking site that connects health care providers and individuals through e-mail, instant messaging, and video chat
Dlife For Your Diabetes Life! http://www.dLife.com	Diabetes patients, consumers, and caregivers social networking site
Athlinks: http://www.athlinks.com	Race results and social network for endurance athletes
Twitter: http://twitter.com	A social networking and micro-blogging service utilizing instant messaging, SMS, or a Web interface

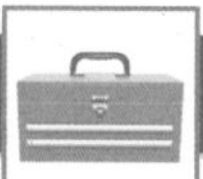

From the Practical Toolbox 6.1

FURTHER RESOURCES FOR USING SOCIAL MEDIA SITES

For more in-depth step-by-step directions, many books are available, including the following:

- *The Twitter Book* by Tim O'Reilly and Sarah Milstein
- *From Facebook to Twitter and Everything in Between: A Step-by-Step Introduction for Social Networks for Beginners and Everyone Else* by Todd Kelsey

There are also many more business-related features on Facebook to help grow your business and build your client base, such as adding Facebook to your Web site. To learn about these features and many more, there are books available that focus on using social networks for professional use, including the following:

- *Reaching Your Online Community with Facebook, LinkedIn, and More* by Tom Funk
- *Doing Business on Facebook* by Vander Veel

Most social media sites also have a user-friendly step-by-step guide on how to get started on their sites and how to use more advanced features, such as the following examples:

- https://support.twitter.com
- http://developers.facebook.com

FACEBOOK

Facebook is arguably the most popular social networking site and can help you reach out to existing or potential clients. Many of the Facebook features described here, such as pages and groups, are also features on other social networking sites. Therefore, much of the information covered in this section applies to other sites as well.

- **Pages:** A "page" is a collection of information about a person, business, or organization. To be a member of Facebook, you need to set up a profile page—it can be a personal and/or professional page. Potential clients can find you by viewing your profile and vice versa. (Tip: You can include a link to your business Web site or other Web sites you think your clients will find useful.)
- **Networks:** A "network" is a group of people with a real-world connection but who might not know each other (*e.g.,* people who are connected through a common school, region, workplace). You can browse through profiles of people in your network to look for potential clients based on various kinds of information, such as age or specific interests. Likewise, others in the network will be able to find and connect with you for your services. The introductions made through your network are safer and less awkward than introducing yourself to people to whom you have no known connection.
- **Groups:** A "group" is a collection of people with the same interests (*e.g.,* clubs, companies, public sector organizations). Groups are a way of enabling a number of people to come together online to share information and discuss specific subjects. You can join one or start your own. This is a great way to network new clients (*e.g.,* participate in industry-related groups, events, discussions) or communicate with current clients (*e.g.,* send messages, exchange ideas, set up meetings).
- **Events:** An "event" is similar to a group, but users RSVP to in-person events. Advertising or promoting an event through Facebook is a quick and easy way to

invite many people at once. For example, you could create an event for Ride Your Bike to Work Day and send invites to your clients.

- **Newsfeeds:** A "newsfeed" is a constantly updated list of the things your Facebook friends are doing on the site (*e.g.,* adding applications, attending events, writing on Walls, commenting on notes and photos, befriending each other). This feature enables you to catch up quickly up on your clients' recent activities.
- **Marketplace application:** This application lets you post and answer want-ads. You can use Marketplace to advertise your business or find those who are looking for a health professional. This application is unique because you can view someone's profile before you contact him or her to conduct business, which makes the transaction safer than want-ad advertisements from the newspaper or sites like Craigslist."

TWITTER

Twitter is another popular social networking site. Twitter is similar to Facebook in many ways, such as users have profiles, it streams updates, and you can meet new people through networking. However, Twitter focuses on communication via short messages of 140 characters or less called "tweets."

- **Tweet:** "Tweets" are similar to text messages because they are short, concise, easy to read and write messages, but they are sent and received in real-time and can be sent through a variety of channels (*e.g.,* computer, phone, tablet). You can choose to have your tweets be public or private.
- **A following:** On Twitter, you choose whose messages you want to subscribe to or follow. You can ask your clients to follow you on Twitter to distribute exercise ideas/comments or news about organized events. Likewise, you can also follow your clients—for instance, you can monitor their physical activity or weight loss progress through their tweets. (Tip: The great thing about Twitter is that you can choose to send public messages and, as such, potential clients can view your conversations with current clients. This offers the opportunity to promote your business because potential clients can see your responsiveness or customer service toward current clients.)
- **Links:** Twitter can be a way to refer potential or current clients to your other sites (*e.g.,* business profile, blog, Facebook page) by posting the link with a creative headline.

SOCIAL NETWORK GROWTH

Whichever social media site you use, the success of your page or group will depend on the social network of people who develops around it. Social networking is about sharing and interaction, so it is important to create a following of users—the more users you have, the faster the social network will develop (53). To create a loyal following of users, the content in your site should be constantly updated so it remains interesting and engaging to your target audience. The more engaging the site, the more users will suggest to other friends to like or subscribe to your site. As a result, your network will grow. Focus on long-term relationship building strategies such as observing the culture and dynamics of the online community that you join. Research what your target audience is interested in and what they find interesting, enjoyable, and valuable (53). Do not be discouraged if at first the response to your site is slow, as you need time to develop a following. See section From the Practical Toolbox 6.1 for more information on social networking tips and strategies (31). Also, From the Practical Toolbox 6.2 provides cautions to health professionals using social networking sites.

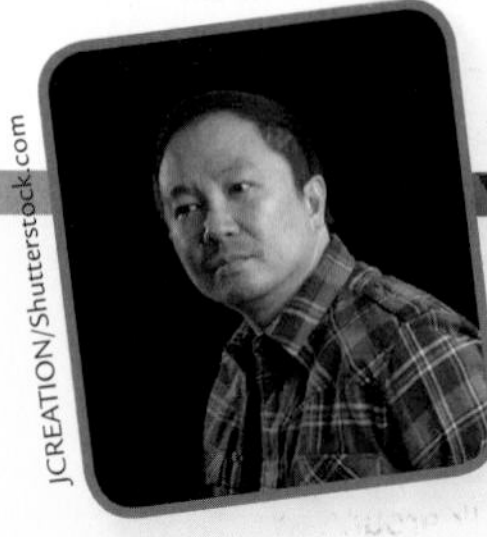

Case Scenario 6.5

This sample scenario presents the use of Facebook and Twitter for physical activity promotion. The scenario demonstrates how Facebook and Twitter can offer individuals social support, provide perceptions of social norms, and influence feelings of empowerment.

Client: Daniel

Client information:

- 33-year-old male
- Diagnosed with Type 2 diabetes mellitus
- Obese (BMI = 31)

Daniel has come to you for help to increase his physical activity levels. He's been feeling depressed lately because of his disease and has lost the motivation to exercise. You suggest that Daniel join Diabetes Daily, an online support group on Facebook for diabetic patients. See Figures 6.1 through 6.3. You also suggest that Daniel follows Everybody Walk, a walking group on Twitter. See Figures 6.4 and 6.5.

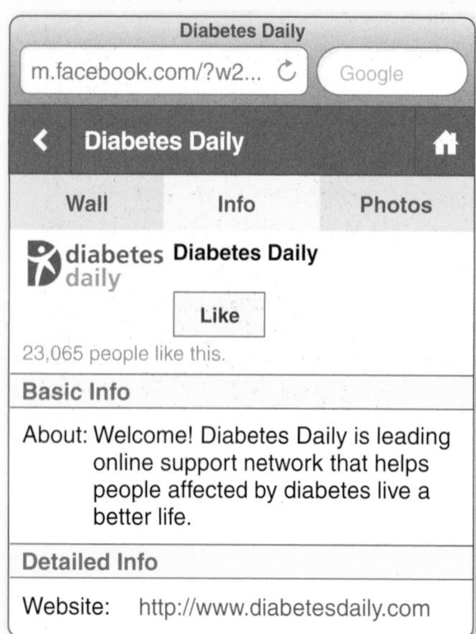

FIGURE 6.1. Facebook Group, Diabetes Daily. (Reprinted with permission from Diabetes Daily.)

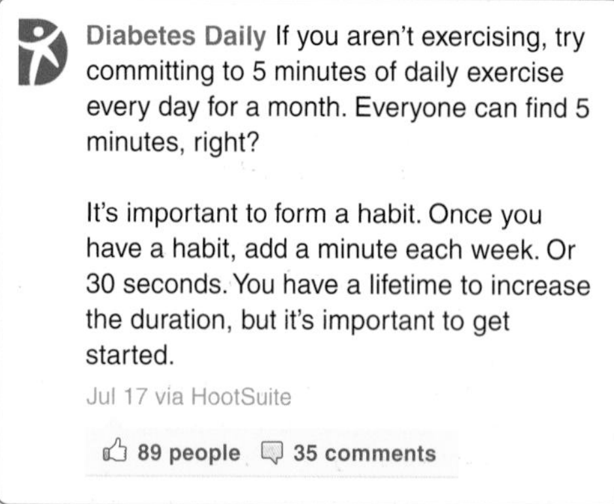

FIGURE 6.2. Sample post from the Diabetes Daily group. (Reprinted with permission from Diabetes Daily.)

Teresa ▇▇▇ You will feel so much better if you incorporate daily exercise into your routine! There is always time... you just have to fit it in. Park your car farther... take the stairs... I read that even 10 minutes a day can make a huge difference.

Jul 17 · 👍 5

Daniel ▇▇▇ I just walk around my neighborhood about twice a day, for about a half-hour each. It lowers my blood sugar (confirmed by measurement) and contributed to my weight loss. It was easy, I didn't have to join a "club", but I am not a candidate for the Olympics!

Jul 17 · 👍 1

Jen ▇▇▇ Good for you Daniel.

Jul 17

FIGURE 6.3. Sample comments on Diabetes Daily from Daniel and other group members (edited for privacy). (Reprinted with permission from Diabetes Daily.)

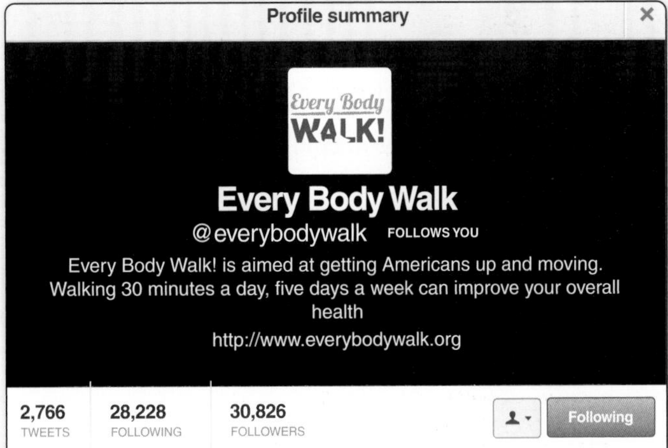
Profile summary
Every Body
WALK!
Every Body Walk
@everybodywalk FOLLOWS YOU
Every Body Walk! is aimed at getting Americans up and moving. Walking 30 minutes a day, five days a week can improve your overall health
http://www.everybodywalk.org
2,766 TWEETS
28,228 FOLLOWING
30,826 FOLLOWERS
Following

FIGURE 6.4. Twitter group, Everybody Walk. (Reprinted with permission from Every Body Walk.)

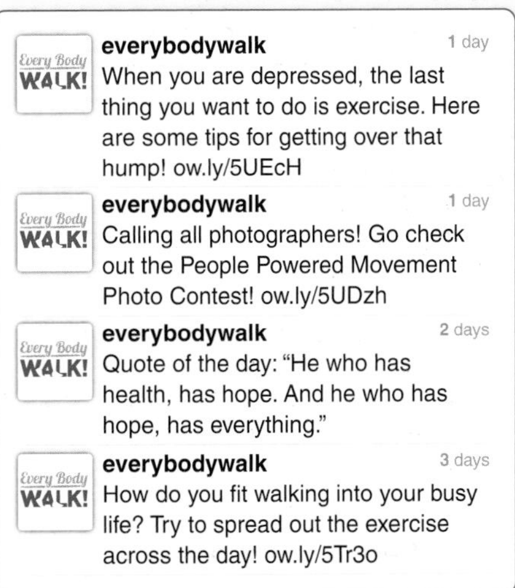
everybodywalk 1 day
When you are depressed, the last thing you want to do is exercise. Here are some tips for getting over that hump! ow.ly/5UEcH
everybodywalk 1 day
Calling all photographers! Go check out the People Powered Movement Photo Contest! ow.ly/5UDzh
everybodywalk 2 days
Quote of the day: "He who has health, has hope. And he who has hope, has everything."
everybodywalk 3 days
How do you fit walking into your busy life? Try to spread out the exercise across the day! ow.ly/5Tr3o

FIGURE 6.5. Sample posts from Everybody Walk. (Reprinted with permission from Every Body Walk.)

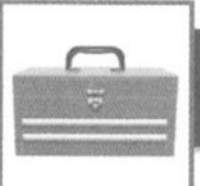

From the Practical Toolbox 6.2

CAUTIONS WHEN USING SOCIAL NETWORKING SITES

When using social network sites as a health professional, there are important considerations to remember.

1. You must remain professional at all times. Be aware that pictures or information you post could be seen by clients and could promote the distortion of boundaries and compromise trust between you and your clients (64). It is recommended that you set up a separate page for your professional use independent of your personal page or use the privacy settings on your personal page (*e.g.*, be selective of who is viewing photos/videos that others "tag" you in).
2. Be mindful of the legal issues surrounding sharing personal information — most importantly, be sure you are in compliance with the Health Insurance Portability and Accountability Act (HIPAA). There have been reports of lawsuits against health providers because of private information appearing on public Web sites (47,76). To be safe, you can guard against hackers by checking if the site is adequately protected against those who may get access to private information.
3. Individuals may misinterpret your online comments (31). In online communication, an array of cues frequently used in face-to-face communication will be absent, such as voice inflections and body gestures. If you need to communicate particularly important or sensitive issues, traditional forms of communication (*e.g.*, phone calls, office visits) may be more appropriate. In general, you should conduct yourself on social network sites as you would in real life, and remember that mishaps can travel fast through your online social network.

PHYSICAL ACTIVITY MONITORING DEVICES

The modern-day health and fitness professional has a distinct advantage over previous generations: the ability to use sensor systems to monitor health behaviors and the outcomes of their clients and give feedback about this information to the client. These kinds of feedback loops can help tailor program goals and keep clients motivated. Sensor-based devices for health behavior monitoring have proliferated over the last decade because of the rise of cheap microelectromechanical systems (MEMS) and rapid improvements in data analytics. Previously if an individual wanted to measure their physical activity or exercise, he or she had to rely on pen and paper, stopwatches, or simple mechanical pedometers. Today, anyone who wants to track their workouts or daily activity can choose from a variety of different tools to meet their needs (also see Chapter 2). Monitoring devices can be a key component of a physical activity program that integrates objective measurement for self-monitoring with information feedback for motivation. This section will describe some of the common sensor systems that can be used to measure, track, and change health behaviors. We will focus mostly on physical activity behaviors, as those sensor systems have been the most widely developed in recent years.

Evidence

PEDOMETERS

Currently, the most common method to determine the extent of daily physical activity is a pedometer. Pedometers are worn on the hip and display the total steps taken for a day, and in some cases the amount of time a person spends moving. The low cost and ease of use make pedometers an ideal tool for a wide range of individuals wishing to start a physical activity program and track their progress. Pedometers do have important limitations that have been addressed by more sophisticated sensing technologies. These limitations include issues related to the accuracy of derived step counts, the inability to discern intensity of movement, and the lack of daily energy expenditure information (108).

Current public health recommendations call for 10,000 steps/day for able-bodied adults, 11,000 for female children, and 13,000 for male children (President's Council on Physical Fitness and Sports, 2002; Hatano, 1993). As with all exercise and activity programs, it is important to take into account the activity and health history of the individual before providing numerical step guidelines (109). A pedometer allows individuals to understand and work toward these activity recommendations. Numerous studies have showed that pedometers are an effective tool for increasing physical activity in adults and youths (17,71). Intervention and observational studies have indicated that the pedometers use can lead to a daily increase of approximately 2,000 steps/day (17) and moderate weight loss (92). It should be noted that pedometer interventions were more effective when used in conjunction with a self-tracking program (*e.g.,* daily step diary), goal setting tied to daily step counts, and when study participants were mostly sedentary at the onset of the intervention. One of the most widely validated low-cost electromechanical pedometers is the Yamax Digiwalker series, which has been shown to be highly accurate (+/− 1%) for assessing step counts (27). One caveat of using electromechanical pedometers is the effect of speed of movement on accuracy. Walking at slower speeds (< 3.0 mph) may not produce the force required to trigger the mechanical lever, and therefore the pedometer will underreport the number of steps (27). This is an important consideration when choosing devices for individuals who are inactive or are of older age.

It is important to note that many modern pedometers use accelerometers instead of electromechanical mechanisms to more accurately assess step counts. Both the New Lifestyles (NL series) and the Omron HJ-710 ITC are validated accelerometer-based pedometers (26,27,45) and have been used in physical activity interventions. These devices are not without drawbacks, as they tend to overestimate energy expenditure (27). A recent study of free-living individuals showed that the Omron pedometer may underestimate steps because of a 4-second filter, which limits the recording of steps to only bouts lasting longer than 4 seconds (101).

ACCELEROMETERS

The proliferation of low-cost accelerometers has changed rapidly the ability of pedometers and other similar sensors to measure human movement. Accelerometers are usually small microchips that contain systems for measuring the gravitational force (g-force) acting on the device. It is important to note that each sensor will have a specific sensitivity to detect a certain range of g-force. Typically, accelerometers measure g-force along a given axis. Uni-axial accelerometers, when oriented correctly, measure g-force along the "y" or vertical axis. A dual-axis accelerometer includes the "y" axis and the horizontal "x" axis, and a tri-axial accelerometer includes the "z" axis in addition to the "y" and "x" axis. Measuring movement only along one axis has limitations as only the vertical displacement of the sensor will be detected. Adding horizontal (x) and sagittal (z) displacement can increase the accuracy of movement detection.

Accelerometers are used in combination with microprocessors in movement-sensing devices. These microprocessors interpret the g-force readings supplied by the accelerometer. Most devices have proprietary algorithms that take the accelerometer data and translate it into useful movement information such as: (a) the number of steps taken, (b) the time spent moving, (c) the intensity of the movement, (d) the distance traveled, and (e) the calorie expenditure of the user. It is important to note that accelerometers are best used when trying to measure primarily leg-based movements that involve a ground reaction force. These movements, such as walking and running, typically make up the majority of daily human movement (107). Movements not captured well are water-based activities, such as swimming, and activities with little to no ground-reaction force, such as cycling (20).

The vast amount of evidence for accelerometers for the measurement of physical activity has focused on research-grade devices like the Actigraph models. Most accelerometers, as mentioned earlier, process the raw gravitational signal and output time-stamped data (typically called a "count") used to determine the activity intensity, the time spent moving, and the time wearing the device (7). Numerous studies have been conducted to determine the validity of different accelerometer models produced by various manufacturers. These studies conduct "side-by-side" comparisons of the proprietary "counts" and research-derived cut-points for translating "counts" into physical activity intensities (96). These devices, although they tend to be more accurate than mechanical pedometers, are more expensive (> $300 for the device and software) and do not have an external display to provide feedback to the user. Therefore, these types of accelerometers manufactured for research purposes are rarely, if ever, used as a tool for feedback in physical activity interventions.

HEART RATE MONITORS

Heart rate monitors are one of the most commonly used activity-related biosensors. Heart rate monitors have sensors that measure the electrical signals derived from heart muscle contraction and relaxation—termed electrocardiography (ECG). Currently available heart rate monitors usually consist of two components, a chest strap and a receiver—typically a watch or other display system. ECG signals can be processed and transmitted to the receiver where the heart rate is displayed. In some cases, raw ECG signals are sent to the receiver, and they are processed into heart rate and other variables like heart rate variability (HRV, the period between R spikes during heart function). Heart rate monitors are an ideal device when real-time feedback about physical activity intensity is needed. This may explain their popularity with trainers or health professionals who are creating personalized training methods to improve the cardiovascular fitness of a client or athlete.

Numerous studies have examined the validity of different heart rate monitors (typically manufactured by Polar Electro) and showed the devices to be consistent with clinical ECG monitors (11,68). Many researchers have examined the use of heart rate monitors for estimating energy expenditure and found variable but positive results (1,25,77). The common theme among studies examining energy expenditure is the valuable increase in accuracy when objective biometric information such as maximal heart rate and VO2 are added to the estimation software.

Heart monitoring is not without its limitations. Typically, all-day wear of heart rate monitors is burdensome to individuals and data quality issues arise during long-term monitoring (14). It is also important to understand that data derived from heart rate monitoring can be affected by many different factors, such as hydration levels, temperature, illness, and altitude (1,2).

GLOBAL POSITIONING SYSTEMS

For users who accurately want to track their outdoor activities, global positioning systems (GPS) are ideal. Personal GPS devices are based on the same technology common in vehicle navigation systems. A small computer chip in the device communicates with GPS satellites orbiting the earth and determines precise location information. This location information is processed and data regarding location (latitude/longitude), speed of travel, and distance traveled is made available. Most commercial GPS units produced for physical activity tracking are used for running and cycling, but they can be used to track most, if not all, outdoor activities. Although stand-alone GPS units are available, most are bundled with additional sensors to measure heart rate or another important variables such as pedal cadence (revolutions per minute) for bicycling.

The objective data (*i.e.*, speed, distance, pace) derived from GPS units do not differ as a function of activity type or individual characteristics. However, the most common concern when using GPS devices is their accuracy. Studies examining commercial GPS units have showed them to be accurate for determining the velocity of running and walking as well as stationary position (95,106,118). These studies have also highlighted a few known issues that may affect data accuracy, including moving in a curvilinear manner (*e.g.*, the curve of a track) and traveling at high speeds (*e.g.*, sprinting). This is in addition to environmental factors external to the movement type that can affect accuracy. These include traveling in or around locations with a high number of tall buildings that can cause signal interference and traveling in locations without clear and unobstructed views of the sky (105).

Step-by-Step

When deciding if using a monitoring system is appropriate for clients or patients, it is best first to understand the relationships among the types of data gathered, the ability to monitor different activities, and the cost of the devices. This information is presented in Table 6.8. Noticeably absent from this list is activity related to strength and resistance training. Compared to aerobic activities, the objective measurement of strength training is currently lacking, although developments in muscle activity sensing are being explored and may prove to be useful for measurement and tracking purposes.

TABLE 6.8 Features of Pedometers, Accelerometers, Heart Rate Monitors, and GPS Devices

	Mechanical Pedometer	Accelerometer	Heart Rate Monitor	GPS
Outputs				
Steps	X	X		
Distance	X	X		X
Intensity		X	X	
Energy Expenditure		X	X	
Speed/Pace		X		X
Activities				
Walking	X	X	X	X
Running (indoors)	X	X	X	
Running (outdoors)		X	X	X

continued

TABLE 6.8 Features of Pedometers, Accelerometers, Heart Rate Monitors, and GPS Devices (Continued)

	Mechanical Pedometer	Accelerometer	Heart Rate Monitor	GPS
Cycling			X	X
Swimming			Some models	Some models
Cost	**\$20–\$50**	**\$50–\$150**	**\$75–\$300**	**\$150–\$350**
Advantages	**Ease of use**	**Higher cost; more accurate**	**More accurate intensity**	**Very accurate speed and distance**
Disadvantages	**Can be inaccurate; no intensity information**	**Proprietary algorithms to calculate outcomes**	**Can be burdensome to wear**	**Costly; only works for outdoor activities**

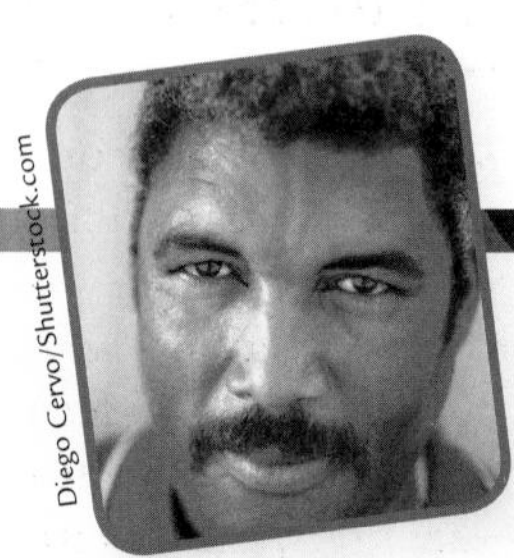
Diego Cervo/Shutterstock.com

Case Scenario 6.6

Client: Jonathan

Client information:

- He is 50 years old
- Recently discharged cardiac surgery patient. He has undergone the typical rehabilitation program administered at the outpatient clinic.
- His doctor has told him that he needs to remain active and try to lose weight.
- He is not comfortable with new technology.
- He does not have access to a gym.

Jonathan has been referred to you to develop an activity plan and stay accountable.

In this scenario, you would most likely use a low-cost pedometer and a daily step goal plan to help encourage Jonathan to be active in his everyday life. You may find it useful to conduct a baseline assessment to understand his current activity levels and create an appropriate plan that gradually increases his step counts. As someone not comfortable with technology, developing a daily step tracking sheet that he can share with you would be ideal.

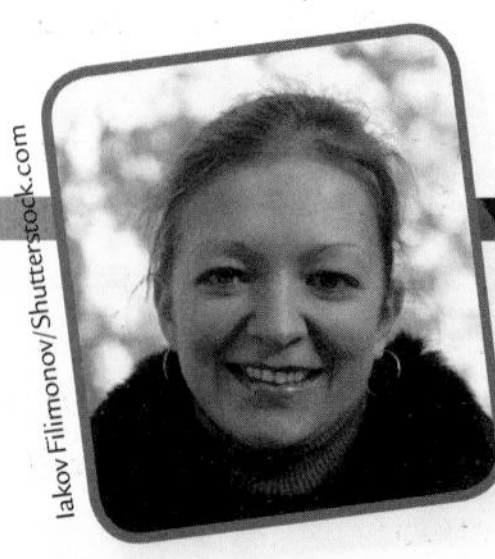
Iakov Filimonov/Shutterstock.com

Case Scenario 6.7

Client: Grace

Client information:

- 35 years old
- Prefers to train indoors at her local gym.
- She is comfortable with technology.

Case Scenario 6.7 *continued*

Grace is moderately physically active and wants to increase her activity and fitness level to train for and compete in an upcoming half-marathon. She has hired you to help her plan her weekly training plan.

In this scenario, you would most likely recommend a heart rate monitor as the best activity monitoring tool. She probably will be participating in aerobic activities using the treadmill and indoor track. A heart rate monitor is the ideal tool for measuring her current fitness state and providing feedback on activity intensity. Many heart rate monitors provide methods for downloading and saving data to a computer or device-specific Web site. You can encourage Grace to share this data with you to better understand if she is following the training program and determine its effect on her fitness level and her recovery from prescribed workouts.

INTEGRATING ACROSS MULTIPLE TECHNOLOGY CHANNELS

Technological advancements such as video streaming, faster processing power, wireless connectivity, and extended battery life and storage capacity have been key contributors in the development of many of the previously mentioned messaging and feedback technologies. As we have presented in this chapter, there are many different types of technologies to measure, track, and give feedback on physical activity. Different combinations of these technologies can be found in some commercially available systems and services. These integrated systems allow users to interact with their data, interact with other users, and receive expert knowledge. The center point or gateway of many integrated systems is the smart mobile phone. This section introduces the smartphone and its features as a way of integrating technologies for physical activity interventions. We describe commercially available integrated systems, and then describe how physical activity and data can be shared across multiple systems to create unique and highly customized interventions.

Smartphones and Their Potential for Physical Activity Interventions

Smartphones have many capabilities that can be harnessed for promoting health (88). Beyond the basic capabilities for two-way communication via voice or text messaging, many mobile phones have built-in cameras, gigabytes of storage, an Internet browser, can transmit data to outside networks, and some even include global positioning systems (GPS), built-in accelerometers, connectivity to WiFi, and wireless communication with external devices via Bluetooth (*e.g.,* heart rate monitors, external accelerometers). These smartphone features are ideal for creating an integrated intervention system.

Current evidence suggests that mobile telephones coupled with Internet services can promote increased physical activity (49). In addition, previous research has suggested that personal digital assistants (PDAs) were effective in increasing physical activity over 8 weeks relative to an assessment-only control (58). Some studies have also demonstrated the potential of using the background of a mobile phone as a "glance-able display" for providing feedback to individuals (23). Beyond this, few studies have explored systematically if these new mobile phone features can be used to promote physical activity.

Consolvo and colleagues (24) identified eight design considerations when developing effective persuasive technology interventions for promoting physical activity: (a) Abstract and Reflective (*i.e.,* do not display raw data but instead abstract that information to something meaningful to the individual and inspires reflection); (b) Unobtrusive (*i.e.,* have the system only be there when wanted/needed and not be bothersome otherwise); (c) Public (*i.e.,* representations of personal information must be done in such a way that it can be displayed in public without making the user uncomfortable), (d) Aesthetic (*i.e.,* to maintain use, the system must fit with a user's sense of style and aesthetic), (e) Positive (*i.e.,* reward good behaviors rather than punish bad ones), (f) Trending / Historical (*i.e.,* provide a sense of past behaviors), and (g) Comprehensive (*i.e.,* take into account the key behaviors that fit into a person's lifestyle). These design considerations are not only conceptually important to interventions, but also can be implemented successfully with smartphones.

Commercially Available Integrated Intervention Systems

Many commercially available integrated systems typically include self-tracking along with interactive Web and/or mobile experiences. The interactive platforms offer more flexible opportunities for *Sources*, *Messages*, *Channels*, *Receivers*, and *Feedback*, which in theory should lead to systems that adapt to the user rather than forcing the individual to adapt to the system. An ideal integrated system: (a) fosters quick and easy communication between multiple devices (*e.g.,* pedometers, Web sites, smartphones) with minimal to no effort for the user; and (b) optimizes each component of the system to perform its role in physical activity promotion without creating additional burden on the user because of technical needs (*e.g.,* feedback is given when and where it is needed, not where it is convenient for the system). The broader goal is the development of systems that integrate into a person's life and daily routine to provide added value with minimal additional burden to the user. Much work is still needed to meet these ideals.

Current systems offer a variety of different tools and capabilities for reaching these mentioned ideals and most often they follow a schema that involves four key functions. First, the platform allows users to upload and view data gathered from a device or sensor system. These data are typically downloaded from the device using a device-specific application or uploaded to a Web site wirelessly. Second, the platform provides ways to visualize data derived from the sensors. Visualizations are meant to be highly interactive, simple to understand, and informative, though it is important to emphasize that highly interactive does not necessarily equate to informative (122). Third, the user can use the system to set a goal, or in some cases multiple goals, that pertain to physical activity, diet, body weight, or sleep. The system then presents feedback to indicate daily and/or weekly progress toward the goal. In some cases, goal attainment is attached to virtual-rewards, such as badges and positive messages. Lastly, the majority of commercial systems have begun integrating a social networking component into their platform. These are often manifested as the platform sending information about the user's behavior to social networking sites, such as Facebook and Twitter on the user's behalf. Some integrated commercial systems enable users to "friend" each other through the platform and engage in friendly competitions and challenges. The most common of these methods is through providing a leaderboard, where a user is compared to their "friends" on a common metric, such as steps per day or calories burned.

One example of an integrated intervention system is the FitBit (Fitbit, Inc., www.fitbit.com). The FitBit is a small accelerometer-based physical activity monitor the size of a typical flash memory stick. It wirelessly syncs physical activity data to a Web interface when it is within range of its USB receiver, which is plugged into a computer. The device has a small display on it to provide feedback on steps taken, miles traveled, calories expended, and activity history. The activity history is a glance-able display of a flower. The flower grows when the person is active and serves as a visual metaphor for the amount of activity achieved in the last three hours. The Web interface allows users to see their current and historical data, set goals, log activities, and see where they rank among their friends who also use a Fitbit. The Web interface can be accessed on a computer or smartphone. Other examples of commercial integrated systems currently available include Garmin Connect (Garmin, Ltd.), Nike+ (Nike, Inc.), and Runkeeper (FitnessKeeper, Inc.).

Data Sharing across Systems and Technologies

Although the aforementioned commercially available integrated systems offer platforms for behavioral tracking and messaging, the true technological strength of many of these systems is the ability to gather and share data, which is critical for an integrated system. Many of the companies that offer physical activity intervention products have begun offering ways for users and other application developers to access data to create additional services or systems that potentially increase the functionality of the core platform. This is possible by using an Application Programming Interface (API) to interact with the platform and user data.

An API is specific programming code that allows for applications to communicate with each other and pass information back and forth. APIs allows for applications to both pull (read) and push (write) data based on the needs of the application. For example, the popular fitness application Runkeeper (FitnessKeeper, Inc.) allows many different applications to read and write data to a user's profile through its own Health Graph API. If a user has a Runkeeper profile, but prefers to use a different mobile phone–based run tracking application, data gathered from it can be pushed (written) to the user's Runkeeper profile. APIs are not limited to product-application-to-product-application communication. Developers can also create their own Web-based applications that pull in user data and use alternative methods of data visualization and feedback that supplements and enhances the user experience. Ideally, this increased connectivity between devices allows for a physical activity system to gather data from multiple sources, aggregate this information, and provide feedback to an individual using the channel of choice for that individual at the appropriate time.

When a company offers an API for its product, it is saying to the world, "take our product and integrate it with your product or make our product better." This access and openness provides others with the opportunity to use products in creative ways and customize products for specific needs. The proliferation of APIs offers an exciting new way to interact with clients and patients who use integrated technology platforms in their training or care. Working with an API requires expertise in computer programming for Web or mobile device applications. Documentation is usually available for an API to illustrate the communication schema and what types of data are accessible.

TAKE-HOME MESSAGE

We hope this chapter served as a useful resource with examples of what is currently possible and how one can start to use the available technology channels to promote physical activity in people's lives. However, we have also raised a note of caution that the scientific evidence to support effectiveness of tailored print and Web-based interventions for physical activity is currently limited, and research is ongoing to determine what factors need to be included in these programs. Even fewer studies have been conducted to evaluate interventions that use mobile and social network technologies to influence physical activity. Using these technologies to deliver physical activity interventions is a rapidly evolving field in both academic research and commercial settings. It is a challenge for researchers and practitioners to keep up with the pace of technology advancements. Ideally, the science and evidence should drive the application of the technology. These technology channels can be used to create persuasive intervention programs by closely following the tenets of behavior change theory. Although new and exciting technologies will continue to offer a variety of communication and persuasion mechanisms, we caution against using such a technology just because it is new and exciting.

Although print materials will likely continue to have a place in physical activity promotion programs, other technologies such as SMS, social networks, and mobile phone applications are likely to be more effective tools to engage individuals daily. These technologies have the potential to transform physical activity interventions because they are easy and convenient to use and have become integrated within the daily lives of most individuals. Print materials can still be considered an important part of a physical activity messaging system. Even when deploying technology-based interventions, there may be the need to prompt individuals to refer to print or online resources for educational or review purposes. Interactive Web sites and Web-based interventions typically provide a location for accessing tailored information and/or materials for "self-paced" learning.

SMS interventions may be of particular interest as a basis for an intervention program because many people have access to this readily used and inexpensive technology. Several studies have shown that SMS helps individuals increase physical activity levels, lose weight, and improve diabetes control. Similarly, online social networks have tremendous potential because they offer the opportunity to facilitate health promotion by increasing communication and accessibility among health care providers, patients, and others who have similar interests. Online social networks may be the ideal technology for fitness professionals without IT support to develop custom pages or IVR systems. Having an online social network as part of a physical activity intervention offers individuals new opportunities for empowerment and helps shape their perceptions of social support and social norms, which are important health behavior determinants.

It is the integration of these different technology channels that can provide individuals with a compelling ongoing user experience for both adoption and maintenance of physical activity. Decisions on which technology channels to use for a physical activity intervention requires a balanced understanding of the needed skills, the resources available, and the level of customizability needed for the development of a particular type of intervention. These factors must be taken into account when deciding among developing a custom *de novo* intervention system, using previously developed devices and systems, or customizing commercial platforms through open APIs. Mobile and wireless technologies are a rapidly changing landscape of devices, systems, and services that will continue to offer many possibilities for delivering physical activity interventions.

REFERENCES

1. Achten J, Jeukendrup AE. Heart rate monitoring: applications and limitations. *Sports Medicine (Auckland, N.Z.)*. 2003;33(7):517–38. Available at: http://www.ncbi.nlm.nih.gov/pubmed/12762827.
2. Ainslie PN, Reilly T, Westerterp KR. Estimating human energy expenditure: A review of techniques with particular reference to doubly labelled water. *Sports Medicine*. 2003;33(9):683–98. Available at: http://www.ingentaconnect.com/content/adis/smd/2003/00000033/00000009/art00004 [Accessed August 31, 2011].
3. Albaina IM, Visser T, van der Mast CAPG, Vastenburg MH. Flowie: a persuasive virtual coach to motivate elderly individuals to walk. In: PervasiveHealth 2009, 3rd International Conference on Pervasive Computing Technologies for Healthcare; April 1–3, 2009:1–7.
4. Anderson RM, Funnell MM, Butler PM, et al. Patient empowerment. Results of a randomized controlled trial. Diabetes Care. 1995;18(7):943–49. Available at: http://care.diabetesjournals.org/content/18/7/943.abstract [Accessed August 11, 2011].

5. Backman D, Scruggs V, Atiedu AA, et al. Using a toolbox of tailored educational lessons to improve fruit, vegetable, and physical activity behaviors among African American women in California. *Journal of Nutrition Education and Behavior.* 2011;43(4 Suppl 2): S75–85. Available at: http://dx.doi.org/10.1016/j.jneb.2011.02.004 [Accessed August 11, 2011].
6. Bahr DB, Browning RC, Wyatt HR, Hill JO. Exploiting social networks to mitigate the obesity epidemic. *Obesity:A Research Journal.* 2009;17(4):723–8. Available at: http://dx.doi.org/10.1038/oby.2008.615 [Accessed July 25, 2011].
7. Bassett DR, Dinesh J. Use of pedometers and accelerometers in clinical populations: validity and reliability issues. *Physical Therapy Reviews.* 2010;15(3):135-142. Available at: http://openurl.ingenta.com/content/xref?genre=article & issn=1083-3196 & volume=15 & issue=3 & spage=135 [Accessed August 10, 2011].
8. Bennett GG, Glasgow RE. The delivery of public health interventions via the Internet: actualizing their potential. *Annual Review of Public Health.* 2009;30:273–92. Available at: http://www.ncbi.nlm.nih.gov/pubmed/19296777 [Accessed July 7, 2011].
9. Bensley RJ, Brusk JJ, Rivas J. Key principles in internet-based weight management systems. *American Journal of Health Behavior.* 2010;34(2):206–13. Available at: <Go to ISI>://000291932800008.
10. Berlo DK. *The Process of Communication:An Introduction to Theory and Practice.* New York: Holt, Reinhart, and Winston; 1960.
11. Bethell H, Letford S, Evans J, et al. Assessing exercise intensity in cardiac rehabilitation: The use of a Polar heart rate monitor. *British Journal of Cardiac Nursing.* 2008;3(11):534–8. Available at: http://www.internurse.com/cgi-bin/go.pl/library/abstract.html?uid=31875.
12. Block G, Sternfeld B, Block CH, et al. Development of Alive! (A Lifestyle Intervention Via Email), and its effect on health-related quality oflife, presenteeism, and other behavioral outcomes: Randomized controlled trial. *Journal of Medical Internet Research.* 2008;10(4):e43. Available at: http://www.pubmedcentral.nih.gov/articlerender.fcgi?artid=2629370 & tool=pmcentrez & rendertype=abstract [Accessed September 7, 2011].
13. Boyd DM, Ellison NB. Social network sites: Definition, history, and scholarship. *Journal of Computer-Mediated Communication.* 2007;13(1):210–30. Available at: http://doi.wiley.com/10.1111/j.1083-6101.2007.00393.x [Accessed July 15, 2011].
14. Brage S, Brage N, Ekelund U, et al. Effect of combined movement and heart rate monitor placement on physical activity estimates during treadmill locomotion and free-living. *European Journal of Applied Physiology.* 2006;96(5):517–24. Available at: http://www.ncbi.nlm.nih.gov/pubmed/16344938 [Accessed August 10, 2011].
15. Bramley D, Riddell T, Whittaker R, et al. Smoking cessation using mobile phone text messaging is as effective in Maori as non-Maori. *The New Zealand Medical Journal.* 2005;118: 1216.
16. Brassington G, Hekler EB, Cohen Z, King AC. Health enhancing physical activity. In: *Handbook of Health Psychology.* Mahwah (NJ): Lawrence Erlbaum Associates Publishers; 2011.
17. Bravata DM, Smith-spangler C, Gienger AL, et al. Using pedometers to increase physical activity and improve health: A systematic review. *Journal of the American Medical Association.* 2007;298(19):2296–304.
18. Brouwer W, Kroeze W, Crutzen R, et al. Which intervention characteristics are related to more exposure to Internet-delivered healthy lifestyle promotion interventions? A systematic review. *Journal of Medical Internet Research.* 2011;13(1):23–41. Available at: <Go to ISI>://000287447100003.
19. Brouwer W, Oenema A, Raat H, et al. Characteristics of visitors and revisitors to an Internet-delivered computer-tailored lifestyle intervention implemented for use by the general public. *Health Education Research.* 2010;25(4):585–95. Available at: <Go to ISI>://000280260200007.
20. Chen KY, Bassett Jr. DR. The technology of accelerometry-based activity monitors: Current and future. *Medicine & Science in Sports & Exercise.* 2005;37(11 Suppl):S490–500. Available at: http://www.ncbi.nlm.nih.gov/entrez/query.fcgi?cmd=Retrieve & db=PubMed & dopt=Citation & list_uids=16294112.
21. Chou W-YS. Social media use in the United States: Implications for health communication. *Journal of Medical Internet Research.* 2009;11(4):e48. Available at: http://www.jmir.org/2009/4/e48/ [Accessed August 11, 2011].
22. Cialdini RB. *Influence: Science and Practice.* 5th ed. Prentice Hall; 2008:272. Available at: http://www.amazon.com/Influence-Practice-Robert-B-Cialdini/dp/0205609996 [Accessed August 11, 2011].
23. Consolvo S, Klasnja P, Mcdonald DW, et al. Flowers or a robot army? Encouraging awareness & activity with personal, mobile displays. *Garden.* 2008:54–63.
24. Consolvo S, Mcdonald DW, Landay JA. Theory-driven design strategies for technologies that support behavior change in everyday life. *Thought, A Review of Culture and Idea.* 2009:405–14.
25. Crouter SE, Albright C, Bassett DR. Accuracy of Polar S410 Heart Rate Monitor to estimate energy cost of exercise. *Medicine & Science in Sports & Exercise.* 2004;36(8):1433–9. Available at: http://content.wkhealth.com/linkback/openurl?sid=WKPTLP:landingpage & an=00005768-200408000-00024 [Accessed June 23, 2011].
26. Crouter SE, Schneider PL, Bassett DR. Spring-levered versus piezo-electric pedometer accuracy in overweight and obese adults. *Medicine and Science in Sports and Exercise.* 2005;37(10):1673–9. Available at: http://www.ncbi.nlm.nih.gov/pubmed/16260966.
27. Crouter SE, Schneider PL, Karabulut M, Bassett DR. Validity of 10 electronic pedometers for measuring steps, distance, and energy cost. *Medicine and Science in Sports and Exercise.* 2003;35(8):1455–60. Available at: http://www.ncbi.nlm.nih.gov/pubmed/12900704.
28. Cugelman B, Thelwall M, Dawes P. Online interventions for social marketing health behavior

change campaigns: A meta-analysis of psychological architectures and adherence factors. *Journal of Medical Internet Research*. 2011;13(1):84–107. Available at: <Go to ISI>://000287447100007.

29. Demark-Wahnefried W, Clipp EC, Lipkus IM, et al. Main outcomes of the FRESH START trial: A sequentially tailored diet and exercise mailed print intervention among breast and prostate cancer survivors. *Journal of Clinical Oncology: Official Journal of the American Society of Clinical Oncology*. 2007;25(19):2709–18. Available at: http://www.ncbi.nlm.nih.gov/pubmed/17602076 [Accessed July 14, 2011].
30. Eakin EG, Lawler SP, Vandelanotte C, Owen N. Telephone interventions for physical activity and dietary behavior change–A systematic review. *American Journal of Preventive Medicine*. 2007;32(5):419–34. Available at: <Go to ISI>://000246416200010.
31. Eckler P, Worsowicz G, Rayburn JW. Social media and health care: An overview. *PM & R: The Journal of Injury, Function, and Rehabilitation*. 2010;2(11):1046–50. Available at: http://www.ncbi.nlm.nih.gov/pubmed/21093840 [Accessed July 25, 2011].
32. Eysenbach G. The Law of Attrition. *Journal of Medical Internet Research*. 2005;7(1):e11. Available at: http://www.ncbi.nlm.nih.gov.laneproxy.stanford.edu/pmc/articles/PMC1550631/.
33. Farzanfar R, Frishkopf S, Migneault J, Friedman R. Telephone-linked care for physical activity: A qualitative evaluation of the use patterns of an information technology program for patients. *Journal of Biomedical Informatics*. 2005;38(3):220–8. Available at: <Go to ISI>://000229494300006.
34. Ferney SL, Marshall AL, Eakin EG, Owen N. Randomized trial of a neighborhood environment-focused physical activity website intervention. *Preventive Medicine*. 2009;48(2):144–50. Available at: <Go to ISI>://000263860600009.
35. Fjeldsoe BS, Marshall AL, Miller YD. Behavior change interventions delivered by mobile telephone short-message service. *American Journal of Preventive Medicine*. 2009;36(2):165–73. Available at: http://www.ncbi.nlm.nih.gov/pubmed/19135907 [Accessed August 7, 2010].
36. Fogg BJ. *Persuasive Technology: Using Computers to Change What We Think and Do*. San Francisco: Morgan Kaufmann Publishers; 2003:51–3.
37. Foster D, Linehan C, Kirman B, Lawson S, James G. *Motivating Physical Activity at Work*. New York: ACM Press; 2010:111. Available at: http://portal.acm.org/citation.cfm?id=1930488.1930510 [Accessed July 25, 2011].
38. Fox NJ, Ward KJ, O'Rourke AJ. The "expert patient": Empowerment or medical dominance? The case of weight loss, pharmaceutical drugs and the Internet. *Social Science & Medicine*. 2005;60(6):1299–309. Available at: http://dx.doi.org/10.1016/j.socscimed.2004.07.005 [Accessed July 8, 2011].
39. Franklin V, Waller A, Pagliari C, Greene S. "Sweet Talk": Text messaging support for intensive insulin therapy for young people with diabetes. *Diabetes Technology & Therapeutics*. 2003;5(6):991–6.
40. Franklin VL, Waller A, Pagliari C, Greene SA. A randomized controlled trial of Sweet Talk, a text-messaging system to support young people with diabetes. *Diabetic Medicine: A Journal of the British Diabetic Association*. 2006;23(12):1332–8. Available at: http://www.ncbi.nlm.nih.gov/pubmed/17116184 [Accessed June 20, 2011].
41. Gerber BS, Stolley MR, Thompson AL, Sharp LK, Fitzgibbon ML. Mobile phone text messaging to promote healthy behaviors and weight loss maintenance: A feasibility study. *Health Informatics Journal*. 2009;15(1):17–25. Available at: http://jhi.sagepub.com/cgi/content/abstract/15/1/17 [Accessed June 13, 2011].
42. Goldman RE, Sanchez-Hernandez M, Ross-Degnan D, et al. Developing an automated speech-recognition telephone diabetes intervention. *International Journal for Quality in Health Care*. 2008;20(4):264–70. Available at: <Go to ISI>://WOS:000257578000005.
43. Greene JA, Choudhry NK, Kilabuk E, Shrank WH. Online social networking by patients with diabetes: A qualitative evaluation of communication with Facebook. *Journal of General Internal Medicine*. 2011;26(3):287–92. Available at: http://www.springerlink.com/content/nrtr7h2254764886/ [Accessed July 25, 2011].
44. Haapala I, Barengo NC, Biggs S, Surakka L, Manninen P. Weight loss by mobile phone: A 1-year effectiveness study. *Public Health Nutrition*. 2009;12(12):2382–91. Available at: http://journals.cambridge.org/abstract_S1368980009005230 [Accessed June 20, 2011].
45. Hasson RE, Haller J, Pober DM, Staudenmayer J, Freedson PS. Validity of the Omron HJ-112 pedometer during treadmill walking. *Medicine and Science in Sports and Exercise*. 2009;41(4):805–9. Available at: http://www.ncbi.nlm.nih.gov/pubmed/19276853.
46. Hatano Y. Use of the pedometer for promoting daily walking exercise. *Journal of the International Committee on Health, Physical Education and Recreation*. 1993;29:4–8. Available at: http://www.new-lifestyles.com/content.php?_p_=10 [Accessed August 31,2011].
47. Hawn C. Take two aspirin and tweet me in the morning: How Twitter, Facebook, and other social media are reshaping health care. *Health Affairs (Project Hope)*. 2009;28(2):361–8. Available at: http://content.healthaffairs.org/cgi/content/abstract/28/2/361 [Accessed June 23, 2011].
48. Hesse BW, Nelson DE, Kreps GL, et al. Trust and sources of health information: The impact of the Internet and its implications for health care providers: Findings from the first Health Information National Trends survey. *Archives of Internal Medicine*. 2005;165(22):2618–24. Available at: http://archinte.ama-assn.org/cgi/content/abstract/165/22/2618 [Accessed July 25, 2011].
49. Hurling R, Catt M, Boni MD, et al. Using Internet and mobile phone technology to deliver an automated physical activity program: randomized controlled trial. *Journal of Medical Internet Research*. 2007;9(2):e7. Available at: http://www.pubmedcentral.nih.gov/articlerender.fcgi?artid=1874722&tool=pmcentrez&rendertype=abstract [Accessed September 13, 2010].

50. Irvine AB, Philips L, Seeley J, et al. Get moving: A web site that increases physical activity of sedentary employees. *American Journal of Health Promotion*. 2011;25(3):199–206. Available at: <Go to ISI>://000286790300009.
51. Jacobs N, Bourdeaudhuij I De, Claes N. Surfing depth on a behaviour change website: Predictors and effects on behaviour. *Informatics for Health & Social Care*. 2010;35(2):41–52. Available at: <Go to ISI>://000282060500001.
52. Joo N-S, Kim B-T. Mobile phone short message service messaging for behaviour modification in a community-based weight control programme in Korea. *Journal of Telemedicine and Telecare*. 2007;13(8): 416–20. Available at: http://jtt.rsmjournals.com/cgi/content/abstract/13/8/416 [Accessed August 25, 2010].
53. Kaplan AM, Haenlein M. Users of the world, unite! The challenges and opportunities of social media. *Business Horizons*. 2010;53(1):59–68.
54. Kaplan B, Farzanfar R, Friedman RH. Personal relationships with an intelligent interactive telephone health behavior advisor system: A multimethod study using surveys and ethnographic interviews. *International Journal of Medical Informatics*. 2003;71(1):33–41. Available at: <Go to ISI>://WOS:000185040100005.
55. Keulen HM van, Mesters I, Ausems M, et al. Tailored print communication and telephone motivational interviewing are equally successful in improving multiple lifestyle behaviors in a randomized controlled trial. *Annals of Behavioral Medicine: A Publication of the Society of Behavioral Medicine*. 2011;41(1):104–18. Available at: http://www.pubmedcentral.nih.gov/articlerender.fcgi?artid=3030742 & tool=pmcentrez &rendertype=abstract [Accessed July 14, 2011].
56. Khaylis A, Yiaslas T, Bergstrom J, Gore-Felton C. A review of efficacious technology-based weight-loss interventions: Five key components. *Telemedicine Journal and E-Health*. 2010;16(9):931–8. Available at: <Go to ISI>://000284576000004.
57. Kim H-S, Song M-S. Technological intervention for obese patients with type 2 diabetes. *Applied Nursing Research: ANR*. 2008;21(2):84–9. Available at: http://www.appliednursingresearch.org/article/S0897-1897(07)00020-1/abstract [Accessed June 20, 2011].
58. King AC, Ahn DK, Oliveira BM, et al. Promoting physical activity through hand-held computer technology. *Am J Prev Med*. 2008;34(2):138–42. Available at: http://www.ncbi.nlm.nih.gov/entrez/query.fcgi?cmd=Retrieve & db=PubMed & dopt=Citation & list_uids=18201644.
59. King AC, Friedman R, Marcus B, et al. Ongoing physical activity advice by humans versus computers: The community health advice by telephone (CHAT) trial. *Health Psychology*. 2007;26(6):718–27. Available at: <Go to ISI>://WOS:000250861700011.
60. Koivusilta LK, Lintonen TP, Rimpelä AH. Orientations in adolescent use of information and communication technology: A digital divide by sociodemographic background, educational career, and health. *Scandinavian Journal of Public Health*. 2007;35(1): 95–103. Available at: http://sjp.sagepub.com/cgi/content/abstract/35/1/95 [Accessed April 28, 2011].
61. Kreuter MW, Strecher VJ, Glassman B. One size does not fit all: The case for tailoring print materials. *Annals of Behavioral Medicine: A Publication of the Society of Behavioral Medicine*. 1999;21(4):276–83. Available at: http://www.ncbi.nlm.nih.gov/pubmed/10721433.
62. Krishna S, Boren S, Balas E. Healthcare via cell phones: A systematic review. *Telemedicine and e-Health*. 2009. Available at: http://www.liebertonline.com/doi/abs/10.1089/tmj.2008.0099 [Accessed June 20, 2011].
63. Kroeze W, Werkman A, Brug J. A systematic review of randomized trials on the effectiveness of computer-tailored education on physical activity and dietary behaviors. *Annals of Behavioral Medicine: A Publication of the Society of Behavioral Medicine*. 2006;31(3): 205–23. Available at: http://www.ncbi.nlm.nih.gov/pubmed/16700634.
64. Krowchuk, HV, Lane, SH, Twaddell JW. Should social media be used to communicate with parents? *American Journal of Maternal Child Nursing*. 2010:6–7. Available at: http://www.mendeley.com/import/ [Accessed August 31, 2011].
65. Bender JL, Jimenez-Marroquin M-C, Alejandro R. Seeking support on Facebook: A content analysis of breast cancer groups. *Journal of Medical Internet Research*. 2011;13(1):e16. Available at: http://www.jmir.org/2011/1/e16/ [Accessed August 11, 2011].
66. Lasica J. The mobile generation: Global transformation at the cellular level: A report of the fifteenth annual Aspen Institute Roundtable on Information Technology. 2007. Available at: http://scholar.google.com/scholar?as_q=the+mobile+generation & num=10 & btnG=Search+Scholar & as_epq= & as_oq= & as_eq= & as_occt=any & as_sauthors=lasica & as_publication= & as_ylo= & as_yhi= & as_sdt=1. & as_sdtp=on & as_sdtf= & as_sdts=5 & hl=en#0 [Accessed June 20, 2011].
67. Latimer AE, Brawley LR, Bassett RL. A systematic review of three approaches for constructing physical activity messages: What messages work and what improvements are needed? *The International Journal of Behavioral Nutrition and Physical Activity*. 2010;7(1):36. Available at: http://www.ijbnpa.org/content/7/1/37 [Accessed October 15, 2011].
68. Laukkanen RMT, Virtanen PK. Heart rate monitors: State of the art. *Journal of Sports Sciences*. 1998;16(4):3–7. Available at: http://www.vivasunsports.com/view_faq.php?article_id=201 [Accessed August 31, 2011].
69. Lee H. Interactive voice response system (IVRS) in health care services. *Nursing Outlook*. 2003;51(6): 277–83. Available at: http://linkinghub.elsevier.com/retrieve/pii/S0029655403001611 [Accessed September 26, 2011].
70. Lenhart A. *Adults and Social Network Sites*. Washington, DC: Pew Internet & American Life Project; 2009. Available at: http://www.pewinternet.org/Reports/2009/Adults-and-Social-Network-Websites.aspx.
71. Lubans DR, Morgan PJ, Tudor-Locke C. A systematic review of studies using pedometers to promote

physical activity among youth. *Preventive Medicine.* 2009;48(4):307–15. Available at: http://www.ncbi.nlm.nih.gov/pubmed/19249328 [Accessed July 23, 2011].

72. Marcus BH, Bock BC, Pinto BM, et al. Efficacy of an individualized, motivationally-tailored physical activity intervention. *Annals of Behavioral Medicine: A Publication of the Society of Behavioral Medicine.* 1998;20(3):174–80. Available at: http://www.ncbi.nlm.nih.gov/pubmed/9989324.
73. Marcus BH, Lewis BA, Williams DM, et al. A comparison of Internet and print-based physical activity interventions. *Archives of Internal Medicine.* 2007;167(9):944–9. Available at: http://www.ncbi.nlm.nih.gov/pubmed/17502536.
74. Marcus BH, Napolitano M A, King AC, et al. Telephone versus print delivery of an individualized motivationally tailored physical activity intervention: Project STRIDE. *Health Psychology: Official Journal of the Division of Health Psychology, American Psychological Association.* 2007;26(4):401–9. Available at: http://www.ncbi.nlm.nih.gov/pubmed/17605559 [Accessed June 20, 2011].
75. Marcus BH, Owen N, Forsyth LH, Cavill NA, Fridinger F. Physical activity interventions using mass, media, print media, and information technology. *American Journal of Preventive Medicine.* 1998;15(4):362–78.
76. McBride D, Cohen E. Misuse of social networking may have ethical implications for nurses. *ONS Connect.* 2009;24(7):17. Available at: http://www.ncbi.nlm.nih.gov/pubmed/19645160 [Accessed July 25, 2011].
77. Montgomery P, Green D, Etxebarria N, et al. Validation of heart rate monitor-based predictions of oxygen uptake and energy expenditure. *Journal of Strength & Conditioning Research.* 2009;23(5):1489–95. Available at: http://journals.lww.com/nsca-jscr/Abstract/2009/08000/Validation_of_Heart_Rate_Monitor_Based_Predictions.18.aspx [Accessed August 10, 2011].
78. Napolitano MA, Fotheringham M, Tate D, et al. Evaluation of an Internet-based physical activity intervention: a preliminary investigation. *Annals of Behavioral Medicine: A Publication of the Society of Behavioral Medicine.* 2003;25(2):92–9. Available at: http://www.ncbi.nlm.nih.gov/pubmed/12704010.
79. Napolitano MA, Marcus BH. Targeting and tailoring physical activity information using print and information technologies. *Exercise and Sport Sciences Reviews.* 2002;30(3):122–8. Available at: http://www.ncbi.nlm.nih.gov/pubmed/12150571.
80. Neve M, Morgan PJ, Jones PR, Collins CE. Effectiveness of web-based interventions in achieving weight loss and weight loss maintenance in overweight and obese adults: A systematic review with meta-analysis. *Obesity Reviews.* 2010;11(4):306–21. Available at: <Go to ISI>://000275885200005.
81. Neve MJ, Collins CE, Morgan PJ. Dropout, nonusage attrition, and pretreatment predictors of nonusage attrition in a commercial web-based weight loss program. *Journal of Medical Internet Research.* 2010;12(4):81–96. Available at: <Go to ISI>://000285637900008.
82. Neville LM, O'Hara B, Milat A. Computer-tailored physical activity behavior change interventions targeting adults: A systematic review. *International Journal of Behavioral Nutrition and Physical Activity.* 2009;6:12. Available at: <Go to ISI>://000267804500001.
83. Newton KH, Wiltshire EJ, Elley CR. Pedometers and text messaging to increase physical activity: Randomized controlled trial of adolescents with type 1 diabetes. *Diabetes Care.* 2009;32(5):813–5. Available at: http://care.diabetesjournals.org/cgi/content/abstract/32/5/813 [Accessed June 20, 2011].
84. Noar SM, Benac CN, Harris MS. Does tailoring matter? Meta-analytic review of tailored print health behavior change interventions. *Psychological Bulletin.* 2007;133(4):673–93. Available at: http://www.ncbi.nlm.nih.gov/pubmed/17592961 [Accessed June 13, 2011].
85. Oake N, Jennings A, Walraven C van, Forster AJ. Interactive voice response systems for improving delivery of ambulatory care. *American Journal of Managed Care.* 2009;15(6):383–91. Available at: <Go to ISI>://WOS:000267292600006.
86. Olsen E, Kraft P. ePsychology: A pilot study on how to enhance social support and adherence in digital interventions by characteristics from social networking sites. *Proceedings of the 4th International Conference on Persuasive Technology–Persuasive '09.* 2009:1. Available at: http://portal.acm.org/citation.cfm?doid=1541948.1541991 [Accessed July 25, 2011].
87. Patrick K, Calfas KJ, Norman GJ, et al. Outcomes of a 12-month web-based intervention for overweight and obese men. *Annals of Behavioral Medicine: A Publication of the Society of Behavioral Medicine.* 2011. Available at: http://www.ncbi.nlm.nih.gov/pubmed/21822750 [Accessed November 17, 2011].
88. Patrick K, Griswold W, Raab F, Intille S. Health and the mobile phone. *American Journal of Preventive Medicine.* 2008. Available at: http://www.ncbi.nlm.nih.gov/pmc/articles/PMC2527290/ [Accessed June 20, 2011].
89. Patrick K, Raab F, Adams M, et al. A text message–based intervention for weight loss: Randomized controlled trial. *Journal of Medical Internet Research.* 2009. Available at: http://www.ncbi.nlm.nih.gov/pmc/articles/PMC2729073/ [Accessed June 20, 2011].
90. President's Council on Physical Fitness and Sports. *The Presidential Active Lifestyle Award (PALA).* Washington, DC 2002. Available at: http://www.fitness.gov/ [Accessed August 31, 2011].
91. Putnam RD. *Bowling alone: The collapse and revival of American community.* New York: Simon & Schuster; 2001:541. Available at: http://books.google.com/books?hl=en & lr= & id=rd2ibodep7UC & pgis=1 [Accessed August 11, 2011].
92. Richardson C, Newton T, Abraham J, et al. A meta-analysis of pedometer-based walking interventions and weight loss. *Annals of Family Medicine.*

2008;6(1):69–77. Available at: http://annfammed.org/cgi/content/abstract/6/1/69 [Accessed August 10, 2011].

93. Riva G, Preziosa A, Grassi A, Villani D. Stress management using UMTS cellular phones: a controlled trial. *Studies in Health Technology and Informatics*. 2005;119:461.
94. Rodgers A, Corbett T, Bramley D, et al. Do u smoke after txt? Results of a randomised trial of smoking cessation using mobile phone text messaging. *Tobacco Control*. 2005;14(4):255–61. Available at: http://www.pubmedcentral.nih.gov/articlerender.fcgi?artid=1748056 & tool=pmcentrez & rendertype=abstract [Accessed July 14, 2011].
95. Rodriguez DA, Brown AL, Troped PJ. Portable global positioning units to complement accelerometry-based physical activity monitors. *Medicine & Science in Sports & Exercise*. 2005;37(Supplement):S572–81. Available at: http://content.wkhealth.com/linkback/openurl?sid=WKPTLP:landingpage&an=00005768-200511001-00010.
96. Rothney MP, Schaefer EV, Neumann MM, Choi L, Chen KY. Validity of physical activity intensity predictions by ActiGraph, Actical, and RT3 accelerometers. *Obesity: A Research Journal*. 2008;16(8):1946–52. Available at: http://www.pubmedcentral.nih.gov/articlerender.fcgi?artid=2700550 & tool=pmcentrez & rendertype=abstract [Accessed August 2, 2011].
97. Sallis JF, Hovell MF. Determinant of exercise behavior. In: *Exercise and Sport Sciences Reviews*. Baltimore (MD): Williams & Wilkins; 1990:307–30.
98. Samoocha D. Effectiveness of web-based interventions on patient empowerment: A systematic review and meta-analysis. *Journal of Medical Internet Research*. 2010;12(2):e23. Available at: http://www.jmir.org/2010/2/e23/ [Accessed August 11, 2011].
99. Shapiro JR, Bauer S, Andrews E, et al. Mobile therapy: Use of text-messaging in the treatment of bulimia nervosa. *The International Journal of Eating Disorders*. 2009;43(6):513–9. Available at: http://www.ncbi.nlm.nih.gov/pubmed/19718672 [Accessed August 14, 2010].
100. Shapiro JR, Bauer S, Hamer RM, et al. Use of text messaging for monitoring sugar-sweetened beverages, physical activity, and screen time in children: A pilot study. *Journal of Nutrition Education and Behavior*. 2008;40(6):385–91. Available at: http://www.pubmedcentral.nih.gov/articlerender.fcgi?artid=2592683 & tool=pmcentrez & rendertype=abstract [Accessed June 8, 2011].
101. Silcott NA, Bassett DR, Thompson DL, Fitzhugh EC, Steeves JA. Evaluation of the Omron HJ-720ITC pedometer under free-living conditions. *Medicine and Science in Sports and Exercise*. 2011;(January). Available at: http://www.ncbi.nlm.nih.gov/pubmed/21311356 [Accessed August 10, 2011].
102. Skinner CS, Campbell MK, Rimer BK, Curry S, Prochaska JO. How effective is tailored print communication? *Annals of Behavioral Medicine: A Publication of the Society of Behavioral Medicine*. 1999;21(4):290–8. Available at: http://www.ncbi.nlm.nih.gov/pubmed/10721435.
103. Spittaels H, Bourdeaudbuij I De, Vandelanotte C. Evaluation of a website-delivered computer-tailored intervention for increasing physical activity in the general population. *Preventive Medicine*. 2007;44:209–17.
104. Stewart J, Quick C. Global mobile—Strategies for growth. *The Nielsen Company*. 2009. Available at: http://blog.nielsen.com/nielsenwire.online_mobile/global-mobile-strategies-for-growth/ [Accessed June 20, 2011].
105. Stopher P, Fitzgerald C, Zhang J. Search for a global positioning system device to measure person travel. *Transportation Research Part C: Emerging Technologies*. 2008;16(3):350–69. Available at: http://linkinghub.elsevier.com/retrieve/pii/S0968090X07000836 [Accessed July 29, 2010].
106. Townshend AD, Worringham CJ, Stewart IB. Assessment of speed and position during human locomotion using nondifferential GPS. *Medicine and Science in Sports and Exercise*. 2008;40(1):124–32. Available at: http://www.ncbi.nlm.nih.gov/pubmed/18091013 [Accessed August 10, 2011].
107. Troiano RP, Berrigan D, Dodd KW, et al. Physical activity in the United States measured by accelerometer. *Medicine and Science in Sports and Exercise*. 2008;40(1):181–8. Available at: http://www.ncbi.nlm.nih.gov/pubmed/18091006.
108. Tudor-locke C, Williams JE, Reis JP, Pluto D. Utility of pedometers for assessing convergent validity. *Sports Medicine*. 2002;32(12):795–808.
109. Tudor-Locke CE, Myers AM. Methodological considerations for researchers and practitioners using pedometers to measure physical (ambulatory) activity. *Research Quarterly for Exercise and Sport*. 2001;72(1):1–12. Available at: http://www.ncbi.nlm.nih.gov/pubmed/11253314.
110. Umberson D. Gender, marital status and the social control of health behavior. *Social Science & Medicine (1982)*. 1992;34(8):907–17. Available at: http://www.ncbi.nlm.nih.gov/pubmed/1604380 [Accessed July 25, 2011].
111. Velicer WF, Prochaska JO, Bellis JM, et al. An expert system intervention for smoking cessation. *Addictive Behaviors*. 1993;18(3):269–90. Available at: http://www.ncbi.nlm.nih.gov/pubmed/8342440.
112. Wanner M, Martin-Diener E, Bauer G, Braun-Fahrlander C, Martin BW. Comparison of trial participants and open access users of a web-based physical activity intervention regarding adherence, attrition, and repeated participation. *Journal of Medical Internet Research*. 2010;12(1). Available at: <Go to ISI>://000274633100003.
113. Waters LA, Galichet B, Owen N, Eakin E. Who participates in physical activity intervention trials? *Journal of Physical Activity & Health*. 2011;8(1):85–103. Available at: <Go to ISI>://000286449700011.
114. Webb TL, Joseph J, Yardley L, Michie S. Using the Internet to promote health behavior change: A systematic review and meta-analysis of the impact of

theoretical basis, use of behavior change techniques, and mode of delivery on efficacy. *Journal of Medical Internet Research*. 2010;12(1). Available at: <Go to ISI>://000274633100004.

115. Webb TL, Sniehotta FF, Michie S. Using theories of behaviour change to inform interventions for addictive behaviours. *Addiction*. 2010;105(11):1879–92. Available at: <Go to ISI>://000282635300006.
116. Wellman B, Wortley S. Different strokes from different folks: Community Ties and Social Support. *The American Journal of Sociology*. 1990;96(3):558.
117. Wilcox S, Dowda M, Leviton LC, et al. Active for life final results from the translation of two physical activity programs. *American Journal of Preventive Medicine*. 2008;35(4):340–51.
118. Witte TH, Wilson AM. Accuracy of non-differential GPS for the determination of speed over ground. *Journal of Biomechanics*. 2004;37(12):1891–8. Available at: http://www.ncbi.nlm.nih.gov/pubmed/15519597 [Accessed August 10, 2011].
119. Wortham J. As older users join Facebook, network grapples with death. *The New York Times*. 2010. Available at: http://www.nytimes.com/2010/07/18/technology/18death.html [Accessed August 11, 2011].
120. Yoon K-H, Kim H-S. A short message service by cellular phone in type 2 diabetic patients for 12 months. *Diabetes Research and Clinical Practice*. 2008;79(2):256–61. Available at: http://www.diabetesresearchclinicalpractice.com/article/S0168-8227(07)00469-X/abstract [Accessed June 20,2011].
121. Young S. What digital divide? Hispanics, African-Americans are quick to adopt wireless technology. *The Wall Street Journal Classroom Edition*. 2006. Available at: http://www.wsjclassroomedition.com/archive/06jan/tech_minoritywireless.htm [Accessed June 20, 2011].
122. Zikmund-Fisher BJ, Dickson M, Witteman HO. Cool but counterproductive: Interactive, web-based risk communications can backfire. *Journal of Medical Internet Research2*. 2011;13(3):e60.

CHAPTER 7

Influencing Policy and Environments to Promote Physical Activity Behavior Change

Adrian E. Bauman, Rona Macniven, and Klaus Gebel

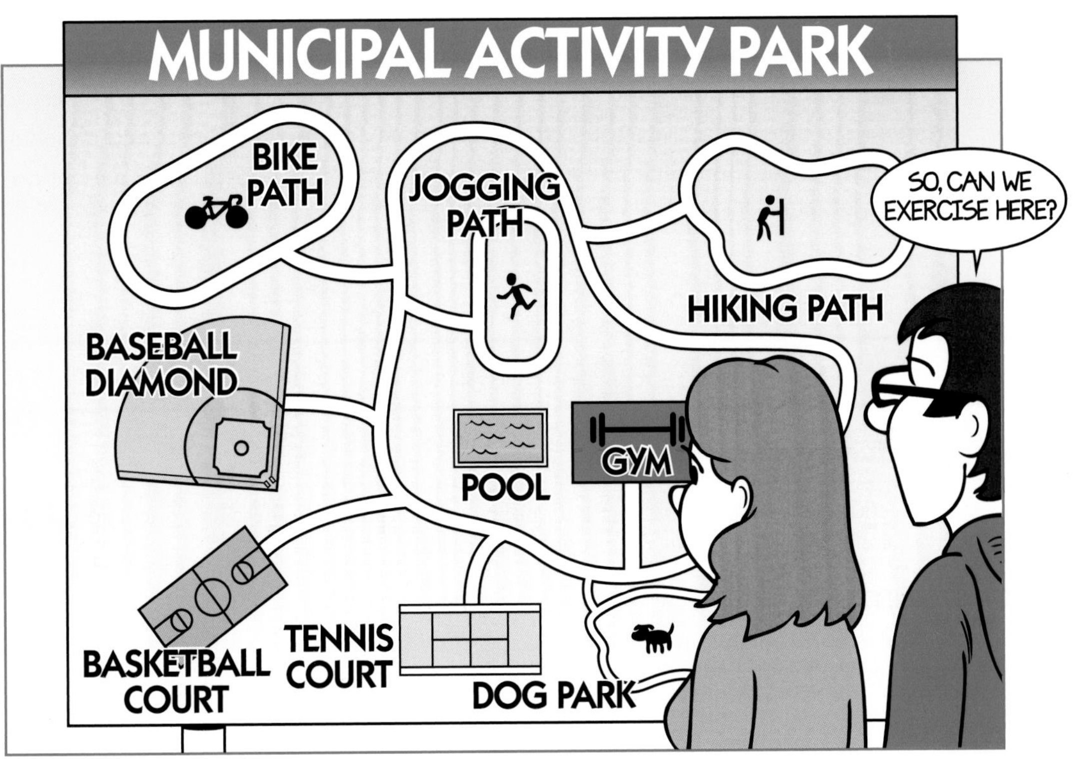

CONCEPT OVERVIEW

This chapter explores the relationship between policy, environmental changes, and physical activity. These areas of work are usually carried out by public health staff in their efforts to increase population levels of physical activity. As such, they are concerned with getting everyone in a community or region to be more physically active, until "health targets" are reached, with all adults and children meeting population recommendations for health-enhancing physical activity (43). These public health actions are far from the individual focus of physical activity counseling, individualized or small-group physical activity programs, or other approaches to change individual behavior regarding activity. This chapter is a link between what public health professionals do, and what individual practitioners do in their daily work.

The objectives of this chapter are to describe the role of policies and the physical environment in physical activity, from a practitioner perspective, rather than from a policymaker or decision-maker perspective. This is seldom done, and the differences between practice and policy are often highlighted. Here, we approach this chapter to minimize the artificial gulf between physical activity policy and practice, and show how an understanding of policy and of the physical environment can help practitioners in their work to increase activity and exercise behaviors among their clients and patients. Terms that may be unfamiliar to some behavioral and exercise scientists and practitioners are defined in Table 7.1.

EVIDENCE

Physical Activity Policy

This section introduces physical activity policy actions and then presents a discussion of the physical environment and its role in physical activity.

POLICY DEFINITIONS

Physical activity policy can be defined in three ways: (i) policy as a set of written rules or regulations, (ii) policy as defined guidelines, and (iii) unwritten social norms (4).

Policy as a Set of Written Rules or Regulations

The most commonly used definition of policy is "written regulations or rules" that facilitate physical activity-related behaviors. This includes rules and regulations, local municipal ordinances, and specific rules in defined settings (27). The range of policy contexts relevant to physical activity is large—ranging from transport and urban design policies, education policy, sport policy through to health sector policies for the health system, primary care and prevention, and community practice. Policy examples include "mandating a specific minimum amount of weekly physical education in schools"; or a municipality developing a possible policy to regulate building codes, such that a "certain amount of green space is mandatory in new urban and housing developments." A key part of this definition of policy is to assess enforcement and uptake; how many agencies or settings adopt and implement the "rule" will influence the impact of the policy on physical activity (45).

TABLE 7.1 Definition of Physical Activity, Policy, and Environment Terms

Term	Definition
Moderate physical activity	Physical activity and exercise performed at moderate intensity, such as walking at 3 mph, cycling at 6 mph, walking during golf, heavy gardening, or household tasks (3.5–5.9 METs)
Vigorous physical activity	Higher energy physical activity or exercise, such as jogging or running, skiing, cycling > 10 mph, swimming laps, singles tennis, gym classes, chopping wood, hiking uphill (≥ 6 METs)
Mixed use	A description of land use, where an urban or town space has a range of types of uses—people live there (residential), there are shops, businesses, schools, public spaces and parks
Pedometer	Small device, worn usually on the hip, to measure steps taken—people can observe their own physical activity in relation to their physical activity counseling advice ("*How much did I walk or how many steps did I take today?*")
Advocate	This is the task of representing a position on an issue to others, to be an "advocate" for physical activity is to promote, recommend, and support physical activity in your community, in your workplace, to your local municipality, and to other decision makers.
Behavior change setting	The places where behavior change occurs; people could be active in different settings—it could be possible at home or at work or in the downtown area, but it may be easier in a park or on a trail (these are more facilitatory settings)
Macro-level micro-level policy or environment	This refers to the physical environment or to a policy; macro level is the city or county level; micro level is your local neighborhood; physical activity is related to both micro- and macro-level environments; for policy, a macro-level policy will impact a large city, county, or state (a micro-level policy will impact local neighborhoods or districts)
Urban design	How cities, towns, or public space is constructed, designed, or used can influence physical activity. Urban design is the process of designing towns and cities to facilitate walking, public transport usage, parks, and open spaces for recreation, and sport and active play. The planners and designers of urban space can help get communities to be more active
Aesthetics	Places where people might be physically active can be appealing, relaxing, full of natural beauty, and have things to look at—such as when walking on a trail along a river; this is the meaning of "aesthetics"—a pleasant place is nicer to run or bike alongside, than is a freeway
Sprawl	Urban sprawl is the growth of residential suburbs a long way from a town center; these suburbs require automobile transport everywhere, are seldom "mixed use" (see earlier) and may not encourage walking for short distances in the community (as the destinations, places people want to go, are too far away to walk)
Residential density	The number of houses, dwellings, apartments in a defined area; where there is medium to high density, there will be more shops, schools, workplaces within walking distance, making it a more "walkable" community (the opposite of "urban sprawl," described earlier)
Negative energy balance	Weight loss or weight gain results from energy imbalance; positive energy balance is eating more than you burn (calorie intake from food is greater than calories burned through activity); negative energy balance is the opposite—move more and expend more energy than you consume.

continued

TABLE 7.1 Definition of Physical Activity, Policy, and Environment Terms (*Continued*)

Term	Definition
"Activity friendly"	"Activity friendly" environments and communities have good facilities for walking, sport, and exercise , and may be (see earlier) any combination of low density, mixed use, high aesthetics, that is well designed for "active living," incorporating physical activity into everyday life
Socio-ecologic models	Models of behavior change that recognize the importance of individual-level, interpersonal, social and physical environmental, and societal-level determinants of behavior such as physical activity; and the interplay between levels of influence in contributing to whether a person is physically active or not.

Clinical exercise physiologists and other clinical practitioners will engage with some policy developments more than others. Every professional providing physical activity advice should become an "advocate" for physical activity, and should be concerned with low population rates of reaching recommended levels of activity for health. Nonetheless, some policies will be more directly relevant to clinical counseling than others. For example, policies that encourage workplace PA programs; others that consider health insurance subsidies for activity programs, and provide other incentives for individuals to be active—these are directly relevant to the behavior change setting (40). Other policies that provide information and support individuals are indirectly important, as they may support individuals trying to change their behavior. These include the policy initiatives that lead to community-wide programs, mass media efforts and social marketing campaigns to inform, persuade, and encourage individuals to be more active. These are complemented by environmental and regulatory macro-level policies around public transport, urban design, park utilization, and mandated school-based programs. These are important for large-scale efforts to achieve population-level physical activity and fitness changes.

An overarching model of the relationship between policy, environments, and individual behavior change is shown in Figure 7.1. The first stage is contributing evidence to make the case; this is shown on the left hand side of the model, and contributes a clear distillation of the evidence for physical activity. In other sectors, physical activity may be a byproduct—for example of increased public transport systems. If more buses or trains are available, active commuting to get to or from transport will increase (32,55), although the transport sector policy objective is primarily growth in transport usage. If there is a clear case for physical activity, which interests the community and political processes, then a planning process may begin to "take action" (see Figure 7.1). The outcome of this is a national, state, or municipal/local-level physical activity plan, which has clear accountability and targets. The development of policy is the mechanism for achieving these targets, and may require partnerships across agencies in sport, health, education, transport, and the environment. In addition, the private sector, nongovernment organizations, and other stakeholder groups may be involved. Policy implementation will require commitment, a sufficient time frame, community support, and appropriate allocation of resources (40).

Policy as Defined Guidelines

A second definition of policy is as "standards" or "guidelines." In the context of physical activity, the development of "physical activity guidelines" has occurred in many countries, including the U.S., and recently, through global physical activity guidelines developed by the World Health Organization (WHO) (13). These guidelines are developed through a thorough review of the epidemiological evidence, and result in clearly specified amounts of physical activity required for health benefits. Separate guidelines have been developed for children and adolescents, for young and middle-aged adults, and for older adults.

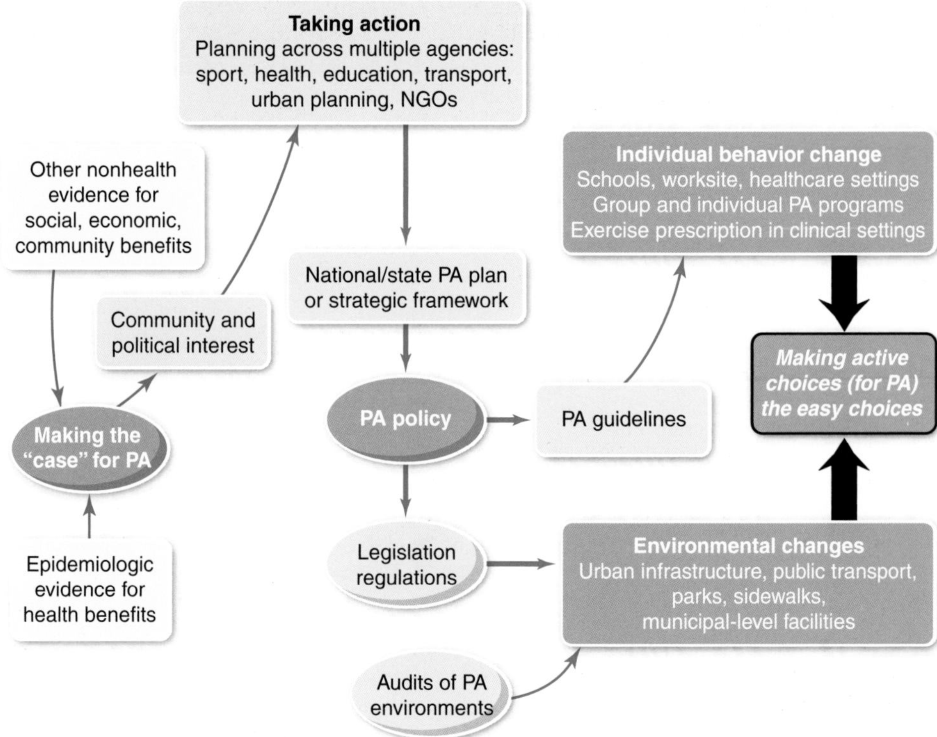

FIGURE 7.1. The link between policy, environments, and individual physical activity programs and behavioral counseling.

These are shown in Table 7.2, adapted from the U.S. and WHO guidelines. Table 7.2 shows the counseling-relevant implications of the guidelines, identifying some of the new messages and communications needed for practitioners. These new messages are updated as the evidence changes, and form the basis for advice from all physical activity practitioners.

The recommendations in Table 7.2 are the key messages only. For further detail, see the original documents (13,43). However, they have substantial implications for clinical practice. This is an example of a guideline that is likely to contribute to adolescent health, and to childhood obesity prevention, so it is useful in providing guidance for clinicians and counselors. Among young people, an hour of physical activity per day is required, and this is difficult to achieve from one source of physical activity only. Hence, recommendations imply some increases in "active living" are needed, so that children and adolescents need to be active at school, in "active after school" programs, through school sport and physical education, and also through active transport to and from school, where possible. Further, some guidelines specify reductions in sedentary time (3), whereas others do not specify a threshold here since the evidence is still developing.

For middle-aged and older adults, a minimum of 30 minutes of moderate intensity physical activity for 5 days per week is the minimum recommended for health (1). This does not need to be performed at vigorous intensity which is important in counseling. Furthermore, physical activity can be accumulated throughout the day, in sessions of at least 10 minutes of activity (1). People who have been inactive for some time should aim for any physical activity, even in small amounts, and increase to the (mostly achievable) 30 minutes per day for 5 days per week, even at moderate intensity. Other U.S. guidelines (42,43) do not specify half an hour daily, but simply ≥150 minutes weekly, suggesting that longer sessions several days per week are sufficient. For both middle-aged and older adults, greater benefits are conferred by ≥300 minutes per week of activity (43). Note that all activity can be moderate-intensity, or that it can be 75 minutes per week of vigorous-intensity activity, which will provide the

TABLE 7.2 Key WHO and U.S. Guidelines for Physical Activity—Implications for Behavioral Counseling (52,55)

Age group	Main recommendation	Other recommendations	Implications for counseling
Children and adolescents 5–17 years	≥60 mins of moderate- to vigorous-intensity physical activity daily	Reduce sedentary time (<2 hours of screen time daily)	Need to promote "active living" across the day for children and adolescents to achieve 60 minutes daily (sport or PE alone will not be sufficient)
Young and middle-aged adults 18–64 years	≥150 mins of moderate-intensity PA / week OR ≥75 mins vigorous PA, or a combination of both	Higher-level PA for additional benefits; ≥300 mins of moderate PA (or ≥150 mins vigorous PA); moderate- or high-intensity muscle strengthening activities on two or more days per week	Moderate-intensity activity is sufficient for many health outcomes, aim to accumulate around half an hour daily; a new "high active" threshold of ≥300 mins/week (around an hour daily)-this high amount will also have a greater role in cancer prevention and in weight maintenance
Older adults ≥ 65 years	≥150 mins of moderate-intensity PA / week OR ≥75 mins vigorous PA , or a combination of both	Muscle-strengthening activities two + days/ week	Same high-active threshold as for middle-aged adults (300 mins/week+), but for older adults, strength training, and resistance training important

same benefits; and is the approximate equivalent to 150 minutes of moderate-intensity activity. These guidelines were generally supported by the 2011 American College of Sports Medicine position statement, indicating that activity can be accumulated in different ways and through different types of activity, as long as the total accumulated meets recommended levels for health and fitness (57). From the counseling perspective, combinations of moderate and vigorous activity are permitted. For example, a client who does 30 minutes of jogging twice a week, and walks the dog for 20 minutes on 2 other days is doing "sufficient activity" (this is above the threshold, as it equates to around 160 "moderate minutes" (30 + 30 vigorous minutes) × 2 + (20 + 20 moderate minutes) (2).

One caveat for practitioners is the contribution of physical activity for weight loss. The behavior change counselor should consider the concept of "active living," especially when clients want to use physical activity to support weight loss. In order to lose weight, substantially more than 150 minutes per week are required; *ACSM's Guidelines for Exercise Testing and Prescription* recommends participation in at least 300 minutes per week of moderate-intensity activity (1). The ACSM Position Stand on physical activity for weight loss and the prevention of weight gain similarly advises participation in at least 250 minutes per week of moderate-intensity activity (38).

In addition to the guidelines in Table 7.2, all adults are encouraged to do strength training activities twice per week. In addition, older adults are encouraged to maintain balance and muscle strength to reduce risk of injurious falls. In summary, any activity is better than none, and the WHO guidelines make this explicit for older adults: "*When adults cannot do the recommended amounts of physical activity due to health conditions, they should be as physically active as their abilities and conditions allow*" (12). This concept is relevant to clinical counseling, as the first behavior change goal is to activate those who are completely sedentary, and encourage them to try, adopt, and maintain at least some regular physical activity.

Policy as Unwritten Social Norms

The third definition of policy encompasses unwritten social norms that influence human behavior. It is apparent that physical activity has strong societal determinants, including the sedentary and pervasive automobile and television cultures in many countries (46). Social influences are strong cues to inactive behaviors. These may be direct peer influences, especially in adolescence. This is a definition of "policy" beyond the scope of this chapter, but it remains important to consider the social context of any client as a cue to inactive choices and role modeling, within their family, peers, and colleagues.

The Physical Environment and Physical Activity

The links between policy and the physical environment are shown in the center and right side of Figure 7.1. Planning processes will lead to policy, which in turn will influence environments to become activity-friendly. The physical environment is important in supporting the adoption and maintenance of active lifestyles among adults and children (54). Recently, the concept of "active living" has emerged to expand the concept of "physical activity" by emphasizing the different domains of physical activity including leisure-time, active travel, household, and work-related activities (37). This has led to the use of socio-ecological models, which emphasize the importance of environmental influences on physical activity (19,39,48).

The built environment encompasses land use patterns, the transportation system, and design features that can all affect physical activity levels (4). At the level of the building, the accessibility of stairwells and other design issues may be relevant to encouraging physical activity (15). Moreover, the provision of showers and storage for bicycles in worksites could facilitate active commuting to work (53).

At the neighborhood level, the provision of sidewalks and cycling paths; access to shops, parks and open space, exercise facilities, and other places of interest; high aesthetics; adequate street lighting; and mixed land use can all contribute to an active lifestyle. On the other hand, sprawl, low street connectivity, and heavy traffic might impede physical activity (16).

At the regional level, the physical environment includes consideration of the distances between where people live and the places where they work, shop, or attend school. Longer distances will make active transport options (traveling to or from work or shops by walking, cycling, or using public transport) more difficult, unless there is a well-connected public transportation system. Even walking to and from public transport stops can contribute to achieving the recommended level of physical activity, particularly among those population groups that are at highest risk of being insufficiently active (10,32).

Evidence Summary

The past two decades have produced hundreds of studies documenting the relationship between the built environment and physical activity. Various literature reviews have synthesized this emerging evidence (11,21,23).

To date, the vast majority of studies have had a cross-sectional research design, and therefore do not provide causal evidence, which is a limitation of the literature (23,34). These studies mostly showed that physical activity was associated with residential density, mixed land use, street connectivity, parks, footpaths, trails, and walkable destinations, such as shops and recreation facilities. The associations for aesthetics and safety from crime and traffic were less consistent (8,28,35,45). In addition, a few relocation studies have examined the influence of an exposure to neighborhoods with different walkability on levels of physical activity (24,25,41). One study (5) found that moving to a more walkable neighborhood was associated with an increase in physical activity. The few studies that have changed or enhanced the environment have shown mixed evidence of effectiveness on physical activity levels (17,29,33,44,51,55,56). Nonetheless, the net sum of this research suggests important links between the environment and whether people are physically active or not.

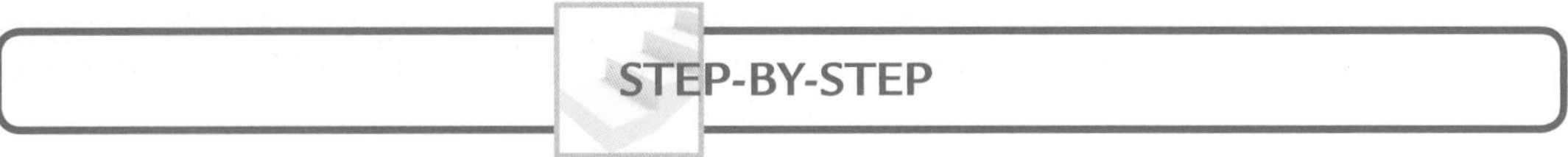

Step 1. Making Sense of Policy from a Practice Perspective

There are several links between policy and physical activity practice.

First, you can become advocates for physical activity in your communities by advocating to your local hospital, health department, municipality or other agency to increase the profile of, and facilities for, physical activity in your community (26). This is an important role for practitioners in supporting and developing community-based integrated programs that encourage people to be more active. This first step in physical activity advocacy is to persuade the community and local decision makers to invest in the program (49).

Policies to promote physical activity may utilize behavior change theories and models that are discussed elsewhere in this book (see Chapter 1 and 4). Health behavior change theory can help decision makers decide if a policy is likely to be effective (47). For example, communication policies to inform populations about becoming more active may have theoretically developed messages (*e.g.*, Theory of reasoned action) (14), or may use diffusion of innovations approaches to reach many people (7). This approach suggests that once a target behavior becomes widely accepted as easy to do, affordable, accessible, and convenient for a population, they will start to change in large numbers, in this case becoming more physically active. Policies that encourage healthy environments may use a socio-ecologic model (34,39), encouraging both the individual change approach provided through counseling and programs, in concert with an improved environment to facilitate active living. Considerable research has shown that both individual and environmental factors, taken together, explain physical activity behavior better than either approach alone (31). This is illustrated in Figure 7.1, where both individual and environmental change together make "active choices the easy choices." These data suggest a link between individual approaches and-facilitatory environments is synergistic. For example, it is not much use encouraging people to walk if their house is surrounded by freeways, there is limited public transportation, and the environment is unsafe. Consideration of these issues may suggest that this person needs to get most of their physical activity in a structured exercise program—for example, at a local YMCA or similar.

Other policy initiatives may also add to individual programs. For example, a policy that offers incentives for public transport, active commuting, decreased health costs, or a group competition to accumulate the most steps in a worksite—all of these can be linked to individual advice. Policies that offer "point of choice decision prompts" to be active—for example, through promoting stair use instead of elevator use—may also help to accumulate small increments of activity across the day (15). Cost-effectiveness analysts suggest this kind of low-cost, high-reach environmental intervention may be very inexpensive, in terms of costs per unit of energy expended (12).

One new dimension of policy relates to those that reduce sitting and sedentary time. It may be that prolonged sitting contributes more to total daily energy expenditure than physical activity time, and hence to the development of obesity (6). Strategies to reduce sitting will probably form part of the policy portfolios of the future, once the epidemiological threshold for risks associated with sitting are identified (52).

Step 2. Using the Physical Environment to Promote Physical Activity

"Active living" need not be difficult or expensive, and should become part of any physical activity regimen. It is simple to integrate physical activities into daily routines, at work, at home, in leisure time, and through the choices we make around transport. Examples

TABLE 7.3 Elements that Contribute to Active Living

Element	Examples
Walkability and connectivity	Improve safe and easy active travel connections to local destinations.
Active travel alternatives	Efficient public transport use, well signposted biking and walking routes and facilities to reduce car dependency and use; safe routes to school for children.
Quality public space, minimal incivilities	Maintain high-quality and safe parks, trails, open space for the community to use.
Social interaction and inclusion	Promote mixed use retail districts that encourage walking and cycling for local trips.
Perceived and objectively safe environments	Well-lit sidewalks, even and well-maintained surfaces (for the elderly, to reduce falls risk)
Domestic environments can be made to be more active	Doing gardening, household chores, and using these as "energy expenditure opportunities" as well as tasks

of active living are shown in Table 7.3. In terms of physical activity counseling, this is a key component of nonstructured physical activity that one could recommend to inactive adults. In addition to attending any structured exercise programs, and especially for those that are unable or unwilling to participate in programs, the active living environment becomes a vital setting for their physical activity. (See also Case Scenarios 7.1 through 7.4 later in this chapter.)

One component of the environment relevant to behavior change is the concept of "walkability." Neighborhood walkability measures how conducive a neighborhood is to walking. A high "walkable" neighborhood contains high residential density, well-connected streets, and mixed land use (workplaces, shops, and facilities, as well as residential dwellings) and is associated with lower body mass index (BMI) and higher physical activity levels (20). Health and fitness practitioners should become aware of the walkability scores in common use, and encourage clients to be active in more walkable local areas. Examples of tools to measure walkability are found in From the Practical Toolbox 7.1. When the walkability of the client's area has been established, the practitioner can then prescribe a program of physical activity which can incorporate the principles of active living. For example, walking to local destinations or in local parks can be specifically integrated into the client's regular routine and activities.

CLINICAL COUNSELING AND COMMUNITY PRACTICE VIGNETTES

Case Scenarios 7.1 through 7.4 are designed to illustrate the kinds of specific roles that practitioners and behavioral scientists could play in promoting physical activity through the built environment. The first involves a practitioner advising a client to better understand their environment and its physical activity opportunities, and to use a pedometer to track their steps each day as a form of behavioral self-monitoring (35). The second scenario focuses on encouraging "active living", building physical activity into everyday life. The third scenario illustrates a public health approach, where a committed

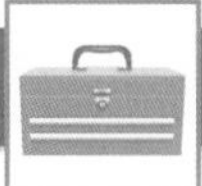

From the Practical Toolbox 7.1

EXAMPLES OF WALKABILITY CHECKLISTS/RESOURCES (12,13,53)

Partnership for a Walkable America Walkability Checklist encourages people to rate an area for walking and identify what can be done to improve the walking score in both the short-term and long-term. This is useful in planning local community walking groups.
Available from http://www.walkableamerica.org/.

Heart Foundation (Australia) Neighbourhood Walkability Checklist is designed to help individuals and groups survey their local walking environment. As well as a checklist, it has a template to use in writing to local municipalities about improving walkability.
Available from http://www.heartfoundation.org.au/SiteCollectionDocuments/HFW-Walkability-Checklist.pdf or with a tiny URL: http://tinyurl.com/3uwcmtb.

Walk Score is an international tool that measures the walkability of any address, providing a score from 0 (car-dependent) to 100 (walker's paradise). The measure is based on the presence of local destinations, but does not include availability and quality of footpaths or public transport infrastructure (12,13).
Available from http://www.walkscore.com.

www.ratemystreet.co.uk allows users to rate streets on a five-star system using eight criteria: Crossing the street; pavement (sidewalk) width; trip hazards; finding your way; safety from crime; safety from traffic; clean/attractive; disabled access. This is a British program.

practitioner in a small-midsized community might work with other agencies to build better infrastructure to encourage the population to be more active (49). The fourth scenario is an example of a "point-of-choice decision prompting" intervention—for example, to encourage stair use rather than elevator use—that is evidence-based, and now should be developed in practice in many settings such as in workplaces, malls, and train stations.

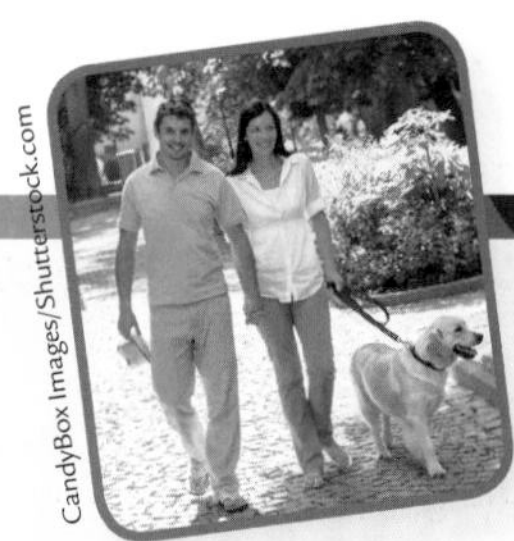

CandyBox Images/Shutterstock.com

Case Scenario 7.1

Belinda is a certified Health Fitness Specialist and uses motivational interviewing techniques to advise clients on how to be more physically active, using behavior change theories when appropriate. Brian is one of Belinda's clients, and he works long hours and often travels long distances on work trips and feels he has little time for physical activity.

Belinda advises Brian to conduct an audit of his local neighborhood for walkability, although he is new to the area and is still unfamiliar with his local surroundings. Belinda helps Brian identify destinations of interest in his local neighborhood and encourages him to have his bicycle serviced so he can travel to local places such as the hardware store. Brian owns a dog, which his wife normally walks, and Belinda suggests he and his wife exercise the dog together in the evenings. Belinda gives Brian a pedometer to help track his progress toward increasing his daily walking by at least 2000 to 3000 more steps.

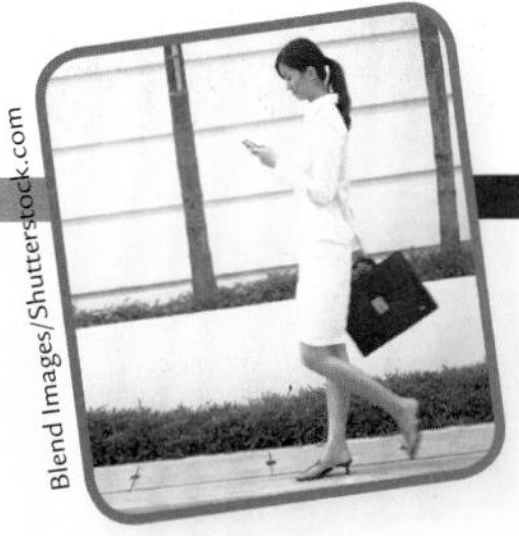
Blend Images/Shutterstock.com

Case Scenario 7.2

Victoria would like to be more physically active and prefers exercising outside in her local neighborhood. Through her health insurance, she makes an appointment to see a wellness consultant, John.

John identifies Victoria's local residential neighborhood has low walkability. However, the neighborhood where her office is located has a higher walkability. John develops a physical activity program for Victoria that includes taking regular lunchtime walks of at least 15 minutes to increase her physical activity and reduce time spent sitting in the workplace. The program also includes opportunities to participate in outdoor activities on weekends and in evenings in the summer, such as cycling.

John also encourages Victoria to help improve her community's walkability score by using some of the suggestions in the Partnership for a Walkable America Walkability checklist (see From the Practical Toolbox 7.1), such as exploring alternative walking routes and reporting unsafe conditions like broken sidewalks to her local authority.

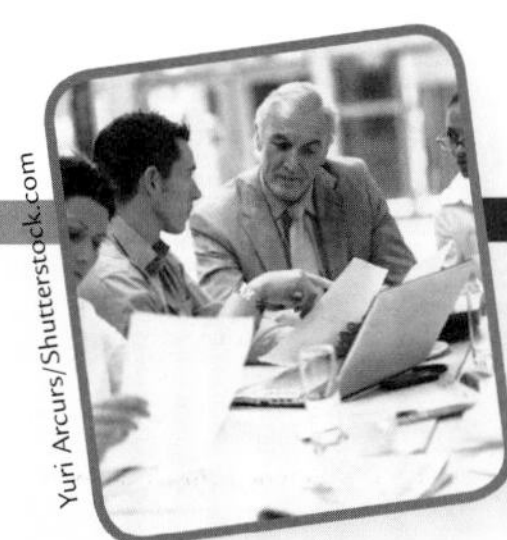
Yuri Arcurs/Shutterstock.com

Case Scenario 7.3

Working with a small to mid-sized local community, an exercise or prevention practitioner has discussions with a range of people interested in promoting physical activity in this municipality or county. These include the local Planning Department, the Mayor's office, the bus company (active transport), the Engineering department (for building trails and infrastructure), and the Hospital Health Education unit. Identifying common needs, the practitioner convenes an initial planning meeting, which may lead to the development of a community taskforce to address physical activity opportunities from a range of agencies and different sector perspectives. Over 12 to 24 months, the taskforce meetings result in an increase in built infrastructure (such as rail trails or park redevelopments), improved mayoral popularity, and increased population participation in health-enhancing physical activity across the community.

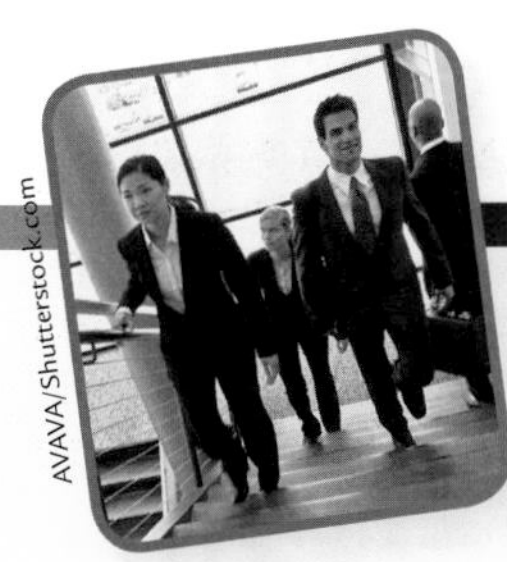
AVAVA/Shutterstock.com

Case Scenario 7.4

This is a generic scenario for behavior change that could be applied in thousands of offices, multi-story shopping malls, train stations, and other settings. The intervention is point-of-choice signage to encourage people in that environment to use the stairs rather than the elevator or escalator. Each day, millions make the "inactive choice" of using the elevator or escalator, and a simple sign to 'use the stairs for health" can encourage people to make the cognitive decision to change to an active mode of moving from one floor to the next.

Intervention studies have documented the efficacy of these interventions in colleges and health centers, but many community settings could benefit. The challenge in practice is to implement these cheap, feasible stair-use motivational signs in buildings, shops, and other facilities to encourage active stair use. This incidental physical activity intervention implemented across the whole population would be of substantial benefit.

TAKE-HOME MESSAGES

Making the links between policy, environments, and individual counseling is not initially obvious. In this area of work, the underlying summary goal for practitioners is to work out how to build physical activity into more of your clients' everyday lives. To do this, you need to know more about your clients' local environments, and opportunities for activity, and help them to make choices about where and what kinds of incidental activity might be suitable for them so as to add to possible structured programs that they might participate in. For many of them, attending structured programs may be difficult or not well maintained in the long term, so to realize optimal health-building physical activity into everyday lifestyles becomes the central behavioral goal.

In summary, policies can support active living opportunities at local or city-wide levels, and physical activity professionals need to contribute here to making their urban environments more physical activity–friendly. Becoming an "advocate" for physical activity is a personal and professional goal, but if enough advocates pressure policy makers at local and national levels, it does contribute to building the supports for population physical activity participation. This kind of advocacy is becoming a public health part of behavior change practice. This has led to the launch of the American National Physical Activity Plan (53), a multistrategy policy initiative to get Americans to become more active. Finally, the release and update of physical activity guidelines allows updated messages for practitioners to understand, define, and explain the amount, intensity, and frequency of activity for health that their clients need.

REFERENCES

1. American College of Sports Medicine. *ACSM's Guidelines for Exercise Testing and Prescription*. 9th ed. Baltimore (MD): Lippincott Williams and Wilkins; 2014.
2. Australian Institute for Health and Welfare (AIHW). *The Active Australia Survey: A Guide and Manual for Implementation, Analysis and Reporting*. Cat. no. CVD 22. Australian Government Canberra: AIHW; 2003.
3. Bauman A, Ainsworth BE, Sallis JF, et al. The descriptive epidemiology of sitting. A 20-country comparison using the international physical activity questionnaire (IPAQ). *Am J Prev Med*. 2011 Aug;41(2):228–35.
4. Bauman A, Allman-Farinelli M, Huxley R, James WP. Leisure-time physical activity alone may not be a sufficient public health approach to prevent obesity—A focus on China. *Obes Rev*. 2008 Mar;9 Suppl 1: 119–26.
5. Bauman A, Reis R, Sallis JF, Wells J, Loos R, Martin BW. Why are some people physically active and others not? Understanding the correlates of physical activity. *Lancet*. 2012 Jul 21;380(9838):258–71.
6. Bauman AE, Nelson DE, Pratt M, Matsudo V, Schoeppe S. Dissemination of physical activity evidence, programs, policies, and surveillance in the international public health arena. *Am J Prev Med*. 2006 Oct;31(4 Suppl):S57–65.
7. Bellew B, Bauman A, Martin B, Bull F, Matsudo V. Public policy actions needed to promote physical activity. *Curr Cardiovasc Risk Rep*. 2011 2011/08/01; 5(4):340–9.
8. Besser LM, Dannenberg AL. Walking to public transit: Steps to help meet physical activity recommendations. *Am J Prev Med*. 2005 Nov;29(4):273–80.
9. Bravata DM, Smith-Spangler C, Sundaram V et al. Using pedometers to increase physical activity and improve health. *JAMA*. 2007 Nov 21;298(19): 2296–304.
10. Brown BB, Werner CM. A new rail stop: Tracking moderate physical activity bouts and ridership. *Am J Prev Med*. 2007 Oct;33(4):306–9.
11. Brownson RC, Eyler AA, King AC, Brown DR, Shyu YL, Sallis JF. Patterns and correlates of physical activity among US women 40 years and older. *Am J Public Health*. 2000 Feb;90(2):264–70.
12. Carr LJ, Dunsiger SI, Marchs BH. Validation of walk score for estimating access to walkable amenities. *Br J Sports Med*. 2011 Nov;45(14):1144–8.
13. Carr LJ, Dunsiger SI, Marcus BH. Walk score as a global estimate of neighborhood walkability. *Am J Prev Med*. 2010 Nov;39(5):460–3.
14. Cope A, Cairns S, Fox K, et al. The UK National Cycle Network: An assessment of the benefits of a sustainable transport infrastructure. *World Transport Policy and Practice*. 2003;9(1):6–17.
15. Davies A, Clark S. Identifying and prioritising walking investment through the PERS audit tool. In:

Proceedings of Walk 21, 10th International Conference for Walking; 2009 Oct 1–12: New York.

16. Ding D, Gebel K. Built environment, physical activity, and obesity: What have we learned from reviewing the literature? *Health Place.* 2012 Jan;18(1): 100–5.
17. Donnelly JE, Blair SN, Jakicic JM, Manore MM, Rankin JW, Smith BK; American College of Sports Medicine. American College of Sports Medicine Position Stand. Appropriate physical activity intervention strategies for weight loss and prevention of weight regain for adults. *Med Sci Sports Exerc.* 2009 Feb;41(2):459–71.
18. Douglas MJ, Watkins SJ, Gorman DR, Higgins M. Are cars the new tobacco? *J Public Health (Oxf).* 2011 Jun;33(2):160–9.
19. Dunton GF, Cousineau M, Reynolds KD. The intersection of public policy and health behavior theory in the physical activity arena. *J Phys Act Health.* 2010 Mar;7 Suppl 1:S91–8.
20. Evenson KR, Herring AH, Huston SL. Evaluating change in physical activity with the building of a multi-use trail. *Am J Prev Med.* 2005 Feb;28(2 Suppl 2): 177–85.
21. Frost SS, Goins RT, Hunter RH, et al. Effects of the built environment on physical activity of adults living in rural settings. *Am J Health Promot.* 2010 Mar–Apr;24(4):267–83.
22. Garber CE, Blissmer B, Deschenes M, et al. Quantity and quality of exercise for developing and maintaining cardiorespiratory, musculoskeletal, and neuromotor fitness in apparently healthy adults: Guidance for prescribing exercise. *Med Sci Sports Exerc.* 2011 Jul;43(7): 1334–59.
23. Gebel K, Bauman A, Owen N. Correlates of non-concordance between perceived and objective measures of walkability. *Ann Behav Med.* 2009 Apr;37(2):228–38.
24. Gebel K, Bauman AE, Bull FC. Built environment: Walkability of neighbourhoods. In: Killoran A, Rayner M, editors. *Evidence-Based Public Health: Effectiveness and Efficiency*. Oxford: Oxford University Press; 2010. p. 298–312.
25. Gebel K, Bauman AE, Petticrew M. The physical environment and physical activity: A critical appraisal of review articles. *Am J Prev Med.* 2007 May;32(5):361–9.
26. Giles-Corti B, Donovan RJ. Relative influences of individual, social environmental, and physical environmental correlates of walking. *Am J Public Health.* 2003 Sep;93(9):1583–9.
27. Giles-Corti B, Knuiman M, Timperio A, et al. Evaluation of the implementation of a state government community design policy aimed at increasing local walking: Design issues and baseline results from RESIDE, Perth Western Australia. *Prev Med.* 2008 Jan;46(1):46–54.
28. Handy SL, Boarnet M, Ewing R, Killingsworth R. How the built environment affects physical activity: Views from urban planning. *Am J Prev Med.* 2002 Aug;23(2 Suppl):64–73.
29. Handy SL, Cao X, Mokhtarian PL. Self-selection in the relationship between the built environment and walking—Empirical evidence from Northern California. *J Am Plann Assoc.* 2006;72(1):55–74.
30. Haskell WL, Lee I-M, Pate RP, et al. Physical activity and public health: Updated recommendation for adults from the American College of Sports Medicine and the American Heart Association. *Med Sci Sports Exer.* 2007;39:1423–34.
31. Heath G, Brownson R, Kruger J, et al. The effectiveness of urban design and land use and transport policies and practices to increase physical activity: A systematic review. *J Phys Act Health.* 2006 Feb;3 Suppl 1:S55–S76.
32. Krizek K. Pretest-posttest strategy for researching neighborhood-scale urban form and travel behavior. *Transp Res Rec.* 2000;1722:48–55.
33. Krizek KJ. Residential relocation and changes in urban travel: Does neighborhood-scale urban form matter? *J Am Plann Assoc.* 2003 69(3):265–81.
34. Librett JJ, Yore MM, Schmid TL. Local ordinances that promote physical activity: A survey of municipal policies. *Am J Public Health.* 2003 Sep;93(9):1399–403.
35. MacDonald JM, Stokes RJ, Cohen DA, Kofner A, Ridgeway GK. The effect of light rail transit on body mass index and physical activity. *Am J Prev Med.* 2010 Aug;39(2):105–12.
36. Merom D, Bauman AE, Vita P, Close G. An environmental intervention to promote walking and cycling—The impact of a newly constructed Rail Trail in Western Sydney. *Prev Med.* 2003 Feb;36 (2):235–42.
37. Painter K. The influence of street lighting improvements on crime, fear and pedestrian street use, after dark. *Landsc Urban Plan.* 1996;35(2–3): 193–201.
38. Pratt M, Macera CA, Sallis JF, O'Donnell M, Frank LD. Economic interventions to promote physical activity: Application of the SLOTH model. *Am J Prev Med.* 2004 Oct;27(3 Suppl):136–45.
39. Reger-Nash B, Bauman A, Booth-Butterfield S, et al. Wheeling walks: Evaluation of a media-based community intervention. *Fam Community Health.* 2005;28(1):64–78.
40. Reger-Nash B, Bauman AE, Smith BJ, Craig CL, Abildso CG, Leyden K. Organizing an effective community-wide physical activity campaign: A step-by-step guide. *ACSM's Health Fit J.* 2011;15(5): 21–27.
41. Saelens B, Sallis JF, Frank LD. Environmental correlates of walking and cycling: Findings from transportation, urban design and planning literatures. *Ann Behav Med.* 2003 Spring;25(2):80–91.
42. Saelens BE, Handy SL. Built environment correlates of walking: A review. *Med Sci Sports Exerc.* 2008 Jul;40(7 Suppl):S550–66.
43. Saelens BE, Sallis JF, Frank LD. Environmental correlates of walking and cycling: Findings from the transportation, urban design, and planning literatures. *Ann Behav Med.* 2003 Spring;25(2):80–91.
44. Sallis JF, Adams MA, Ding D. Physical activity and the built environment. In: Cawley J, editor. *The Oxford*

Handbook of the Social Science of Obesity. Oxford: Oxford University Press; 2011. p. 433–51.

45. Sallis JF, Bauman A, Pratt M. Environmental and policy interventions to promote physical activity. *Am J Prev Med.* 1998 Nov;15(4):379–97.
46. Sallis JF, Cervero RB, Ascher W, Henderson KA, Kraft MK, Kerr J. An ecological approach to creating active living communities. *Annu Rev Public Health.* 2006;27:297–322.
47. Sallis JF, Owen N, Fisher EB. Ecological models of health behavior. In: Glanz K, Rimer BK, Viswanath K, editors. *Health Behavior and Health Education: Theory, Research, and Practic.*4th ed. San Francisco: Jossey-Bass; 2008. p. 465–86.
48. Shilton T. Advocacy for physical activity—From evidence to influence. *Promot Educ.* 2006;13(2):118–26.
49. Tester J, Baker R. Making the playfields even: Evaluating the impact of an environmental intervention on park use and physical activity. *Prev Med.* 2009 Apr;48(4):316–20.
50. Transportation Research Board. *Does the Built Environment Influence Physical Activity? Examining the Evidence.* Washington D.C.: Transportation Research Board; 2005.
51. Tremblay MS, Leblanc AG, Janssen I, et al. Canadian sedentary behaviour guidelines for children and youth. *Appl Physiol Nutr Metab.* 2011 6(1):59–64; 65–71.
52. U.S. Department of Health and Human Services. *2008 Physical Activity Guidelines for Americans.* Washington D.C.: U.S. Department of Health and Human Services. 2008.
53. U.S. National Physical Activity Plan Web site [Internet]. Washington, D.C.: May 2010. National Physical Activity Plan: [cited 2011, July 1]. Available from: http://www.physicalactivityplan.org/.
54. Vuori I, Oja P, Paronen O. Physically active commuting to work: Testing its potential for exercise promotion. *Med Sci Sports Exerc.* 1994;Jul;26(7):844–50.
55. World Health Organization. *Global Recommendations on Physical Activity for Health.* Geneva: World Health Organization; 2010.
56. Wu SY, Cohen D, Shi YY, Pearson M, Sturm R. Economic analysis of physical activity interventions. *Am J Prev Med.* 2011 Feb;40(2):149–58.
57. Zimring C, Joseph A, Nicoll GL, Tsepas S. Influences of building design and site design on physical activity: Research and intervention opportunities. *Am J Prev Med.* 2005 Feb;28(2 Suppl 2):186–93.

CHAPTER 8

Promoting Physical Activity Behavior Change: Population Considerations

Lauren Capozzi and S. Nicole Culos-Reed

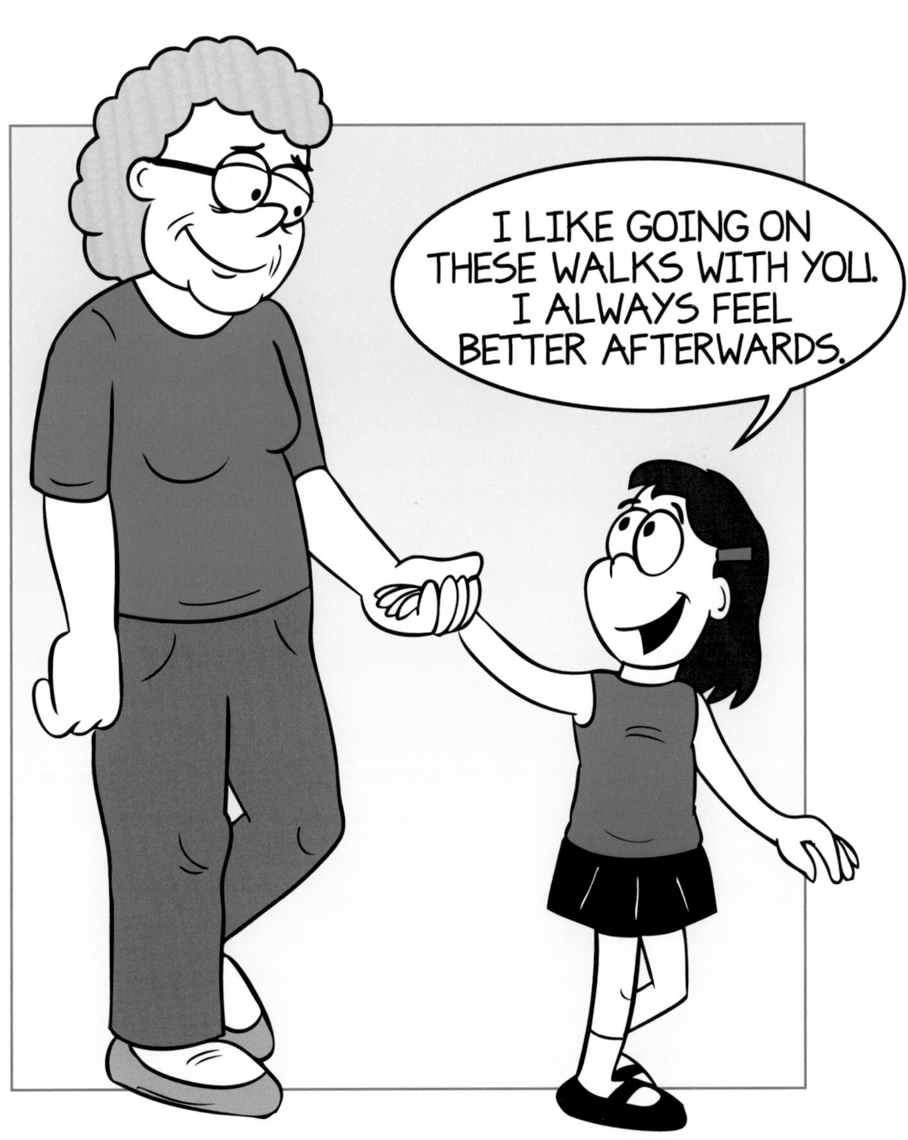
I LIKE GOING ON THESE WALKS WITH YOU. I ALWAYS FEEL BETTER AFTERWARDS.

In the preceding chapters, you have learned about behavior change from theory to practice, including how to use the many valuable tools and strategies for the successful promotion of physical activity interventions. In this chapter, we discuss the evidence for intervening within targeted groups—children, the elderly, and within chronic disease populations—and provide the tools and resources to tailor the intervention to those you are working with.

CONCEPT OVERVIEW

Physical activity (PA) has been well documented as an important contributor to overall health and well-being (20,39). However, the latest numbers in the United States suggest that only 48.8% of the population is currently meeting physical activity recommendations of at least 150 minutes of moderate- to vigorous-intensity activity distributed over 3 to 5 days per week (1,7). Moderate-intensity activity is defined as activity producing small increases in breathing and heart rate, and these recommendations of at least 150 minutes of moderate-intensity activity per week are associated with improved overall health outcomes (43). With over one third of the population reporting insufficient levels of activity (37.7%), and 13.5% of the population remaining completely inactive, a total of 51.2% of people in the U.S. are not participating in enough activity to receive the associated health benefits (7). This issue of inactivity becomes even more important when we consider populations that have potentially "more to gain" from being active—or "more to lose" from an inactive lifestyle. Such populations include, but are not limited to, children, the elderly, and those with various medical conditions.

The specific population is essentially the first level of "tailoring" for effective intervening, allowing for the values, traditions, and cultural and demographic norms to be reflected in PA promotion (48). Effective PA promotion at the population level further necessitates tailoring of more specific variables, including the needs of the particular group or individual within the given population, the training of the given fitness instructor or coach, and the content of the PA intervention, including the psychosocial and behavioral components. Consideration of the population is particularly important since varying populations experience different perceptions of, and barriers to, PA (48,26). Given that PA adoption and adherence are so poor in the general population and may be even more pronounced in specific populations, the tailoring of the PA prescription within the intervention needs to specifically examine determinants of, and barriers to, PA, including physiological, psychosocial, and environmental factors (19). Current research strongly advocates for the translation of evidence on the benefits of PA into optimal models of behavior change in which determinants of PA, including exercise preferences and barriers, are incorporated into interventions (11). See also From the Practical Toolbox 8.1.

As a professional in the exercise and fitness industry, it is important to recognize the principles of PA promotion and behavior change and how to apply these principles to different populations and individuals (see Chapters 1 to 5). In each section, we will provide population-specific tips to help improve activity adoption and maintenance.

These suggested techniques can help you promote improved client confidence and self-efficacy (the belief that your client can accomplish the exercise goals he or she has set), and improve the likelihood that your client will adhere to and maintain the exercise recommendations that you provide. As discussed in Chapter 3, we will consider personal factors, behavioral factors, environmental factors, and program-related factors.

The following sections consider the rationale and evidence for intervening with the following populations:

1. Children and youth
2. The elderly
3. Chronic medical conditions, including a spotlight on PA interventions for cancer survivors

CHILDREN AND YOUTH

The Evidence

In children, recent numbers indicate very high levels of inactivity, despite the recommended 60 minutes or more of PA each day (see Table 8.1 for recommendations) (7). The U.S. Youth Risk Behavior Surveillance conducted in 2009 showed that among high school students (grade 9–12), only 17.3%–19.5% reported participating in PA for at least 60 minutes 7 days a week, and only 35.2%–38.8% reported participating in PA for at least 60 minutes 5 days a week (6). Between 21.5%–24.8% of high school students reported not participating in at least 60 minutes of PA on any day of the week (6).

PA participation among children and youth has been linked to health benefits associated with development, mental abilities, school behavior, and academic achievement (42). Concern with childhood inactivity is on the rise, and the prevalence of overweight children is increasing rapidly (7,12,40). This associated increase in overweight and other chronic conditions including obesity, heart disease, and musculoskeletal conditions, is now reported at younger ages and is linked to diminished quality of life, premature illness and death, and increased health care costs as these children age (12,32). Since PA levels in children are a strong predictor of PA levels into adulthood, developing successful interventions for children is a necessity to improve health outcomes as well as increase lifelong PA participation (41).

Recommendations

Children between the ages of 6 and 17 should be getting at least 60 minutes of physical activity each day (7). See Table 8.1.

Step-by-Step

See Table 8.2 for step-by-step instructions on implementing PA interventions for children and youth, and Table 8.3 for a summary of successful interventions in this population.

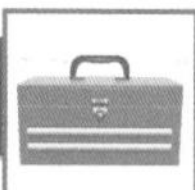

From the Practical Toolbox 8.1

EXPLORE EXERCISE PREFERENCES

One of the most important predictors of long-term PA adherence is whether or not the exercise program is specifically designed to meet the client's goals, personal preferences, and lifestyle and environmental factors. It is important to first evaluate your client's lifestyle, and exercise preferences before creating a PA program. It is also important to evaluate current barriers to exercises and personal characteristics that will motivate the client to adopt an active lifestyle.

The Healthy Physical Activity Participation Questionnaire
This questionnaire evaluates frequency, intensity, and perceived fitness and gives a total "heath benefit" score.
http://www.getactivepenticton.com/gap/assets/thehealthyphysicalactivityparticipationquestionnaire.pdf

The Fantastic Lifestyle Checklist
This is a simple checklist which provides clients with a "health benefit" rating based on various lifestyle habits.
http://hk.humankinetics.com/AdvancedFitnessAssessmentandExercisePrescription/IG/App_A5.pdf

TABLE 8.1 PA Recommendations for Children and Youth (1,7,43)

Activity Type	Recommended Weekly Frequency, Intensity, and Time	Examples
Aerobic	Moderate Intensity Activity should make up the majority of the recommended minimum 60 minutes per day.	• Activities like brisk walking, cycling, hiking, rollerblading, skateboarding. • Games like baseball and golf
	Vigorous Intensity Activity: Include at least 3 days per week.	• Activities that include running, cycling, jumping, dancing, skiing • Games like hockey, basketball, swimming, soccer
Strength Training	At least 3 days per week as a part of the minimum 60 minutes per day.	• Activities that include pulling or pushing, supporting bodyweight • Games like tree climbing, swinging on playground equipment, or playing tug-of-war • Resistance exercises using body weight or resistance bands may be performed
Bone Strengthening	At least 3 days per week as a part of the minimum 60 minutes per day.	• Activities that include hopping, skipping, and jumping • Games like jump rope, and hopscotch • Running

Source: *Physical Activity Guidelines for Americans, U.S. Department of Health and Human Services*, 2008; *Physical Activity for Everyone,* CDC, 2011; American College of Sports Medicine. *ACSM's Guidelines for Exercise Testing and Prescription*. 9th ed. Baltimore (MD): Lippincott Williams and Wilkins; 2014.

TABLE 8.2 Implementing PA Programs for Children and Youth (1)			
Steps	**Recommendation**	**Considerations**	**Tools**
1. Screen for safety.	• Assess for safety and whether clearance is needed from physician (*i.e.*, if current signs of illness, injury, or advanced deconditioning).	• Make sure to discuss participation in activities that are fun for the individual and group.	
2. Explore and educate: Discuss motivations and goals, health beliefs, and preferences.	• Discuss health beliefs and provide education on the importance of PA.	• PA participation must be meaningful to children.	• Decisional balance sheets (see Ch. 3) • Stages of Change (see Ch. 4) • Goal setting worksheet and exercise contract (see Ch. 3) • Physical Activity Calendar (see From the Practical Toolbox 8.2)
3. Test.	• Utilize tests with established normative data.	• Generally, standard adult testing applies to children, however response to testing will differ. • Children may also require additional support and guidance during testing.	• See From the Practical Toolbox 8.3 and ACSM's Guidelines for Exercise Testing and Prescription.
4. Prescribe exercise and implement the plan.	• Implement PA intervention and use appropriate tools for adherence. • Provide continuous feedback and encouragement	• Promote activities that are fun, interactive and encourage longitudinal participation in PA. • Make efforts to decrease sedentary activities. • Children and youth should exercise in thermoneutral environments and be properly hydrated. • Activity should be promoted as something positive, and not used for punishment.	• PA Journals (see From the Practical Toolbox 8.4) • For older children, online PA logs may be appropriate. (See From the Practical Toolbox 8.4.)
5. Actively evaluate and progress.	• Follow up with individual or group. • Assess for enjoyment. • Progress.	• Children who are overweight or new to activity will need to progress at a slower rate than active children. • Many children & youth sports have built in progression.	

Source: American College of Sports Medicine. *ACSM's Guidelines for Exercise Testing and Prescription*. 9th ed. Baltimore (MD): Lippincott Williams and Wilkins; 2014.

TABLE 8.3 Successful Interventions and Strategies: PA Interventions for Children and Youth

Intervention	Methods	Outcomes	Practical Strategies
The VERB Campaign, 2002–2004—A marketing campaign addressed to children ages 9 to 13 years living in the U.S. (22)	• Developed the VERB brand to market PA as cool, fun, and a chance to have a good time with friends. • Advertised on television, the radio, in print, and through promotion on the Internet, in schools and greater community.	• Measurements after 2 years indicated a dose response with regard to the number of VERB messages viewed and PA behaviors and associated positive attitude. • After 2 years, 81% of U.S. children reported seeing the VERB campaign and were engaging in at least one session of PA per week.	• Market PA as cool, fun, and a chance to have a good time with friends. • If possible, implement marketing strategies over popular media or at schools and in the greater community. • Create a "brand" for PA that children will recognize.
The Sports, Play, and Active Recreation for Kids (SPARK) program (35)	• Compared three physical education class conditions. 1. Certified Physical Education specialists implemented the program. 2. Classroom teachers were trained to implement the intervention. 3. Usual physical education class. The intervention groups focus on promoting regular physical activity outside of school.	• Students in specialist-led classes spent more minutes per week being physically active (40 mins) than the teacher-led classes (33 mins), and both were significantly higher than the regular PA class (18 mins). • The increased number of minutes of activity in the intervention classes translated into increased fitness level 2 years post-intervention.	• Provide training for physical education teachers to help them implement effective strategies to promote increased exercise minutes in the classroom.
Promoting Lifestyle Activity for Youth (PLAY) (31)	1. Taught children healthy lifestyle habits and encouraged 30–60 minutes of moderate to vigorous PA daily. 2. Techniques included 12-minute activity breaks during the school day to teach new PA concepts, and self-monitoring of total PA participation.	• PA participation in children increased with the PLAY intervention.	• Promote attitudes and behaviors in children that will translate into a lifetime of PA participation. • Encourage children to record PA on a calendar or to schedule activity with their friends and family.

From the Practical Toolbox 8.2

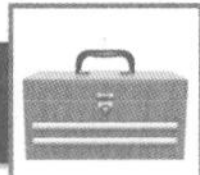

PHYSICAL ACTIVITY CALENDAR

Planning and scheduling PA is a great way to increase PA participation. Using a calendar to plan activities for the next month is a simple yet effective way to start recording activity. See the following calendar for an example.

Let's Move! Healthy Family Calendar

Day of the Week		Type of Activity	What Time of the Day	Who Will Participate	Did We Do It?
(For Example) Monday	*Your Fun Activity*	Walk 15 minutes	7 a.m. and 5 p.m.	Mom and Sally	★
	Your Healthy Food	Fruit	Lunch	Sally and John	★
Monday	Your Fun Activity				
	Your Healthy Food				
Tuesday	Your Fun Activity				
	Your Healthy Food				
Wednesday	Your Fun Activity				
	Your Healthy Food				
Thursday	Your Fun Activity				
	Your Healthy Food				
Friday	Your Fun Activity				
	Your Healthy Food				
Saturday	Your Fun Activity				
	Your Healthy Food				
Sunday	Your Fun Activity				
	Your Healthy Food				
	How many stars did you give yourself?				

(Adapted from http://www.letsmove.gov/sites/letsmove.gov/files/Family_Calendar.pdf.)

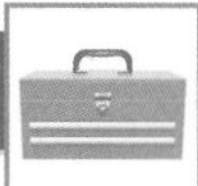

From the Practical Toolbox 8.3

FITNESS TESTING

Fitness testing must be adapted to suit the population and individual you are working with.

ACSM's Guidelines for Exercise Testing and Prescription
This resource offers a clear and specific approach to exercise testing. More fitness testing resources can be found at http://www.acsm.org/.

Rated Perceived Exertion Scale
Before beginning fitness testing, it is important to teach clients about the Rated Perceived Exertion Scale so they are able to clearly communicate their level of exercise intensity throughout testing and future physical activity participation. The Borg Rated Perceived Exertion Scale can be found at http://www.cdc.gov/physicalactivity/everyone/measuring/exertion.html.

Barriers

Current barriers to PA participation include lack of time due to other obligations, lack of interest or motivation, body-related barriers (*e.g.*, body self-consciousness), social barriers, and environmental barriers (*e.g.*, no equipment, unsuitable weather) (49).

Adherence and Maintenance Considerations

Improving parental, school, and community support, and providing access to environments that promote PA, are helpful at improving adherence. Table 8.4 highlights important PA adherence and maintenance techniques for children and youth. Enhancing children's knowledge of PA benefits, improving motivation and time management skills, and offering

TABLE 8.4 Techniques to Improve Children's PA Adherence and Maintenance

Factor	Techniques for Adherence/Maintenance
Personal	• Always consider PA history, personal abilities, preferences, and personal resources.
Behavioral	• Encourage children to set realistic and achievable PA goals. • Plan for rewards once activity goals are reached. • Ensure PA is used as a reward, and not as a punishment (*i.e.*, going for a family walk vs. having to run laps for punishment). • Encourage children to practice self-monitoring techniques (*i.e.*, journaling).
Environmental	• Promote activity that is safe, accessible, and affordable.
Program	• Encourage children to try different types of activities to prevent boredom and improve overall fitness skills.

From the Practical Toolbox 8.4

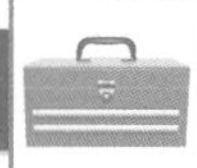

ADHERING TO EXERCISE: PHYSICAL ACTIVITY JOURNAL

While interventions, when well-designed, can clearly provide numerous positive physical and psychosocial benefits to the target population, our greater concern is the "next step." Specifically, what must be done to ensure that individuals maintain activity after the completion of a formal PA intervention?

A journal can help to evaluate the frequency of exercise, intensity, duration, and type of activity. Journals can be "paper and pencil" or can be kept electronically on one of the many online lifestyle recording Web sites.

- A sample journal and tracking log can be found in From the Practical Toolbox 3.6.
- An example of an online tracking Web site is: http://www.mypyramidtracker.gov/.
- Check out the Center for Disease Control's online PA tracking tool: http://www.bam.gov/sub_physicalactivity/physicalactivity_activitycalendar.html.

For more on setting and maintaining exercise goals, refer to Chapters 2 and 3.

a variety of exercise opportunities are all useful strategies (30). Further strategies to overcome these barriers are important and research into effective interventions is ongoing (see Table 8.3).

Useful Links

Refer to the following Web sites on this topic for more information:

- Active Healthy Kids Canada: http://www.activehealthykids.ca/
- American Academy of Pediatrics: http://www.healthychildren.org/English/healthy-living/Pages/default.aspx
- Center for Disease Control and Prevention: Physical Activity for Everyone: http://www.cdc.gov/physicalactivity/everyone/guidelines/children.html

Case Scenario 8.1

v.s.anandhakrishna/Shutterstock.com

Name: Steven Johnston

Age: 15

Presentation: Steven and his mom visit a local fitness center in search of an exercise program that will help Steven feel more comfortable participating in physical education class at school. His mom is worried because Steven's teacher reports very poor participation and lack of attendance in class. Steven says that if he could keep up with the other children in class, he would be more likely to actively participate.

continued

Case Scenario 8.1 *continued*

Case Scenario 8.1 Step-by-Step

Screen	Evaluate and Educate	Test	Implement	Progress
Steven does not report any physical symptoms that would indicate exercise to be unsafe. Therefore, move on to evaluate goals and motivations for PA participation.	Steven is frustrated because he finds it difficult to keep up with his friends in the schoolyard. He reports decreased motivation for PA participation due to a lack of skill in common sports. Steven's goal is to be able to participate in activities with children his own age and to avoid feeling uncomfortable or inadequate.	General assessment of ability. Formal fitness testing determined to be not necessary.	Prescription: • Two days/week with trainer to work on basic aerobic endurance, muscular strength, and agility. • Practice catching, throwing, and running activities with family members twice/week. • Register for a soccer class with kids at his ability level. • Steven will practice planning weekly PA on a calendar, which will be placed on his fridge at home. • Steven will record his activity in an online log.	• Steven will hand in journal log to trainer each week and reflect on overall enjoyment, difficulty, and progress. • Once Steven has established adherence, training sessions can decrease to once per week to encourage Steven to become an independent exerciser. • Program will be progressed accordingly to continue to produce overload.

TAKE-HOME MESSAGE

Both the physical and psychological health benefits of PA for children and youth are well documented, but with activity participation levels remaining low, improving ways to effectively promote PA is crucial (40,42). Decreasing perceived barriers to PA participation and improving PA accessibility is our responsibility as parents, teachers, coaches, personal trainers, and policy makers. As indicated earlier in Table 8.3, successful interventions focus on increasing PA participation minutes during regularly scheduled physical education class (the SPARK campaign) (35), utilizing marketing techniques so as to brand PA as "cool" and "fun" (the VERB campaign), and promoting lifestyle PA adoption (PLAY campaign) (31). Utilizing these tools to help improve children and youth's perception of PA, accessibility to sport and active playtime, and to effectively adopt active lifestyles will provide meaningful benefits to children and effectively encourage lifelong PA participation.

OLDER ADULTS

The Evidence

The 150 weekly minutes of moderate-intensity activity for older adults (65 years plus) is not currently met by over 60% of older adults in the U.S. (1,7) (see Table 8.5 for complete recommendations). While there is a decline in activity as a natural part of aging, the literature clearly supports that promotion of activity can be successful in older adults and lessen many of the negative side-effects associated with aging, including decreased health and functional independence (24). Participation in regular PA also improves cardiovascular function in older adults, reduces risk factors associated with disease states, improves body composition and bone health, improves quality of life and cognition, and extends life expectancy (10). Table 8.6 outlines key steps necessary to the implementation of a successful PA program for older adults.

A second reason for promoting PA interventions in older adults comes from the increase in our aging population. Older adults are the least physically active of any age group and yet are the most rapidly growing age group, with this population expected to double by 2030 (13). Creating mass interventions that promote moderate-intensity aerobic activity, muscular strengthening, flexibility, balance, and risk management is meaningful for a large portion of this population.

Recommendations

Adults aged 65 years and older are recommended to participate in 150–300 minutes of moderate-intensity activity every week (1). Alternatively, older adults can accumulate 75–100 minutes of vigorous intensity activity every week (1). In addition to this aerobic exercise, 2 or more days of muscle strengthening activities are recommended. (See Table 8.5.)

Step-by-Step

See Table 8.6 for steps for implementing physical activity programs for older adults, and Table 8.7 references effective interventions and practical, evidence-based behavior change strategies.

Barriers

Barriers to PA participation among older adults may include, but are not restricted to, a past inactive lifestyle and decreased understanding of PA benefits, physical frailty and/or health issues that may restrict mobility, fear of injury or falling, lack of guidance, and the cost of transport or access to exercise facilities (5,9). Furthermore, if older adults are residing in long-term care facilities, they may face increased barriers to PA, including limited access to exercise space or equipment (9).

Adherence and Maintenance Considerations

Strategies to increase PA options for the elderly can be seen in Table 8.8.

TABLE 8.5 PA Recommendations for Older Adults (1,3,10)

Activity Type	Recommended Weekly Frequency, Intensity, and Time	Type Examples
Aerobic	Moderate Intensity Activity: at least 5 days per week for 30–60 minutes per day, totaling 150–300 minutes per week.	• Activities like walking, golf, cycling, gardening, house cleaning
	Vigorous Intensity Activity: for at least 3 days per week for at least 20 to 30 minutes per day, totaling 75–100 minutes per week.	• Activities that include jogging, dancing, aerobics or water aerobics, swimming, cycling • Games like tennis
Strength Training	At least 2 days per week at moderate intensity (60%–70% 1RM) or low intensity (40%–50% 1RM) for older adults beginning a resistance training program.	• Activities that include pulling or pushing, supporting bodyweight • Exercises using hand weights, weight machines, resistance bands • Resistance exercises using body weight or calisthenics-type exercises • Activities of daily living including carrying groceries, getting up and down from a chair or the floor
Balance Exercises	At least 3 days per week as a part of the minimum 60 minutes per day.	• Exercises that progressively reduce the base of support, dynamic movements that challenge the center of gravity, exercises that stress postural muscles, or exercises that reduce sensory input (*i.e.*, stand or balance with eyes closed) • Balance on one leg, balance on toes or heels • Activities such as walking backward or in circles • Activities such as yoga or tai chi
Flexibility	At least 2 days per week	• Performing static stretches from a prone, seated, or standing position • Holding stretches for at least 30–60 seconds and maintaining stretch below point of discomfort

Source: American College of Sports Medicine. *ACSM's Guidelines for Exercise Testing and Prescription*. 9th ed. Baltimore (MD): Lippincott Williams and Wilkins; 2014; ACSM's Exercise Management for Persons with Chronic Diseases and Disabilities, 3rd edition, 2009 (3); Chodzko-Zajko et al., 2009 (10).

TABLE 8.6 Implementing PA Programs for Older Adults (7)

Steps	Recommendation	Considerations	Tools
1. Screen for safety.	• Assess for safety and whether clearance is needed from physician (*i.e.*, if current signs of illness, injury, or advanced deconditioning).	• Current health status: Existing disability? Presence or signs of cardiovascular, pulmonary or metabolic disease? Use of walking aids? • History of health condition or injury? • Explore contraindications for exercise.	• PAR-Q (see Ch. 2) • PARmed-X (see Ch. 2) • AHA/ACSM Health/Fitness Facility Preparticipation Screening Questionnaire (see Ch. 2) • Informed Consent (see Ch. 2)
2. Explore and Educate: Discuss motivations and goals, health beliefs, and preferences.	• Discuss health beliefs and provide education on the importance of PA for older adults.	• PA participation must be meaningful, accessible, and modifiable depending on contraindications.	• Decisional balance sheets (see Ch. 3) • Stages of Change (see Ch. 4) • Goal setting worksheet and exercise contract with strategies to overcome barriers (see Ch. 3) • PA Calendar (see From the Practical Toolbox 8.2)
3. Test.	• Most older adults do not require exercise testing before beginning a moderate-intensity exercise program. • For people with known risk factors, a clinical exercise test is recommended. • Utilize tests with established normative data.	• Ensure the testing environment is safe and necessary assistance is provided. • Handrails on treadmill may be required. • A cycle ergometer test may be recommended for those with poor balance. • Adjust workload accordingly.	• See From the Practical Toolbox 8.3 and ACSM's Guidelines for Exercise Testing and Prescription.

continued

TABLE 8.6 Implementing PA Programs for Older Adults (7) (*Continued*)

Steps	Recommendation	Considerations	Tools
4. Prescribe exercise and implement the plan.	• Establish safe exercise environment • Implement the PA intervention and use appropriate tools for adherence	• Make efforts to decrease sedentary activities. • Plan for activities that are accessible and offer the necessary support and guidance. • For highly deconditioned older adults, intensity and duration should be low at the beginning. • Supervise initial strength training sessions for safety.	• PA Journals (see From the Practical Toolbox 8.4) • Online PA logs may be appropriate if client has access to a computer. (see From the Practical Toolbox 8.4) • Encourage social support. • Promote self-efficacy.
5. Actively evaluate and progress.	• Follow-up with individual or group. • Assess for enjoyment. • Progress when necessary. • Provide continued encouragement and feedback.	• May progress at a slower rate due to contraindications and limited mobility. • Progression should always be individualized and should meet satisfaction of client.	

Source: American College of Sports Medicine. *ACSM's Guidelines for Exercise Testing and Prescription*. 9th ed. Baltimore (MD): Lippincott Williams and Wilkins; 2014.

TABLE 8.7 Successful Interventions and Strategies: PA Interventions for Older Adults

Intervention	Methods	Outcomes	Practical Strategies
Long-Term Follow-up of PA Behavior in Older Adults (27)	• Following a six-month randomized, controlled PA trial, participants were evaluated at 2 and 5 years postintervention. • The primary outcome was to evaluate PA levels over time. • Researchers examined previous behavior, self-efficacy and effect, and evaluated how these factors impacted future PA participation.	• PA at two years was a strong predictor of PA at five years. • Self-efficacy and affect at two years was also associated with PA at 5 years.	• Implement strategies that promote self-efficacy and positive self-affect. • Educate clients on the importance of adherence, and that adherence can promote future PA participation.
Interventions to Promote PA by Older Adults (24)		• Studies indicate the importance of environmental interventions to promote PA and adherence. It is reported that environments that are accessible, attractive, safe, and low cost are the best at promoting PA adherence.	• Help to put signs and information promoting PA in accessible work environments. • Provide easy-to-use maps for people who want to cycle or walk along trails.

TABLE 8.8 Techniques to Improve Older Adults' PA Adherence and Maintenance

Factor	Techniques for Adherence/Maintenance
Personal	• Always consider PA history, personal abilities, medical conditions, preferences, and personal resources.
	• The older adult should feel safe and well monitored during exercise.
Behavioral	• Encourage older adults to set realistic and achievable PA goals. • Plan for rewards once activity goals are reached. • Encourage older adults to practice self-monitoring techniques (*i.e.*, journaling, keeping a calendar).
Environmental	• Promote activity that is safe, accessible, and affordable. • Encourage group-based activities since the social aspect may improve accountability and enjoyment.
Program	• Encourage older adults to try different types of activities to prevent boredom and improve overall fitness.

Useful Links

Refer to the following Web sites on this topic for more information:

- Active Aging Partnership: http://www.agingblueprint.org/partnership.cfm
- Center for Disease Control and Prevention: Physical Activity for Everyone: http://www.cdc.gov/physicalactivity/everyone/guidelines/olderadults.html
- Elder Gym: http://www.eldergym.com/exercises.html
- Elderly Activities: http://www.elderlyactivities.co.uk/
- Senior Exercise and Fitness Tips: http://www.helpguide.org/life/senior_fitness_sports.htm

Jan Mika//Shutterstock.com

Case Scenario 8.2

Name: Ellie Jones

Age: 72

Presentation: Ellie is a 72-year-old widower, living independently. She enjoys social activities with friends, but currently does not participate in any regular physical activity. Her doctor has recommended beginning an exercise program, in part to deal with her osteoporosis and weight gain issues. However, Ellie does not know where to begin!

Case Scenario 8.2 Step-by-Step

Screen	Evaluate and Educate	Test	Implement	Progress
Ellie's doctor completes the PARmed-X. Osteoporosis and being currently inactive necessitate a gentle progression for both weight-bearing and aerobic activities.	Ellie is educated on the goal of including body-resistance activities (prior to the implementation of further weights or resistance) in her daily lifestyle. The importance of being active with friends is highlighted and a network of active ladies and walking opportunities is developed. Barriers to staying active are discussed and plans for overcoming barriers are realized.	Initial screening (ACSM exercise testing for older adults) is performed. Results indicate Ellie is okay to begin with a mild exercise program, with gradual progression. Consideration should be given to balance-based activities, thereby reducing the likelihood of future falls.	Gentle, weight-bearing, and aerobic activities are recommended. A progressive walking program, with a home journal for record keeping, is implemented. Prescription: 2d/week for resistance; 3–5 d/week for aerobic	Ellie sets weekly and monthly goals, and a weekly journal is used to track activity and results (energy levels, feeling states). Progress is monitored and evaluated every 2 weeks, with readjustment of weekly PA levels as necessary.

TAKE-HOME MESSAGE

Older adults have much to gain from participating in regular PA, including maintaining current physical functioning, managing current chronic disease and preventing further medical conditions, and enhancing quality of life (29). Unfortunately, older adults are at a high risk for living sedentary lifestyles (24). Significant predictors of long-term adherence to active lifestyles in older adults include more positive affect and higher self-efficacy (27). Overall, interventions designed to promote PA among older adults have been promising, confirming many health benefits for participants who engage in an active lifestyle long term (24).

Increased health concerns in an aging population make the necessity of intervening with older adults a priority. Initiatives must consider how to make active living part of the natural aging process. Consideration of personal barriers including health and mobility, motivation, as well as social support and environmental barriers such as accessibility to safe exercise environments is essential.

OVERVIEW OF COMMON CHRONIC CONDITIONS

Numerous chronic diseases may be managed effectively with PA interventions. While it is outside the scope of the current chapter to provide details on PA interventions for all conditions, this section of the chapter provides a brief overview of chronic conditions that have substantial evidence for the role of PA in disease management. In addition, with recent advancements in our understanding of the benefits of PA for cancer survivors, we chose to highlight this condition in greater depth.

With all chronic conditions, it is extremely important to engage the appropriate health care professionals to ensure the safety and appropriateness of the intervention for the particular population. Simple screening tools, such as the Par-MEDX (see Chapter 2) should be employed to ensure physician clearance prior to the start of the PA program. Additional tools for screening, evaluation, and feedback should be utilized as specific to the chronic conditions as possible. See the From the Practical Toolbox features in this chapter and other chapters of this book for examples of these resources.

Behavioral strategies to promote PA adoption, adherence, and maintenance are extremely important for people with chronic conditions. These individuals may be apprehensive about starting a new PA program or addressing activity levels following changes in health status. These issues highlight the need for tailored PA interventions that include effective behavior change strategies.

Adherence and Maintenance Considerations

Table 8.9 highlights key behavior change strategies when working with people with varying chronic conditions. These strategies can be further tailored to the individual's condition and tailored based on health history, need, interests, and preferences.

COMMON CHRONIC CONDITIONS

Overweight and Obesity

Worldwide obesity rates are reported to be at epidemic proportions, with over 1.5 billion adults considered overweight, and of these, 500 million considered obese (47). Obesity is

TABLE 8.9 Techniques to Improve PA Adherence and Maintenance

Factor	Techniques for Adherence/Maintenance
Personal	• Consider PA history, personal abilities, other medical conditions, preferences, and personal resources. • The person should feel safe and be well monitored during exercise. • The medical team should be aware and grant permission for the person to participate in activity and promote exercise adherence and maintenance. This can be promoted through personal fitness reports generated by the fitness professional for the medical team.
Behavioral	• Encourage people to set realistic and achievable PA goals. • Remind people currently being treated for their condition to adjust total activity minutes and intensity based on treatment side-effects. • Encourage people to practice self-monitoring techniques (*i.e.*, journaling, keeping a calendar). • Plan for rewards once activity goals are reached.
Environmental	• Promote activity that is safe, accessible, affordable, and lead by exercise practitioners with specific experience in the necessary field. • Encourage group-based activities as the social aspect may improve accountability, enjoyment, and support.
Program	• Disease-specific programs may provide increased peace of mind for individuals. • People can start slowly in activities like yoga, and increase total activity minutes and intensity from there.

linked to a multitude of lifelong physical and psychological health complications, yet PA holds significant value in terms of an effective treatment option in helping to burn calories and manage energy imbalances (18). PA also plays a key role in psychological well-being, cardiovascular fitness, and maintaining weight loss (18). See Table 8.10 for recommendations and considerations for overweight and obese individuals and populations.

Cardiovascular Disease

Cardiovascular disease remains the leading cause of death and disability among adult men and women in the United States, and physical inactivity is well defined as an independent risk factor for this disease (8,44). The benefits of PA extend beyond prevention and management of heart disease, aiding weight management, the prevention of further disability, and reducing depression and anxiety—all of which are closely associated with cardiovascular disease (46,50). See Table 8.11 for recommendations and considerations for individuals and populations with cardiovascular disease.

Cancer: The Role of Physical Activity for Cancer Survivors

EVIDENCE

The rapidly accumulating research clearly indicates a beneficial role of PA for cancer survivors, both during and after treatment (21,36,37). PA improves a variety of physical, psychosocial, and health outcomes in cancer survivors, both during and after cancer treatment,

TABLE 8.10 PA Recommendations and Considerations for Overweight and Obese Individuals and Populations (1,7,14)

Recommendations	• Exercising at least 5 days per week • At least 150 minutes per week progressing to at least 300 minutes per week of moderate-intensity activity, or 150 minutes of vigorous-intensity activity per week. • Intensity: Moderate to vigorous-intensity physical activity should be encouraged. • Focus should be on aerobic activity that utilizes large muscle groups. Resistance training at least 2 days per week should be included.
Barriers	• Feelings of insecurity and discomfort when exercising • Tiredness • Fear of injury • Low self-esteem, diminished self-efficacy for being active • Diminished self-worth and decreased perceived control • Higher prevalence of comorbidities
Interventions	• Weight loss of at least 5% to 10% of initial body weight over a three- to six-month period will provide significant health benefits. • For adequate weight loss, energy intake must be addressed. Patient should consult with dietitian and together with exercise programming, a deficit of 500 to 1000 kcal / day should be achieved. • Reference Table 8.9 for effective behavior change techniques.
Take-Home Message	• Helping someone who struggles with excessive weight to adopt a more active lifestyle can help to significantly improve physical and psychological well-being as well as decrease the risk for comorbidities (18). • Creating a safe exercise environment for someone who may have body image issues, comorbidities, and fear of injury is extremely important and can directly affect long-term adherence (34).
Web links	• World Health Organization: http://www.who.int/dietphysicalactivity/childhood/en/ • Centers for Disease Control and Prevention: Physical Activity for a Healthy Weight: http://www.cdc.gov/healthyweight/physical_activity/index.html • Scope–Healthy Choices: Physical Activity: http://www.childhood-obesity-prevention.org/live5210/resources/healthy-choices-physical-activity/ • How to Begin an Exercise Routine for Overweight People, The Livestrong Foundation: http://www.livestrong.com/article/16350-begin-exercise-routine-overweight-people/

Source: American College of Sports Medicine. *ACSM's Guidelines for Exercise Testing and Prescription*. 9th ed. Baltimore (MD): Lippincott Williams and Wilkins; 2014.

TABLE 8.11 Recommendations and Considerations for Individuals and Populations with Cardiovascular Disease (1,4)

Recommendations	• Exercising between three to seven times per week for 20 to 60 minutes per session. Following a cardiac event, 1- to 10-minute sessions are recommended, followed by progression in duration. • Exercise sessions can be split up into multiple shorter sessions per day to accommodate patients with limited exercise capacity. • Intensity between 11 and 16 on a 6 to 20 RPE scale. • Activities that include large muscle groups with an emphasis on caloric expenditure are encouraged. These may include use of the arm ergometer, cycle ergometer, elliptical, rower, or treadmill for walking.
Barriers	• Lack of time to exercise • Lack of motivation • Poor health • Fear of injury
Interventions	• Patients should participate in a medically supervised Cardiac Rehabilitation Program to ensure safety and promote lifestyle change adherence. • Promote independent exercise once patient reports stable or absent cardiac symptoms, appropriate physiological response to exercise, demonstrates a knowledge and confidence with exercise principles, and demonstrates motivation to continue exercise. • Light resistance training programs should be introduced with slow progression. • For return to work, implement exercise training aimed at improving necessary energy systems used for occupational tasks. • Reference Table 8.9 for effective behavior change techniques
Take-Home Message	• PA is a well-established factor in the prevention and management of heart disease (44). • People with cardiovascular disease should be appropriately cleared for exercise and be assigned to an individualized program that is progressive in nature. • There is a very important need to promote PA among adults who may be at risk for cardiovascular disease or who may be in the early stages of the disease. Beginning a progressive PA program can help to prevent the disease and manage related risk factors.
Web links	• The Heart and Stroke Foundation: http://www.heartandstroke.on.ca/site/c.pvI3IeNWJwE/b.5264885/k.F930/Position_Statements__Physical_Activity_Heart_Disease_and_Stroke.htm • The American Heart Association: http://www.heart.org/HEARTORG/GettingHealthy/PhysicalActivity/Physical-Activity_UCM_001080_SubHomePage.jsp

Source: Booth, Bauman, Owen, Core, 2007 (4); American College of Sports Medicine. *ACSM's Guidelines for Exercise Testing and Prescription*. 9th ed. Baltimore (MD): Lippincott Williams and Wilkins; 2014.

including the management of the potential negative long-term effects of treatment (25,38). Research indicates that the sooner cancer survivors reestablish or improve upon prediagnosis PA levels, the more likely they are to report both physical and psychosocial benefits. These individuals may also exhibit fewer symptoms, less comorbidities, and decreased all-cause mortality (17,23).

BARRIERS

Despite the evidence mentioned earlier, there is a notable decrease in PA across the cancer continuum (11). This decreased PA may be associated with increased perceived barriers to participation, both similar to those seen in the general population (*e.g.,* lack of motivation and time, limited access) as well as health-related barriers such as pain and stiffness from surgery, treatment-related side-effects such as fatigue and nausea, self-consciousness related to surgery (*e.g.,* mastectomies), and a fear of overdoing it without proper direction (45). Offering cancer survivors an individualized exercise program in a supportive environment can alleviate many of these potential barriers. See Table 8.9 for additional behavior change techniques.

RECOMMENDATIONS

The recent ACSM roundtable on Exercise Guidelines for Cancer Survivors concluded that exercise is both safe and potentially beneficial during and after cancer treatments (36). Current recommendations from ACSM can be seen in Tables 8.12 through 8.14. These guidelines should be implemented within tailored exercise programs, based on the individual's current health and treatment status. Table 8.15 outlines effective interventions and evidence-based strategies for PA adoption among cancer survivors.

In addition, the research suggests that the timing of the exercise intervention is important. It is suggested that while regular exercise may improve outcomes during treatment, it may provide greater noticeable benefits to the survivor when performed post-treatment (11). This may be a reflection of patients' treatment completion and the removal of barriers (*i.e.,* medical demands, time, and fatigue). ACSM roundtable guidelines suggest that cancer survivors, regardless of where they are in the treatment continuum, should avoid inactivity and that any level of PA carries with it some benefit (36). It has been further suggested that interventions should include multiple options based on participant preferences (33).

Useful Links

Refer to the following Web sites on this topic for more information:

- ACS Guidelines on Nutrition and Physical Activity for Cancer Prevention: http://www.cancer.org/Healthy/EatHealthyGetActive/ACSGuidelinesonNutritionPhysicalActivityforCancerPrevention/nupa-guidelines-toc
- Canadian Society of Exercise Physiology: Older Adult Cancer Survivors and Exercise: http://www.csep.ca/english/view.asp?x=724 & id=181
- The National Cancer Institute: Physical Activity and Cancer http://www.cancer.gov/cancertopics/factsheet/prevention/physicalactivity

TABLE 8.12 ACSM Guidelines for PA Levels for Cancer Survivors: Preexercise medical assessments and exercise testing

Cancer Site	Breast	Prostate	Colon	Adult Hematologic (No HSCT)	Adult HSCT	Gynecologic
General medical recommended before exercise	Recommend evaluation for peripheral neuropathies and musculoskeletal morbidities secondary to treatment regardless of time since treatment. If there has been hormonal therapy, recommend evaluation of fracture risk. Individuals with known metastatic disease to the bone will require evaluation to discern what is safe before starting exercise. Individuals with known cardiac conditions (secondary to cancer or not) require medical assessment of the safety of exercise before starting. There is always a risk that metastasis to the bone or cardiac toxicity secondary to cancer treatments will be undetected. This risk will vary widely across the population of survivors. Fitness professionals may want to consult with the patient's medical team to discern this likelihood. However, requiring medical assessment for metastatic disease and cardiotoxicity for all survivors before exercise is not recommended because this would create an unnecessary barrier to obtaining the well-established health benefits of exercise for the majority of survivors, for whom metastasis and cardiotoxicity are unlikely to occur.					
Cancer site-specific medical assessments recommended before starting an exercise program	Recommend evaluation for arm/shoulder morbidity before upper body exercise.	Evaluation of muscle strength and wasting.	Patient should be evaluated as having established consistent and proactive infection prevention behaviors for an existing ostomy before engaging in exercise training more vigorous than a walking program.	None	None	Morbidly obese patients may require additional medical assessment for the safety of activity beyond cancer-specific risk. Recommend evaluation for lower extremity lymphedema before vigorous aerobic exercise or resistance training.
Exercise testing recommended	No exercise testing required before walking, flexibility, or resistance training. Follow ACSM guidelines for exercise testing before moderate to vigorous aerobic exercise training. One-repetition maximum testing has been demonstrated to be safe in breast cancer survivors with and at risk for lymphedema.					
Exercise testing mode and intensity considerations	As per outcome of medical assessments and following ACSM guidelines for exercise testing.					
Contraindications to exercise testing and reasons to stop exercise testing	Follow ACSM guidelines for exercise testing.					

Reprinted with permission from Schmitz et al., 2010 (36), see also American College of Sports Medicine. *ACSM's Guidelines for Exercise Testing and Prescription.* 9th ed. Baltimore (MD): Lippincott Williams and Wilkins; 2014.

TABLE 8.13 ACSM Guidelines for PA Levels for Cancer Survivors: Exercise Prescription for Cancer Survivors

	Breast	Prostate	Colon	Adult Hematologic (No HSCT)	Adult HSCT	Gynecologic
Objectives/goals of exercise prescription	1. To regain and improve physical function, aerobic capacity, strength, and flexibility. 2. To improve body image and QOL. 3. To improve body composition. 4. To improve cardiorespiratory, endocrine, neurological, muscular, cognitive, and psychosocial outcomes. 5. Potentially, to reduce or delay recurrence or a second primary cancer. 6. To improve the ability to physically and psychologically withstand the ongoing anxiety regarding recurrence or a second primary cancer. 7. To reduce, attenuate, and prevent long-term and late effects of cancer treatment. 8. To improve the physiologic and psychological ability to withstand any current or future cancer treatments. These goals will vary according to where the survivor is in the continuum of cancer experience.					
General contraindications for starting an exercise program common across all cancer sites	Allow adequate time to heal after surgery. The number of weeks required for surgical recovery may be as high as 8. Do not exercise individuals who are experiencing extreme fatigue, anemia, or ataxia. Follow ACSM guidelines for exercise prescription concerning cardiovascular and pulmonary contraindications for starting an exercise program. However, the potential for an adverse cardiopulmonary event might be higher among cancer survivors than age-matched comparisons given the toxicity of radiotherapy and chemotherapy and long-term/late effects of cancer surgery.					
Cancer-specific contraindications for starting an exercise program	Women with immediate arm or shoulder problems secondary to breast cancer treatment should seek medical care to resolve those issues before exercise training with the upper body.	None	Physician permission recommended for patients with an ostomy before participation in contact sports (risk of blow) and weight training (risk of hernia).	None	None	Women with swelling or inflammation in the abdomen, groin, or lower extremity should seek medical care to resolve these issues before exercise training with the lower body.
Cancer-specific reasons for stopping an exercise program. (Note: General ACSM guidelines for stopping exercise remain in place for this population.)	Changes in arm/shoulder symptoms or swelling should result in reductions or avoidance of upper body exercise until after appropriate medical evaluation and treatment resolves the issue.	None	Hernia, ostomy-related systemic infection.	None	None	Changes in swelling or inflammation of the abdomen, groin, or lower extremities should result in reductions or avoidance of lower body exercise until after appropriate medical evaluation and treatment resolves the issue.

continued

TABLE 8.13 ACSM Guidelines for PA Levels for Cancer Survivors: Exercise Prescription for Cancer Survivors (*Continued*)

	Breast	Prostate	Colon	Adult Hematologic (No HSCT)	Adult HSCT	Gynecologic
General injury risk issues in common across cancer sites	Patients with bone metastases may need to alter their exercise program concerning intensity, duration, and mode given increased risk for skeletal fractures. Infection risk is higher for patients who are currently undergoing chemotherapy or radiation treatment or have compromised immune function after treatment. Care should be taken to reduce infection risk in fitness centers frequented by cancer survivors. Exercise tolerance of patients currently in treatment and immediately after treatment may vary from exercise session-to-exercise session about exercise tolerance, depending on their treatment schedule. Individuals with known metastatic disease to the bone will require modifications and increased supervision to avoid fractures. Individuals with cardiac conditions (secondary to cancer or not) will require modifications and may require increased supervision for safety.					
Cancer-specific risk of injury and emergency procedures	The arms/shoulders should be exercised, but proactive injury prevention approaches are encouraged, given the high incidence of arm/shoulder morbidity in breast cancer survivors. Women with lymphedema should wear a well-fitting compression garment during exercise. Be aware of risk for fracture among those treated with hormonal therapy, a diagnosis of osteoporosis, or bony metastases.	Be aware of risk for fracture among patients treated with ADT, a diagnosis of osteoporosis or bony metastases	Advisable to avoid excessive intra-abdominal pressures for patients with an ostomy.	Multiple myeloma patients should be treated as if they have osteoporosis.	None	The lower body should be exercised, but proactive injury prevention approaches are encouraged, given the potential for lower extremity swelling or inflammation in this population. Women with lymphedema should wear a well-fitting compression garment during exercise. Be aware of risk for fractures among those treated with hormonal therapies, with diagnosed osteoporosis, or with bony metastases.

Reprinted with permission from Schmitz et al., 2010 (36), see also American College of Sports Medicine. *ACSM's Guidelines for Exercise Testing and Prescription*. 9th ed. Baltimore (MD): Lippincott Williams and Wilkins; 2014.

TABLE 8.14 ACSM Guidelines for PA Levels for Cancer Survivors: Review of US DHHS PAG for Americans and Alterations Needed for Cancer Survivors

	Breast	Prostate	Colon	Adult Hematologic (No HSCT)	Adult HSCT	Gynecologic
General statement	Avoid inactivity; return to normal daily activities as quickly as possible after surgery. Continue normal daily activities and exercise as much as possible during and after nonsurgical treatments. Individuals with known metastatic bone disease will require modifications to avoid fractures. Individuals with cardiac conditions (secondary to cancer or not) may require modifications and may require greater supervision for safety.					
Aerobic exercise training (volume, intensity, and progression)	Recommendations are the same as age-appropriate guidelines from the PAG for Americans.				Ok to exercise everyday: lighter intensity and lower progression of intensity recommended.	Recommendations are the same as age-appropriate guidelines from the PAG for Americans. Morbidly obese women may require additional supervision and altered programming.
Cancer site-specific comments on aerobic exercise training prescriptions	Be aware of fracture risk.	Be aware of increased potential for fracture.	Physician permission recommended for patients with an ostomy before participation in contact sports (risk of blow).	None	Care should be taken to avoid overtraining given immune effects of vigorous exercise.	If peripheral neuropathy is present, a stationary bike might be preferable over weight bearing exercise.
Resistance training (volume, intensity, and progression)	Altered recommendations. See below.		Recommendations are the same as age-appropriate PAG.	Altered recommendations. See below.	Recommendations are the same as age-appropriate PAG	Altered recommendations. See below.

continued

TABLE 8.14 ACSM Guidelines for PA Levels for Cancer Survivors: Review of US DHHS PAG for Americans and Alterations Needed for Cancer Survivors (*Continued*)

	Breast	Prostate	Colon	Adult Hematologic (No HSCT)	Adult HSCT	Gynecologic
Cancer site-specific comments on resistance training prescription	Start with a supervised program of at least 16 sessions and very low resistance; progress resistance at small increments. No upper limit on the amount of weight to which survivors can progress. Watch for arm/shoulder symptoms, including lymphedema, and reduce resistance or stop specific exercises according to symptom response. If a break is taken, back off the level of resistance by 2 wk worth for every week of no exercise (e.g., a 2-wk exercise vacation = back off to resistance used 4 wk ago). Be aware of risk for fracture in this population.	Add pelvic floor exercises for those who undergo radical prostatectomy. Be aware of risk for fracture.	Recommendations are the same as age-appropriate PAG. For patients with a stoma, start with low resistance and progress resistance slowly to avoid herniation at the stoma.	None	Resistance training might be more important than aerobic exercise in bone marrow transplant patients. See text for further discussion on this point.	There are no data on the safety of resistance training in women with lower limb lymphedema secondary to gynecologic cancer. This condition is very complex to manage. It may not be possible to extrapolate from the findings on upper limb lymphedema. Proceed with caution if the patient has had lymph node removal and/or radiation to lymph nodes in the groin.

Flexibility training (volume, intensity, and progression)	Recommendations are the same as age-appropriate PAG for Americans		Recommendations are the same as age-appropriate PAG, with care to avoid excessive intraabdominal pressure for patients with ostomies.	Recommendations are the same as age-appropriate PAG for Americans		
Exercises with special considerations (e.g., yoga, organized sports, and Pilates)	Yoga seems safe as long as arm and shoulder morbidities are taken into consideration. Dragon boat racing not empirically tested, but the volume of participants provides face validity of safety for this activity. No evidence on organized sport or Pilates.	Research gap	If an ostomy is present, modifications will be needed for swimming or contact sports. Research gap.	Research gap	Research gap	Research gap

Reprinted with permission from Schmitz et al., 2010 (36), see also American College of Sports Medicine. *ACSM's Guidelines for Exercise Testing and Prescription*. 9th ed. Baltimore (MD): Lippincott Williams and Wilkins; 2014.

TABLE 8.15 Successful Interventions and Strategies: PA Interventions for Cancer Survivors

Intervention	Methods	Practical Strategies
PA and nutrition guidelines and recommendations for cancer survivors (15)	• Overview of the literature in nutrition and PA interventions; provides recommendations	• ACS guidelines for nutrition and PA cancer prevention also recommended in survivorship • Precautions/contraindications to exercise provided
Rationale and strategies for promoting PA within the medical system (23)	• Provides rationale for PA interventions and approaches to promote successful adoption and maintenance of PA	• Give PA counseling during treatment, by health care providers (HCPs), and oncologists in particular. • Tailor exercise programs—start (during or after treatment); group versus alone; home versus supervised; delivery options (mail, phone, Web-based). • Increase oncologist knowledge and discussion of PA for cancer survivors. • Increase insurance coverage. • Increase number of certified fitness professionals to counsel/exercise cancer survivors.

Oleg Mikhaylov/ Shutterstock.coma

Case Scenario 8.3

Name: Michael Johnson

Age: 45

Presentation: Michael was diagnosed with a carcinoma on the base of his tongue 3 months ago, and finished chemotherapy and radiation treatments 3 weeks ago. Michael reports extreme fatigue, a lack of energy, and a total weight loss of 45 lbs. He notices large deficits in his muscular strength and endurance and says that he even struggles to get up from a chair due to the great muscle wasting in his legs. His pain management is improving, but he struggles with frequent dry mouth due to treatment-related salivary gland damage. Michael wants to increase his strength and energy, but is concerned that he will increase his fatigue with exercise and produce more stiffness in his neck.

Case Scenario 8.3 *continued*

Case Scenario 8.3 Step-by-Step

Screen	Evaluate and Educate	Test	Implement	Progress
Michael has been cleared by a physician to participate in progressive exercise. He brought a signed and completed PARmed-X form to his initial assessment. Therefore, move on to evaluate goals and motivations for PA participation.	Michael's goal is to increase his energy levels, manage his fatigue, and improve his muscular strength and endurance so he can return to work. He is provided with education pertaining to safe exercise for cancer survivors and is told that much of the weight he lost was muscle, and with commitment, he can regain his strength and improve his energy levels.	Michael has general anthropometric measurements taken, and his muscular strength and endurance is evaluated using a handgrip dynamometer and a 30-second sit-to-stand test. Michael's predictive aerobic capacity is measured with a 6-minute walk test.	Prescription: • Michael will begin with a progressive strength training and stretching program to help him rebuild wasted muscle and regain range of motion in his neck and shoulders. • Michael begins with a trainer two times per week and does his strength training and stretching once/week at home. • Michael will record activity in an online log. • He is encouraged to bring water to exercise to prevent excessive dry mouth.	• Michael will hand in journal log to trainer each week. • Program will be

TAKE-HOME MESSAGE

The research on PA for cancer survivors clearly indicates both physical and psychosocial benefits. The majority of the evidence supports the role of PA for after treatment completion. However, during-treatment programs of low to moderate intensity may be beneficial in mitigating many of the detrimental treatment-related side-effects. Exercise practitioners are highly encouraged to work within a multidisciplinary health care team when delivering PA interventions to cancer survivors.

ADDITIONAL POPULATION CONSIDERATIONS—SOCIAL INFLUENCES ON EXERCISE

Numerous social influences, from social support and the role of influential others to the role of social norms, may impact individuals' PA behavior, including both the initiation and maintenance of PA. At the individual level, the role of social support on PA behavior should be considered when tailoring an intervention. Specifically, the social support needs and preferences for an individual (*e.g.,* working out with others or alone; having instrumental support for getting started) should be considered. Second, consideration should be given to the role of influential others for the targeted population. For example, peers are an important source of significant others for children. For older adults as well as for individuals with chronic disease, health care professionals can play an influential role in both prescribing and advocating for PA. Third, at a population level, cultural norms are an important consideration when planning PA interventions. The cultural norm, or what is considered acceptable behavior for a population, along with group customs and values, can greatly impact PA participation rates. Different cultures may also require translation services, or access to programming within a culture's geographic environment (*i.e.,* delivery of a PA program for Hispanic seniors in a Spanish Cultural Center). When working with specific cultural populations, it is important to take these values and societal norms into consideration in order to develop the most appropriate intervention. Finally, the social environment, including the role of the PA leader and the cohesiveness within a group exercise environment, can be important considerations when delivering population-based PA interventions. Well-trained leaders, with expertise/certification in working with a specific population and utilizing positive and socially supportive leadership styles, will positively impact PA adherence.

CONCLUSIONS

Every population will experience different barriers to PA participation, but it is important to remember that many barriers are modifiable. An exercise specialist can help to tailor a PA program so it is manageable, safe, and tolerated, and help clients create strategies to overcome perceived barriers.

Due to the well-documented benefits of PA for various populations, future interventions focused on strategies that promote PA maintenance are required to help people adopt long-term active lifestyles, therefore improving quality of life, decreasing disease-related risk factors, and benefiting from the associated cost-effectiveness of a long-term physically active lifestyle (16,28).

REFERENCES

1. American College of Sports Medicine. *ACSM's Guidelines for Exercise Testing and Prescription*. 9th ed. Baltimore (MD): Lippincott Williams and Wilkins; 2014.
2. Baranowski T, Bouchard C, Baror O, et al. Assessment, prevalence, and cardiovascular benefits of physical activity and fitness in youth. *Medicine & Science in Sports & Exercise*. 1992;24:237–47.
3. Bayles CM, Chan S, Robare J. Frailty. In: Durstine JL, Moore GE, Painter PL, Roberts SO, editors. *ACSM's Exercise Management for Persons with Chronic Diseases and Disabilities*. 3rd ed. Champaign (IL): Human Kinetics; 2009. p. 201–8.
4. Booth M, Bauman A, Owen N, Core C. Physical activity preferences, preferred sources of assistance, and perceived barriers to increased activity among physically inactive Australians. *Preventative Medicine*. 1997;26:131–7.
5. Borschmann K, Moore K, Russell M, Ledgerwood K, Renehan E, Lin X. Overcoming barriers to physical activity among culturally and linguistically diverse older adults: a randomized controlled trial. *Australasian Journal on Aging*. 2010 Jun;29(2):77–80.
6. Centers for Disease Control and Prevention. *Youth Risk Behavior Surveillance–United States, 2009*. Department of Health and Human Services, Centers for Disease Control and Prevention, 2010. 26 p. Available from: http://www.cdc.gov/mmwr/pdf/ss/ss5905.pdf.
7. Centers for Disease Control and Prevention Web site [Internet]. Atlanta (GA): Centers for Disease Control and Prevention; [cited 2011 August 15]. Available from: http://www.cdc.gov/physicalactivity/everyone/guidelines/index.html.
8. Ibid.
9. Chen YM. Perceived barriers to physical activity among older adults residing in long-term care institutions. *Journal of Clinical Nursing*. 2010; 19: 432–9.
10. Chodzko-Zajko WJ, Proctor DN, Singh, MAF, et al. Exercise and physical activity for older adults. *Medicine & Science in Sports & Exercise*. July 2009;41(7):1510–30.
11. Courneya KS, Friedenreich CM. Physical activity and cancer control. *Seminars in Oncology Nursing*. 2007;23(4):242–52.
12. De Onis M, Blossner M, Borghi E. Global prevalence and trends of overweight and obesity among preschool children. *American Journal of Clinical Nutrition*. 2010;92:1257–64.
13. Department of Health and Human Services Web site [Internet]. Washington (D.C.): Administration on Aging; [cited 2011 August 10]. Available from: http://www.aoa.gov/AoARoot/Aging_Statistics/index.aspx.
14. Donnelly JE, Blair SN, Jakicic JM, Manore MM, Rankin JW, Smith BK. Appropriate physical activity intervention strategies for weight loss and prevention of weight regain for adults. *Medicine & Science in Sports & Exercise February*. 2009;41(2):459–71.
15. Doyle C, Kushi L, Byers T, Courneya, K, et al. Nutrition and physical activity during and after cancer treatment: An American Cancer Society guide for informed choices. *CA Cancer J Clin*. 2006;56:323–53.
16. Fjeldsoe B, Neuhaus M, Winkler E, Eakin E. Systematic review of maintenance of behavior change following physical activity and dietary interventions. *Health Psychology*. 2011;30(1):99–109.
17. Gillison FB, Skevington SM, Sato A, Standage M, Evangelidou S. The effects of exercise interventions on quality of life in clinical and healthy populations: A meta-analysis. *Soc Sci Med*. 2009;68(9):1700–10.
18. Gourlan MJ, Trouilloud DO, Sarrazin PG. Interventions promoting physical activity among obese populations: A meta-analysis considering global effect, long-term maintenance, physical activity indicators and dose characteristics. *Obesity Reviews*. 2011;12: e633–45.
19. Hacker E. Exercise and quality of life: Strengthening the connections. *Clin J Oncol Nurs*. 2009 Feb;13(1):31–9.
20. Haskell WL, Lee IM, Pate RR, et al. Physical activity and public health: Updated recommendation for adults from the American College of Sports Medicine and the American Heart Association. *Med Sci Sports Exercise*. 2007;39(8):1423–34.
21. Hayes SC, Spence RR, Galvao, Newton, RU. Australian Association for Exercise and Sport Science position stand: Optimising cancer outcomes through exercise. *J Sci Med Sport*. 2009;12(4):428–34.
22. Huhman M, Potter L, Duke J, Judkins D, Heitzler C, Wong F. Evaluation of a national physical activity intervention for children: VERB campaign, 2002–2004. *American Journal of Preventative Medicine*. 2007;32:38–43.
23. Irwin ML. Physical activity interventions for cancer survivors. *Br J Sports Med*. 2009 Jan;43(1):32–38.
24. King A. Interventions to promote physical activity by older adults. *Journal of Gerontology*. 2001;58A:36–46.
25. Knobf MT, Musanti R, Dorward J. Exercise and quality of life outcomes in patients with cancer. *Semin Oncol Nurs*. 2007 Nov;23(4):285–96.
26. Kumanyika S. Obesity treatment in minorities. In: Wadden TA, Stunkard AJ, editors. *Obesity: Theory and Therapy*. 3rd ed. New York: Guilford Publications, Inc.; 2002. p. xiii–377.
27. McAuley E, Morris K, Motl R, Hu L, Konopack J, Elvasky S. Long-term follow-up of physical activity behavior in older adults. *Health Psychology*. 2007;26:375–80.
28. Muller-Riemenschneider F, Reinhold T, Willich SN. Cost-effectiveness of interventions promoting physical activity. *British Journal of Sports Medicine*. 2009;43:70–6.
29. Nelson ME, Rejeski WJ, Blair SN, et al. Physical activity and public health in older adults: recommendations from the American college of sports medicine and the American heart

association. *Medicine & Science in Sports & Exercise.* 2007;39(8):1435–45.

30. O'dea JA. Why do kids eat healthful food? Perceived benefits of and barriers to healthful eating and physical activity among children and adolescents. *Journal of the American Dietetic Association.* 2003;103(4):497–500.
31. Pangrazi R, Beighle A, Vehige T, Vack C. Impact of promoting lifestyle activity for youth (PLAY) on children's physical activity. *Journal of School Health.* 2003;73:317–21.
32. Pate R, Pfeiffer K, Trost S, Ziegler P, Dowda M. Physical activity among children attending preschools. *Pediatrics.* 2004;144:1258–63.
33. Rogers LQ, Markwell SJ, Verhulst S, McAuley E, Courneya KS. Rural breast cancer survivors: Exercise preferences and their determinants. *Psychooncology.* 2009 Apr;18(4):412–21.
34. Sallinen J, Leinonen R, Hirvensalo M, Lyyra TM, Heikkinen E, Rantanen T. Perceived constraints on physical exercise among obese and non-obese older people. *Preventative Medicine.* 2009;49:506–10.
35. Sallis JF, McKenzie TL, Alcaraz JE, Kolody B, Faucette N, Hovell MF. The effects of a 2-year physical education program (SPARK) on physical activity and fitness I elementary school students. *American Journal of Public Health.* 1997;87:1328–34.
36. Schmitz KH, Courneya KS, Matthews C, et al. American College of Sports Medicine roundtable on exercise guidelines for cancer survivors. *Med Sci Sports Exercise.* 2010 Jul;42(7):1409–26.
37. Speck RM, Courneya KS, Masse LC, Duval S, Schmitz KH. An update of controlled physical activity trials in cancer survivors: A systematic review and meta-analysis. *Journal of Cancer Survivorship.* 2010;4(2):87–100.
38. Speed-Andrews AE, Courneya KS. Effects of exercise on quality of life and prognosis in cancer survivors. *Curr Sports Med Rep.* 2009 Jul–Aug;8(4):176–81.
39. Stone W. Physical activity and health: Becoming mainstream. *Complementary Health Practice Review.* 2004;9:118–28.
40. Strauss RS, Pollack HA. Epidemic increase in childhood overweight, 1986–1998. *Journal of the American Medical Association.* 2001;286(22):2845–48.
41. Telama R, Yang X, Laakso L, Vikari J. Physical activity in childhood and adolescence as predictor of physical activity in young adulthood. *American Journal of Preventative Medicine.* 1997;13:317–23.
42. Tomporowski P, Lambourne K, Okumura M. Physical activity interventions and children's mental function: An introduction and overview. *Preventative Medicine.* 2001;52:S3–S9.
43. U.S. Department of Health and Human Service Web site [Internet]. Washington (D.C.): 2008 Physical Activity Guidelines For Americans; [cited 2011 August 15]. ODPHP Publication No. U0036. Available from: www.health.gov/paguidelines/.
44. Wang G, Pratt M, Macera CA, Zheng XJ, Heath G. Physical activity, cardiovascular disease, and medical expenditures in U.S. adults. *Ann Behav Med.* 2004;28(2):88–94.
45. Whitehead S, Lavelle K. Older breast cancer survivors' views and preferences for physical activity. *Qualitative Health Research.* 2009;19:894–906.
46. Williams MA, Haskell WL, Ades PA, et al. Resistance exercise in individuals with and without cardiovascular disease: 2007 update: A scientific statement from the American heart association council on clinical cardiology and council on nutrition, physical activity, and metabolism. *Circulation.* 2007;116:572–84.
47. World Health Organization Web site [Internet]. Geneva (Switzerland): Obesity and Overweight: Fact sheet number 311; [cited 2011 August 15]. Available from: http://www.who.int/mediacentre/factsheets/fs311/en/index.html.
48. Yancey A, Ory M, Davis S. Dissemination of physical activity promotion interventions in underserved populations. *American Journal of Preventative Medicine.* 2006;31:82–91.
49. Zabinski MF, Saelens BE, Stein RI, Hayden-Wade HA, Wilfley DE. Overweight children's barriers to and support for physical activity. *Obesity Research.* 2003;11:238–56.
50. Zoeller RF. Physical activity: Depression, anxiety, physical activity and cardiovascular disease: What's the connection? *American Journal of Lifestyle Medicine.* 2007;1:175–80.

CHAPTER 9

Evaluating Physical Activity Behavior Change Programs and Practices

Paul A. Estabrooks, Kacie Allen, Erin Smith, Blake Krippendorf, and Serena L. Parks

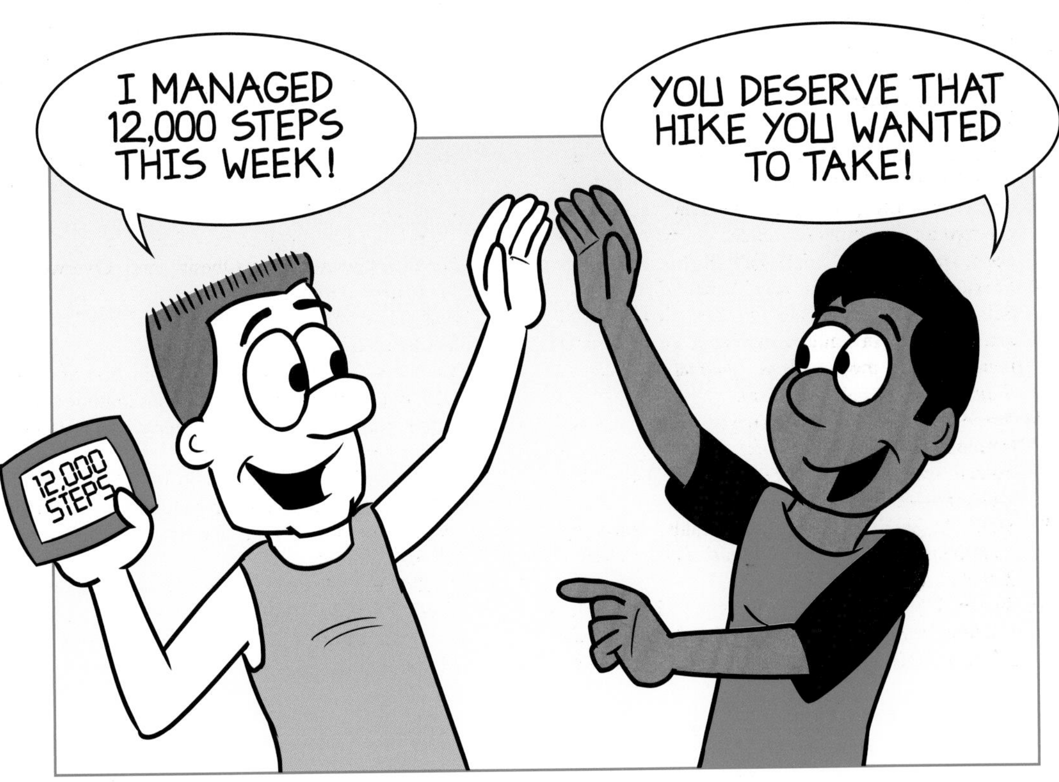
I MANAGED 12,000 STEPS THIS WEEK!
YOU DESERVE THAT HIKE YOU WANTED TO TAKE!
12,000 STEPS

CONCEPT OVERVIEW

As you have progressed through this book, you have read about a number of key factors to be considered when developing a program to change physical activity behavior. It's likely that you've identified a number of new strategies that you are going to put into practice with your own clients. It's also possible you may want to try some new things that require more resources than you currently have, that require approval from a supervisor, or might make your work a little more time-intensive. In these cases, it is critical to have a good evaluation to demonstrate that your changes make a big difference in your work.

This chapter is intended to help you, as you move forward, with your physical activity promotion plans, and demonstrate the value of any changes you are intending to implement, or to simply demonstrate the value of your current approach. You may notice that the use of the term "value of your program" rather than a term like "effectiveness of your program." Whether you are in business for yourself, working for a public health organization, or delivering care in a clinic or rehabilitation center, you will want to demonstrate your ability to be effective. However, while demonstrating the effectiveness of a physical activity program is necessary, it is not always sufficient to ensure that a community or clinical strategy will be adopted and sustained by the organizations or health professionals that are interested in delivering it (2,23).

This chapter focuses on planning and evaluating your work based on the RE-AIM framework, and will highlight program aspects (including effectiveness) that, if optimized, will greatly improve your chances of ongoing success (22,31,38). As depicted in Figure 9.1, running a program usually involves a number of steps beginning with determining need, planning program characteristics and targets based upon that need, implementing the program, and evaluating it for success. In most cases, these steps can be approached in a linear way when developing a new program or when activity updating an existing program. A useful source for physical activity program planning is "Exercise is Medicine" (see http://exerciseismedicine.org/fitpros.html). The Web site

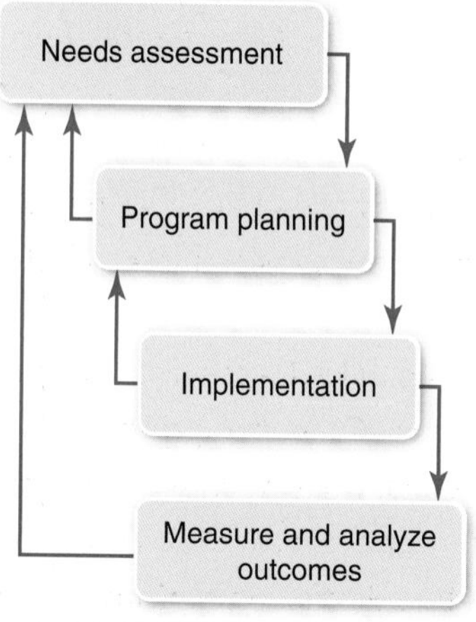

FIGURE 9.1. Running a program.

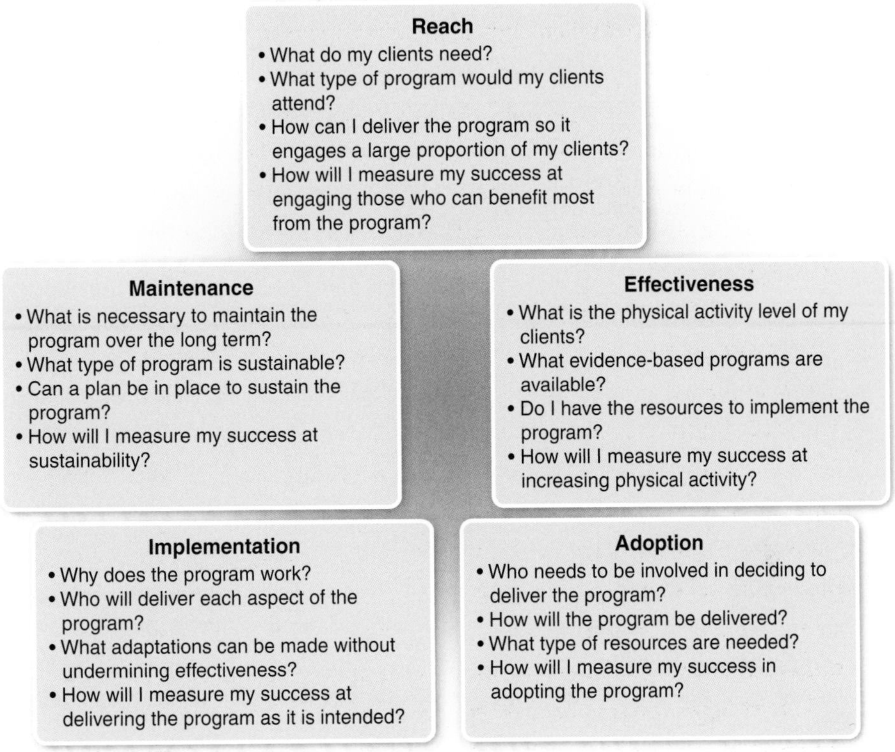

Reach
- What do my clients need?
- What type of program would my clients attend?
- How can I deliver the program so it engages a large proportion of my clients?
- How will I measure my success at engaging those who can benefit most from the program?

Maintenance
- What is necessary to maintain the program over the long term?
- What type of program is sustainable?
- Can a plan be in place to sustain the program?
- How will I measure my success at sustainability?

Effectiveness
- What is the physical activity level of my clients?
- What evidence-based programs are available?
- Do I have the resources to implement the program?
- How will I measure my success at increasing physical activity?

Implementation
- Why does the program work?
- Who will deliver each aspect of the program?
- What adaptations can be made without undermining effectiveness?
- How will I measure my success at delivering the program as it is intended?

Adoption
- Who needs to be involved in deciding to deliver the program?
- How will the program be delivered?
- What type of resources are needed?
- How will I measure my success in adopting the program?

FIGURE 9.2. RE-AIM and program development questions.

includes resources for marketing, planning exercise programs with a client, and other materials for both clients and organizations.

The RE-AIM framework (Figure 9.2) has been developed for both research and practice professionals who are interested in determining the public health impact of their work. It outlines that practitioners should assess the *R*each of their work, its *E*ffectiveness, how well it can be *A*dopted in other settings or by professionals with differing levels of expertise, the degree to which it can be *I*mplemented appropriately (and its cost), and finally, the degree to which the strategies can be *M*aintained in your practice. Table 9.1 includes a definition of each of the dimensions and gives an example of the type of information that is necessary to evaluate your physical activity program. It also includes an example from some of our previous research that depicts how the information could be reported.

You will notice that some of the RE-AIM dimensions, like Reach and Effectiveness, focus on the clients who would benefit from your expertise. Other components, like Adoption and Implementation, focus on organizational factors, while Maintenance can pertain to either the individual level (*i.e.*, how long the effects of an intervention last) or organizational level (*i.e.*, how long the program or practice can be delivered or implemented over time).

TABLE 9.1 RE-AIM Definitions, Data Requirements, and Examples from Research

Dimension and Definition	Data Requirements	Example Study and Outcomes
REACH: The number, percent of target audience, and representativeness of those who participate.	Denominator—number of eligible people contacted for potential participation Numerator—number of eligible people that participate Comparative information on target population	Improving the Reach of Move More (2) Goal: To increase participation in a clinic-based physical activity program using physician prompts. Denominator—11 patient referrals/week Numerator—8 patients agreed to participate/week Participation Rate—72% Representativeness—Based on census data of the clinical catchment area, the participants were older and more likely to be women.
EFFECTIVENESS: Change in primary outcome; impact on quality of life; any adverse outcomes	Before and after assessments of primary outcome (PO), quality of life (QOL), and potential negative outcomes (PNO)	Family Connections to Reduce Childhood Obesity (23,46) Goal: To reduce weight status of obese children by providing parents with automated telephone counseling that promoted changes to the home environment. PO: Significant reductions in BMI z-score. QOL: Improvement in quality of life with lower weight status. PNO: No evidence of heightened eating disordered symptoms
ADOPTION: Number, percent, and representativeness of settings and practitioners who participate	Denominator—number of eligible sites/practitioners Numerator—number of eligible sites/practitioners that participate Comparative information on target population of sites/practitioners	Walk Kansas (19,20) Goal: To increase physical activity through a group-based physical activity program delivered at the county level. Denominator—105 counties in Kansas Numerator—48 counties delivered the program Participation rate—46%

TABLE 9.1 RE-AIM Definitions, Data Requirements, and Examples from Research (*Continued*)

Dimension and Definition	Data Requirements	Example Study and Outcomes
		Representativeness—smaller population counties, more likely to deliver. Health educators who personally participate in physical activity more likely to deliver.
IMPLEMENTATION: Extent to which a program or policy is delivered consistently, and the time and costs of the program	Information on program components and essential elements Information on resource use	Fit Extension Goal: To increase physical activity in a community. 100% of program components were delivered as intended Approximately 2.5 hours of health educator time per participant over 8 weeks.
MAINTENANCE: Long-term effects on primary outcome Program sustainability at the organizational level.	Primary outcome assessment 6 months postintervention Documented sustained delivery	Family Connections demonstrated decreased BMI z-scores that were sustained 6 months after the intervention was completed Walk Kansas documented that the percent of counties that maintained delivery of program up to 5 years postresearch studies was well over 90%.

Each of the RE-AIM dimensions can be used for both planning and evaluation purposes, so this chapter was formed around planning and evaluation information. First, issues to consider when planning and evaluating a physical activity program, practice, or policy intervention are provided, with successful examples from the research literature. Second, you will walk through the methods necessary to evaluate your physical activity program to determine the degree to which your strategies are influencing the RE-AIM metrics.

EVIDENCE

The RE-AIM framework is relatively new from a scientific perspective, introduced by Dr. Russell Glasgow and his colleagues in 1999 (31). Introductory work included a number of systematic reviews of the scientific literature to determine the degree to which researchers were providing information across the RE-AIM dimensions. Over the past 12 years, the reviews have remained consistent (14,21,30,51): Researchers are good at reporting the degree to which behavioral interventions are efficacious (*i.e.,* the degree to which an intervention works under optimal conditions), but don't do a very good job reporting information such as the representativeness of participants, characteristics and training of those delivering the interventions, time and financial costs, or the setting in which the intervention took place. Physical activity research was included in a number of these reviews and the findings were confirmed in a recent review of literature examining theory-based physical activity interventions (3). Essentially, researchers weren't reporting information that could tell practitioners if the research-based interventions and outcomes could be generalized to typical community or clinical settings, or to typical client or patient populations.

Fortunately, things are changing and, based on current research databases, approximately 30 articles have been published in the last 3 years that have explicitly used the RE-AIM framework within physical activity promotion initiatives. This chapter employs a number of these studies to summarize different strategies that can improve different dimensions of RE-AIM within different practice settings, and when possible, will distinguish between the following three general types of physical activity promotion strategies. First, and most common, are physical activity programs, which may be most beneficial to the physical activity promotion practitioner. These programs include sessions or interactions for an individual to engage in for a finite period of time. They can include, for example, in-person sessions with a personal trainer (52), small group meetings (40), Internet or print-based materials (33), or telephone counseling (16). Second, are strategies aimed at changing the environment to promote physical activity. While it is clear that many communities are in the process of adding park or trail space, improving sidewalks, or using traffic calming strategies to improve physical activity, there are relatively few experimental tests of these strategies (6,50). Third, are strategies aimed at changing policy to promote physical activity. Policy approaches represent another emerging area in physical activity promotion. Policy approaches can include the implementation of medical guidelines (17), changes to school wellness policies (4), or zoning laws (44). Few experimental studies exist that examine policy changes. In fact, if you are implementing policy and environmental changes, you can aid in the creation of evidence using the RE-AIM framework.

In each of the following sections is a list of planning strategies to optimize each of the RE-AIM dimensions in your physical activity promotion program. It is important to note, that some of the ideas for improving one dimension could have negative consequences on another dimension. A good example of this is the suggestion that program Reach can be improved by making the intervention less intensive (*e.g.*, lower frequency of meetings; low time commitment). Conversely, it has been suggested that more intensive interventions are needed to see large changes in behavior (53). More specifically, a physical activity promotion program that requires only one initial in-person meeting and follow-up telephone calls could be delivered to a lot more people than one that requires exercise classes three times per week, a 2-hour group problem-solving session every other week, and follow-up telephone calls. On the other hand, the intervention with all the exercise classes and group meetings will probably result in bigger changes in behavior but reach fewer people. We anticipate that you will encounter some of these issues as you plan your program, and our advice is to plan what you or your organization values most (*e.g.*, reach vs. effectiveness)—while still trying to optimize across dimensions when possible.

Reach

Working from the definition of Reach provided in Table 9.1, the first decision that needs to be made when planning your program is: What aspect of Reach is most important to you? In research settings, it is likely that the most important aspect of Reach is representativeness. For research evidence to be applicable to practice settings, the people that are included in a study should be representative (*i.e.*, share the same motivational, demographic, and behavioral characteristics) of those typically served in practice. In practice settings, an initiative's success is often based (a) on the appropriateness of the initiative in responding to community needs, and (b) on the total number of people that participate regardless of their current level of physical activity, race/ethnicity, or socioeconomic status, so the context of your intervention will contribute to your decision about what aspects (maybe all of them!) of Reach to target for improvement.

Think about a physician in a clinic who has 1000 patients who are not meeting the recommended guidelines for physical activity. Her goal is to get all 1000 patients to participate or benefit from her physical activity strategy. Alternatively, a community health worker may be required to have a certain quota of clients at any one time and may, therefore, focus solely on the number and characteristics of the people he works with to ensure meeting his quota. Finally, if you are offering a fee-for-service program, then understanding how to increase numbers and track characteristics to identify groups that may not be responding to your recruitment efforts is critical.

An obvious starting point to increasing Reach is to consider how you will advertise your initiative. Mass media approaches are often quite successful in bringing in participants to a physical activity program (49), but their success often depends on your resources and setting. If you are looking to be efficient with your resources, and are recruiting for your program in cities, the mass media approach can work very well; however, if you are recruiting in rural areas, often more personal (and strategic) word-of-mouth strategies work better (49). Similarly, when you are trying to recruit minority populations or groups that have health disparities, strategies that are place-based (*e.g.*, going to where the participants are) and reaching out directly to potential participants is better than flyers, posters, or other less interactive recruitment strategies (39). Furthermore, when considering the cost per participant that enrolls in your program, holding events where your target audience already aggregates is one of the least expensive ways to successfully recruit participants (36).

A less obvious approach to improving Reach is to consider the characteristics of your facility or program. In one of the authors' ongoing studies, two community-based physical activity programs were compared (26). One of the programs included an evidence-based approach where participants met as a group for 90 minutes each week for 12 weeks. The other program didn't include weekly meetings, but focused on group goal setting that was intended to bring all participants to the recommended 150 minutes per week of physical activity over an 8-week period. Results showed that the second program recruited nearly four times the number of participants when similar advertising strategies were used. The implication is that a program that has regular classes, allows participants to do activities when they want, and encourages setting goals with friends and families is more attractive (and may have less obstacles) than a program that has regular weekly meetings at a set time and location. Even more drastic improvements in Reach can be achieved by implementing policy and environmental changes. The key to improving your likelihood of a strong Reach is to determine who will consistently be exposed to the changes. For example, in the Healthy Youth Places program (an intervention that targeted increased physical activity and healthy eating in middle school children), changes in policy around a health education curriculum ensured that all students in the intervention sessions were exposed to effective strategies to promote physical activity (15).

How do you evaluate the Reach of your program? Determining the Reach includes tracking the number of participants or clients, the proportion of the target population that participates, and ensuring that you are getting participants from all sub-groups of your target population—especially those who could benefit most from your intervention or expertise. While tracking the number of participants is a straightforward process, identifying the proportion and representativeness of program participants can be a little more complex. To determine the proportion of the target population that participates, understanding the denominator is key. This can be relatively easy if your program or policy is being implemented in a defined setting (*e.g.*, health care clinic, school, church) where there is a concrete record of the number of people that could participate. In one trial to promote healthy eating, physical activity, and weight control for people at risk for diabetes, all of the patients in a health care system were included as the denominator and found that about 8% (approximately 1000 patients) were reached by our diabetes prevention efforts (1). Calculating the denominator becomes a little more challenging when your program is promoted through mass media or word-of-mouth. Still, even a reasonable estimate is valuable information, and can help to identify what types of strategies are best for getting a large proportion of your target population to participate. For example, when using newspaper or television advertisements, working with a media representative to get estimates of reader/viewership numbers can be used as a reasonable estimate for a denominator. In fact, most media outlets publish this information online to encourage advertising. An alternative method is to simply determine the number of people in your community who are eligible for your program and use that as the denominator. In Walk Kansas, a community-based physical activity program, the total adult population in the counties where the program was delivered was used as the denominator (20). In the first year the program was delivered, approximately 1% of the population (approximately 6000 people) participated. These two examples are provided to demonstrate that proportional Reach in community and clinical interventions may be very small (*e.g.*, 1%, 8%) but still indicate successful recruitment when specific participant numbers are considered.

From an environmental or policy perspective, it may be hard to deduce exactly how many individuals are affected by environmental changes (34,37); however, Reach can be estimated by determining the number of the target population exposed to the policy or environmental change. This can be calculated with a number of tools (*e.g.*, observational audits, market surveys, land use audits, etc.) (34,37,35). To determine the denominator, you can measure the total target population within a certain buffer zone of the environmental change. An example for policy change would be to identify the number of children who are in schools with a certain local wellness policy. Many databases, like the U.S. Census and geographic information systems, can provide population estimates regarding buffer zones and, in settings like schools, publicly available data on school size and child eligibility for free or reduced-price lunch (an indicator of economic status) can be used (34,37,45). Finally, to determine representativeness, completing comparisons of key characteristics of those in the targeted intervention area with those who are exposed to the environmental or policy change can help to uncover any potential gaps (see Table 9.2 for examples).

TABLE 9.2 Key Characteristics to Determine Representativeness

Demographic Characteristics	Behavioral or Health Characteristics
Age	% Moderately and Vigorously Active
Gender	% Sedentary
Race and Ethnic Background	Fitness and Strength Level
Socioeconomic Status	General Health
Education	% with or at risk of chronic conditions that can be improved through physical activity
Health Literacy Level	

Effectiveness

Within RE-AIM, the "E" can represent either efficacy or effectiveness. Efficacy refers to how well an intervention works when it is tested under optimal conditions (*e.g.*, in a university medical center). Effectiveness refers to how well an intervention works in real-world settings. Because this book is targeted toward health professionals working with participants, we will stick with the real-world version and use the term Effectiveness. Effectiveness includes not only how well your program can increase physical activity, but also the degree to which it influences the quality of life for your participants. In addition, focusing on safety is key when promoting physical activity. Recently, the American College of Sports Medicine (ACSM) published a position statement that outlines not only the recommended amount of physical activity, but also strategies to improve safety and avoid injury across different segments of the population (29). Practitioners are encouraged to review that position stand for detailed information on safety issues related to physical activity prescriptions (24).

There have been a number of systematic reviews on the Effectiveness of physical activity promotion interventions over the previous decade (7,18,35,48). Findings suggest that interventions that use behavioral approaches to tailor intervention content to participants are more successful than those that do not use tailoring. Similarly, social support or group dynamics–based interventions consistently lead to increases in physical activity. There is less evidence for physician-based counseling, unless it is partnered with community resources to support physical activity.

Related to this, improving access to physical activity resources also has a positive influence on behavior. In fact, many of the chapters in this book highlight the cutting edge of effective interventions for increasing physical activity. Understanding the relationship between policies to promote physical activity and an increase in the behavior reflects a gap in the current research base. As with Reach, when planning what strategies to employ to increase physical activity in your target population, it is important to align your activities with your organizational mission and resources. There are many effective physical activity strategies available. Take the time to find the one that is best for your situation.

As with Reach, there are a number of ways to measure the Effectiveness of your program or initiative. Your job is to determine the type of information that is likely to be sufficient for your key stakeholders (*e.g.*, funders, administrators, participants). No doubt you will want to assess changes in physical activity. But how is this done? Most community programs use self-report measures of activity before and after the program. To try and reduce the burden to participants or clients, physical activity measures (32) can be included as part of the registration documents. You may also want to introduce a direct measure of physical activity on a randomly selected subset of your participants (see Table 9.3 for examples), though this may not be practical if you are reaching a large number of participants and have limited resources.

Measuring quality of life and potential negative consequences can also be completed with brief self-report measures. Using the Center for Disease Control and Prevention's Healthy Days measure (see From the Practical Toolbox 9.1 for the measure and www.cdc.gov/hrqol/pdfs/mhd.pdf for a full description) is a good selection as it is brief (four items), and allows you to compare your program outcomes to a national sample (42). This measure can also be integrated into a registration form and follow-up assessment for your clients. Measures for potential negative outcomes can include simply tracking client injuries or changes in other health behaviors. One example could be adding physical activity promotion to an ongoing nutrition program. Measuring nutritional changes in clients before and after the new physical activity strategies are implemented can help to determine if the additions reduced the Effectiveness of the nutrition education components of the program (12).

TABLE 9.3 Possible Measures to Include When Assessing Effectiveness

Measures	Examples
Direct Physical Activity Measures	Pedometers Accelerometers
Self-reported Physical Activity Measures	International Physical Activity Questionnaire (IPAQ) Godin Leisure-Time Exercise Questionnaire (GLTEQ) Physical Activity Survey for the Elderly (PASE) Yale Physical Activity Survey (YPAS)
Quality of Life Measures	CDC Healthy Days SF-36v2 (RAND-36) Quality of Well Being Scale (QWB, QWB-SA-self-administered) Health Utilities Index (HUI)

Follow-up assessments are ideal but often difficult for community and clinical groups to complete. Your goal should be to obtain follow-up on as high a proportion of clients who begin the program as possible (*e.g.*, >70%). One way to aid in getting higher response rates to follow-up assessments is to build physical activity assessment into the intervention itself. For example, most programs include developing some form of goal setting and feedback process that includes having participants report physical activity levels periodically through the program. By using the same physical activity measure that was used on a registration form, a program can be evaluated by comparing client reports over time. The authors have found in their work that making the evaluation easy to complete by offering different methods like paper and pencil, Web-supported measures, and telephone interviews can lead to high follow-up rates. Using a stepped approach to getting follow-up assessments using these different methods always works well.

For the ongoing program, Fit Extension, all participants get a paper version of the follow-up evaluation and a link to an online version during the last week of the program. Over the 3 years this approach has been used with this first step resulting in approximately a 50% response rate. Those who don't respond receive a second step that includes an e-mail prompt with a link to the follow-up assessment. The e-mail expresses appreciation for participation, the value of evaluation to improve the program, and recognition that the participant may not have time to complete the assessment online. In the latter case, participants are told they can complete the evaluation during a follow-up telephone call that will come in a few days. This message gets on average an additional 15% of participants (up to 65%). Finally, telephone contacts are made to the remaining 35% of the participants, and an additional 10% respond, for a total response rate of about 75% of the participants.

For environmental and policy approaches, measuring Effectiveness is more difficult, but not impossible. If possible, identify an appropriate physical activity measure and observe and map the population behavior occurring before and after the environmental change (a pre- and postassessment) (37). For example, observations of community resident walking patterns can be monitored before and after a sidewalk development and improvement initiative.

For policy changes, random samples from the population exposed to the policy could be used to assess physical activity levels before and after the policy is implemented. A drawback to the random sampling is that you may miss legitimate changes in physical activity if the policy or environmental change has influenced some but not all of the population.

From the Practical Toolbox 9.1

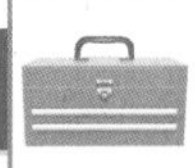

CORE HEALTHY DAYS MEASURES

1. Would you say that in general your health is excellent, very good, good, fair, or poor?
2. Now thinking about your physical health, which includes physical illness and injury, for how many days during the past 30 days was your physical health not good?
3. Now thinking about your mental health, which includes stress, depression, and problems with emotions, for how many days during the past 30 days was your mental health not good?
4. During the past 30 days, for about how many days did poor physical or mental health keep you from doing your usual activities, such as self-care, work, or recreation?

Reprinted from www.cdc.gov/hrqol/pdfs/mhd.pdf.

It may be appealing to do more strategic prepost assessments with groups that the policy or environmental change is most likely to impact. Going this route has its drawbacks, too, but as long as you document how you did the evaluation and why you made the strategic decision, you will get a clearer picture of who was (and wasn't) influenced by your change.

Planning for Adoption

Adoption is about designing an intervention to enhance its potential to be disseminated and used by various settings and delivered by staff with certain levels of expertise. If you work in an organization with multiple health professionals who could implement your intervention, then understanding how you can get each person to adopt and begin delivering the program is an important aspect of RE-AIM for you to consider. There has been very little experimental research to determine factors that influence Adoption of physical activity programs; however, there is a large body of literature that summarizes Adoption decisions in other organizational contexts (Table 9.4) (43). For some practitioners, Adoption may be a RE-AIM dimension that is of lesser relevance. Many practitioners are concerned

TABLE 9.4 Program Characteristics that Positively Influence Adoption [5]
• Low complexity (*i.e.,* not lots of different parts)
• Ease of understanding
• Compatibility with organizational norms and values
• Low need for a large organizational time commitment
• Associated with a strong evidence base that limits the risk of poor or uncertain results
• Observable in terms of results
• Easy to test out and stop if necessary
• Able to be updated and modified over time

about their own practice and focus on how to make their programs work better, reach more people, and be sustainable in their specific setting.

Adoption is also more likely to occur when incentives, training, and organizational structures are addressed (5). Aligning your physical activity program with the specific workflow of your organization will also improve Adoption. For example, adding prompts within the electronic medical record to cue physician referrals to physical activity resources in the community could improve Adoption (2). Finally, current research documents that collaborative development of a physical activity initiative with health professionals from the systems where the program is ultimately to be adopted can increase Adoption rates significantly. The underlying principle is that if the people who deliver an intervention contribute to its design, it is likely that the design will fit well in that setting and those who deliver it will feel a sense of ownership for the initiative.

When instituting an environmental or policy change, it may be helpful to consider planning and approval stages (37). Many of these changes require advanced planning, and it will be helpful to track how many organizations, residents, and members of the target population are included in the initial planning. Also, understanding what agencies and organizations approve the change, and engaging them in action steps to complete the changes, is critical. Finally, although this may go without saying, it is key in making environmental or policy changes that all those who will be influenced by the change, or needed to implement it, are included in the planning and approval process (37).

Evaluating Adoption includes many of the same considerations that were used to assess Reach—with the caveat that Adoption is at the level of the organizations and health professionals delivering a program or implementing a policy or environmental change. The 10,000 Steps Rockhampton project provides a good example of examining both practice and health professional Adoption of a physical activity program delivered through primary care practices, and also demonstrates the dynamic nature of evaluating physical activity programs (17). The researchers identified that there were 66 general practitioners in 23 clinics in Rockhampton as potential individuals and locations to deliver the program. Of course, over the course of the project new general practitioners took up practice, some ceased practice, and by the time Adoption was assessed using in-person visits to the clinics, there were 55 total general practitioners employed.

The clinical Adoption rate was very high for the project in that 21 of the 23 clinics participated. Within clinics, the proportion of general practitioners that had adopted the program was 58% (*i.e.,* 32/55). To determine representativeness of the general practitioners and clinics, the research team compared those clinics and physicians who participated on the only two publicly available characteristics, the number of physicians per clinic, and the gender of the physicians. They found that the number of physicians per clinic was the same for those that participated versus those that did not. They also showed that male and female physicians were just as likely to offer the program (17).

It is somewhat more difficult to determine the rate of Adoption and representativeness of organizations or individuals who adopt policy and environmental changes. Indeed, as noted earlier, if your focus is on a single community, a single location, or a single organization, your rate of Adoption doesn't have much meaning (*i.e.,* it will always be 100%). In these situations, it will be much more important to focus on Implementation as described in the next section. Some have suggested that the denominator in each stage of an environmental or policy intervention should be the total number of agencies and organizations invited to contribute to making the change happen, rather than those that will ultimately be responsible for implementing the strategy (37).

For instance, a researcher may invite the following organizations to help plan, approve, and implement the addition of a public playground in low-income housing: mayor's office, city legislative body, city public housing manager/department, affected citizen coalitions, residents, playground manufacturers, etc.; however, only three (the city public housing manager, residents, and playground manufacturers) may be interested in participating in each Adoption stage. The actual number of agencies participating will be the numerator (37). In these cases, it may be most helpful to divide partners into those who can contribute to planning (*e.g.*, all six contacted as the denominator; 6/6 for planning), those who can generate resources (*e.g.*, four of the six, but only three do so; 3/4 for resource generation), and those who will be involved in the implementation (*e.g.*, 3/3 as described earlier).

Implementation

Implementation is sometimes confused with organizational Adoption. The best way to distinguish between the two is to consider Adoption to be the process of deciding whether or not to deliver a program or institute a policy and initiating the first action to do so. Alternatively, Implementation is the ongoing process associated with program delivery or monitoring of policy adherence. Using the Rockhampton example from earlier, Adoption was based on the clinics and physicians that agreed to participate in each aspect of the program (17). Implementation was assessed as the degree to which they followed through on that agreement (17). The key concept associated with Implementation is that it reflects the extent to which your initiative gets put into action the way it was intended.

In one simple example, the Implementation of the WellingTONNE Challenge Toolkit—a step-by-step toolkit for health professionals and community groups to describe how to develop and implement a healthy lifestyle community intervention—was simply reported as 98% of the health professionals who received the toolkit indicated they were using it to encourage healthy lifestyle behaviors in the community (8). A more complex description of Implementation comes from the Exercise Your Options program that reported 86% of teachers indicated they delivered all eight lessons, and classroom observations confirmed that teachers were delivering between 81% and 100% of the content in each lesson (13).

There is a large body of literature on factors that facilitate or inhibit successful program Implementation (see Table 9.5) (9). Within the physical activity domain, the Well for Life trial used external program evaluators to determine positive and negative influences on program Implementation (41). In their program, which targeted older adults, they found that the presence of champions who encouraged participation, high commitment from management and staff, preexisting relationships between the Well for Life developers and health care systems, and access to funds to purchase equipment all improved Implementation. Similar to Adoption, if the benefits of Well for Life were promoted, it may have improved Implementation. Not surprisingly, time constraints and lack of staff continuity were negatively associated with Implementation (41).

School-based environmental change and policy interventions all seem to have similar barriers to successful Implementation. In the JUMP-in school-based physical activity intervention, Implementation was reduced when teacher workloads were high, there was little cooperation between schools, physical education teachers were unqualified, and when the intervention guidelines were not well understood (11). When considering environmental change interventions, it is necessary to identify standards and guidelines of the environmental change (37). This includes anticipating community concerns and backlash, barriers, and any delays that might affect costs (37).

To evaluate Implementation, you need to have a strong understanding of the specific components of your intervention or program, the resources used, and the amount of staff and time dedicated to delivering the program. The primary components of assessing Implementation are the degree to which the program is delivered as intended and the costs associated with that Implementation. At the broadest assessment of Implementation, you can simply track if all of your intervention sessions were completed. If you are using small group sessions, you could report, for instance, that 10 of 10 planned sessions were offered at the designated time. If you are using mail support or education, you could track

TABLE 9.5 Factors that Can Facilitate or Inhibit Implementation

Factors	Examples
Intervention Characteristics	The perceptions of key stakeholders regarding internally/externally developed intervention
	The quality of evidence arguing the intervention's success
	The relative advantage of implementing the intervention versus an alternative
	The adaptability of the intervention
	The perceived difficulty to implement the intervention
	The design quality and packaging of the intervention
	Intervention costs
Organization's Outer Setting	The ability of the organization to meet patient needs
	The organization's ability to network with external organizations
	Peer pressure to implement the intervention
	External policies and incentives that can spread the intervention
Organization's Inner Setting	Structural characteristics of the organization (age, size, and maturity)
	The quality of informal and formal networks within an organization:
	Organizational culture
	The implementation climate of the organization
	The readiness of the organization for program implementation
Individual Characteristics within an Organization	Attitudes and values of individuals regarding the intervention
	The individual self-efficacy to execute aspects of the program
	The individual's relationship with the intervention (which stage of use is the individual at)
	The individual's relationship with the organization
	Other attributes like personal motivation, competence, capacity, and learning styles
Process Elements	Degree of planning involved to implement the intervention, and;
	The engagement of appropriate individuals (opinion leaders, formally appointed implementation leaders, program champions, external change agents) to implement the intervention;
	The execution of the implementation according to plan
	Quantitative and qualitative feedback regarding implementation progress

the number of mailings that were delivered when intended and report the proportion of those that were not returned unopened (*e.g.*, if the address was incorrect or changed). Occasionally, this information may not be all that helpful or informative. From the authors' experience with community partners, if sessions are set up they are delivered unless there are extraordinary circumstances (*e.g.*, a snowstorm that closes roads; a printer breakdown at the office). You may find it more helpful to track the degree to which participants actually receive the program materials as indicated through class attendance or reports of getting the mailed intervention content.

Another important aspect to track in Implementation is the degree to which each program session or contact contains the content that was intended. In the Gimme 5 intervention conducted in Georgia, the Implementation evaluation involved determining how much of the intervention curriculum was delivered as intended. This determination can be completed using self-reports from the people delivering the intervention or randomized observations of classroom sessions. In Gimme 5, they found that only half of the curricular activities intended to be delivered in schools were actually implemented (10). Parents were also a key in the intervention and very few parents received the information delivered during evening classes (<10%) (10).

Tracking costs and resource use can provide useful information on areas that you may focus on to increase the efficiency of your program offerings. Cost data can be gleaned by converting salaries to per-hour costs of those implementing the intervention, determined through tracking material costs, and monitoring indirect costs (*e.g.*, space rental, air conditioning). By monitoring the cost of each program component and implementing a good effectiveness evaluation, practitioners can test out different delivery models that reduce costs without reducing effectiveness.

Evaluating the Implementation of policy and environmental changes focuses on the degree to which the environmental change is conducted according to planning documents, and a policy is applied as intended. For an environmental change, while ongoing monitoring and upkeep will likely be necessary, Implementation evaluation is typically concurrent with the completion of the environmental change. Policies, however, include plans for enforcement and ongoing compliance with the core components of the policy (34). Though somewhat burdensome, local audits in areas where the policy has been adopted can be used to determine the degree to which the policy has been implemented. Monitoring of policy evaluation language and interviews with key stakeholders can also be used to assess the degree of compliance related to policy components.

Maintenance

As with Effectiveness, there are now emerging systematic reviews on the Maintenance of individual levels of physical activity once an intervention is complete. Most recently, Fjeldsoe and colleagues examined the degree to which physical activity and dietary interventions result in maintained behavior change at least 3 months after the initial program was complete (27). About a third of all studies since 2000 included data on Maintenance and the primary findings suggested that there are a number of characteristics of interventions that could be modified to improve Maintenance. Interventions that lasted 6 months or more were more likely than shorter programs to result in maintained physical activity.

Somewhat related to this, programs that included follow-up prompts once the formal program was complete were more likely to lead to behavioral Maintenance. In addition, while interactive technology–based interventions were often effective in maintaining behavior changes, any intervention (including interactive technology–based ones) that included some face-to-face contact with those delivering the program were significantly more likely to result in longer-term changes in physical activity. Interventions that target women carefully screen volunteers so as to include only those most likely to adhere and are also more likely to result in maintained behaviors. Although both of these factors are more likely due to the motivational characteristics of the final sample than due to program content (27).

As with Effectiveness, the use of brief physical activity and quality of life measures and, when practical, direct measures on a subsample of the population can provide the data necessary to document Maintenance of physical activity changes. You can also apply similar follow-up assessment methods that use a stepped-approach (as previously mentioned in the Effectiveness section of this chapter). To assess the maintained influence of environmental and policy approaches, it is appropriate to use the same measures and methods that were completed to assess the Effectiveness immediately post-implementation. A good timeline for program, policy, and environmental change assessments is every 6 months after the program ended or after the policy or environmental change was implemented.

There is much less information on organization-level Maintenance of physical activity program delivery, but based on research in other areas there are a few key strategies to improve sustainability in community or clinical organizations (25). Specifically, generating evidence that your program can reach a broad cross-section of participants and effectively increase physical activity can be very helpful in highlighting success with key stakeholders. This information can be adapted into materials that can promote the program to future participants and organizational decision makers who can determine if a program is offered in the future or not. As sustainability is often jeopardized by reductions in funding (41), the development of a funding development committee and integrating the program into existing operations are important for sustained programs. Community engagement and the support of program champions can also significantly improve the chances of sustainability (25).

One of the benefits for using ongoing implementation evaluation is that it can double as an assessment of program sustainability. If a program continues to be implemented, it is an indicator of sustainability. Using the Implementation assessment can also provide indications of adaptations that were necessary to improve the likelihood of sustainability. The timing of sustainability assessment should probably occur on an annual or semi-annual basis.

STEP-BY-STEP RE-AIM EVALUATION

The authors have developed this step-by-step process for completing a RE-AIM evaluation of your physical activity initiative, keeping in mind that your initiative could be a program, environmental change, or policy. They also direct readers to the RE-AIM Web site (www.re-aim.org) for general information about the framework and clarification. The Web site includes detailed descriptions and evaluation examples as well as some checklist and calculation tools that may be helpful for you. When appropriate, in the following sections, specific links to relevant content are provided. RE-AIM was initially titled the ARI-EM framework to align with a practical assessment of programs from Adoption, to Reach within the adoption sites, to Implementation, to Effectiveness as a result of Implementation, and then finally focusing on Maintenance once effectiveness is achieved (28). The following instructions will follow this pragmatic order.

Step 1: Adoption

a. Determine if you need to monitor Adoption. If you are a sole operator in your organization (*e.g.*, health educator in a community health center) and you are trying to improve your effects with your clients, you will not need to track Adoption and you could move on to Reach.
b. Identify the total number of settings where you think your program could be delivered. To help with this estimate, go to http://www.re-aim.hnfe.vt.edu/tools/links/index.html#data where you will find links to databases for estimating schools, worksites, health care, civic, and community organizations that are in your particular area.
c. Determine if there are characteristics of those settings that could influence the likelihood of program delivery and locate available information on those settings. For many settings, the client/health professional ratio, the number of health professionals per setting, the socio-economic make-up of the census tracts that reflect the catchment

area for the setting, and the time the setting has been operating are all variables that could influence Adoption. See the link in part b earlier for data resources to obtain this type of information.

d. Invite the representatives from local settings to participate in delivering your intervention. Count the number that agree and the number that do not. Create a proportional indicator for Adoption.
e. Compare the settings that agree to deliver the intervention to the information you gathered on all eligible settings (*i.e.*, point "c"). This does not have to include sophisticated statistics, just simple comparisons (*e.g.*, those churches that agreed to participate had congregation sizes of approximately 150 compared to congregation sizes of approximately 300, on average, for those that declined).
f. For each setting that agrees to participate, determine if there are multiple health professionals that will be expected to implement the strategies. If so, determine the denominator of health professionals in each participating setting. Identify specific characteristics about the health professionals (on average is fine). Age, gender, physical activity status (if available), race, ethnicity, years in the field, and level of expertise are all useful characteristics. Invite all health professionals to deliver the program; track the number that agree and the number that do not to create a proportional health professional Adoption measure. Again, compare characteristics of those that agree to participate with the average characteristics in each setting.
g. For policy or environmental changes, identify and invite various organizations that have interest in the environmental change (public works, parks and recreation, etc.), and the agencies / key stakeholders that could participate in the planning, approval, and implementation stages. To measure the rate of Adoption, use the total number of agencies invited to the planning, approval, and implementation stages as the denominator and those that engage as the numerator. Rather than comparing to an aggregated group of similar agencies (as we did with settings earlier), determine representativeness based upon the degree to which you were able to attract all of the key stakeholders necessary to make the Adoption decision.
h. To complete the assessment of Adoption, record the number of settings and health professionals that agreed to deliver your program or participate in planning/ implementation of your environmental or policy change. Record the percent of those eligible that engaged at both the setting and health professional level (see http://www.re-aim.hnfe.vt.edu/resources_and_tools/calculations/adoption_calculator/index.html for an Adoption calculator to help with this). Report the degree to which you were successful in getting a representative sample based on the available setting and health professional information.

Step 2: Reach

a. Identify the total number of people who would be eligible for your intervention or program that receive services or interact with the settings where access to the intervention is offered. Use the information found at http://www.re-aim.hnfe.vt.edu/tools/calculations/reach_calculator/finding_numbers_to_estimate_reach.html to aid in estimating your denominator. The Web site also provides a description of methods to estimate the proportion of people who were exposed to your recruitment activities.
b. Determine the basic characteristics of your target population using census data or other locally available data (*e.g.*, de-identified data from a clinic's electronic medical record). Basic demographic information is appropriate, but other behavioral or health status information can also help you determine if there are subsamples in the population that are either over- or under-represented in your intervention.

c. Determine the number of people who respond to your recruitment efforts and begin your program.
d. Compare those that agree to participate in the intervention to the information you gathered on all eligible people in your settings. As with Adoption, this does not have to include sophisticated statistics, just simple comparisons (*e.g.*, there is a smaller proportion of Latinos in our intervention than there is at the worksite where we offered the program).
e. For policy or environmental changes, estimate the total number of people living and/or working within a specific buffer zone around the proposed environmental change. Use intercept surveys to determine the place of origin of individuals and observe and describe visitors during various times of day after implementation of environmental change. For a government policy like tax breaks for children participating in youth sports, the denominator would be all children in the area eligible for the breaks, and the numerator would be those that actually took advantage of them. Use this setting-level data as a proxy to track changes of Reach over time.

To complete the assessment of Reach, record the number of people that agreed to participate in your program or interacted with your environmental or policy change. Record the percent of those eligible that engaged with your intervention (see http://www.re-aim.hnfe.vt.edu/resources_and_tools/calculations/reach_calculator/index.html for a Reach calculator to help with this). Report the degree to which you were successful in getting a representative sample based on the information available.

Step 3: Implementation

a. Identify the components of your intervention (*e.g.*, small group session, followed by three tailored mailings, and six motivational interviewing based calls). Identify the key content in each of the intervention components.
b. Track the extent to which each component of the intervention is delivered on time according to the intervention delivery schedule. Use a checklist for health professionals to indicate the content that was or was not covered during each intervention contact.
c. Calculate the proportion of the intervention that was delivered as intended (*i.e.*, what was delivered as the numerator and what was intended as the denominator).
d. When determining the Effectiveness of the program, examine differences based on the percent of the program that was delivered as intended. Similarly, track all costs associated with the intervention and use this to consider potential areas to create efficiency without reducing key content.
e. Track any adaptations to the intervention that were completed to make it more suited to your setting, the expertise of the staff, or the interests of potential participants. Include Effectiveness assessments before and after any significant adaptations.
f. For environmental or policy changes, identify standards or guidelines for your changes as well as develop and use planning documents. Determine the degree to which the change aligned with planning documents and guidelines. Similar to program implementation evaluation, track all costs associated with the change.

Step 4: Effectiveness

a. Select an appropriate measure of physical activity. Ensure that the measure aligns with the type of physical activity you are promoting and includes an assessment of frequency, intensity, and duration. Use a validated measure rather than making up your own. On a subsample of your group, when possible, use a direct measure of physical activity.

b. Select appropriate measures for quality of life (see CDC Healthy Days measure) and unintended consequences (this can simply be the tracking of minor and major adverse events).
c. Assess physical activity and quality of life before the program begins and when the program ends. For more accurate accounts, collect reports of physical activity on a weekly basis using telephone or online tracking. Compare changes in physical activity changes in quality of life and potential negative outcomes.
d. Track participant attrition (*i.e.*, what proportion of those that began the program dropped out before it ended).
e. If a large proportion of your participants do not complete the follow-up assessment (*e.g.*, >30%), use a simple procedure that uses the baseline value as the follow-up value for those that didn't complete the assessment to give a more conservative estimate of your program's effectiveness. This is a form of an intention to treat analysis.
f. Using data collected for Reach, determine if there are differential effects of the intervention for different subgroups in your sample. Also examine if participants who dropped out were different than those that did not. In particular, examine differences based on initial physical activity level, gender, race/ethnicity, and economic status.
g. Using data collected for Implementation, determine if effectiveness is influenced by the degree to which key content was delivered as intended to the participants.
h. For environmental or policy changes, replace individual assessments with physical activity audits in the setting where the change occurred. When possible, also assess before and after to determine if the change is influencing different groups within the target population.

Step 5: Maintenance

INDIVIDUAL LEVEL

a. At the individual level, Maintenance assessment is a continuation of effectiveness assessment. It includes assessing participants some time after the formal intervention is completed, usually 6 months after it is completed.
b. Follow steps e–h of Effectiveness 6 months after the program is complete or the environmental or policy change has been in place.

ORGANIZATIONAL LEVEL

a. Maintain contact with those who are delivering the intervention over time. Track the number of times a program is offered and continued Reach as an indicator of sustainability.
b. Conduct brief interviews with those implementing the intervention to determine if adaptations have occurred, if there are plans to continue delivery, and if there have been expansions or contractions in delivery.
c. Brief interviews can occur on a pragmatic schedule. If a program is 6 months long, tracking on a semi-annual basis would make sense. If a program is 8 weeks long, tracking would need to occur more frequently.
d. Record the ongoing number of times the program is offered and the Reach of each specific offering.

e. For environmental or policy approaches, determine if there have been plans for upkeep or enforcement and the degree to which those plans have been followed to determine setting or organizational sustainability.

There are so many different types of physical activity initiatives that can be evaluated using the RE-AIM framework. Case Scenario 9.1 presents a realistic, community-wide approach. It can include program, policy, and environmental change strategies, is recommended as an evidence-based approach to improving physical activity, and has been the focus of RE-AIM evaluations previously (35,47).

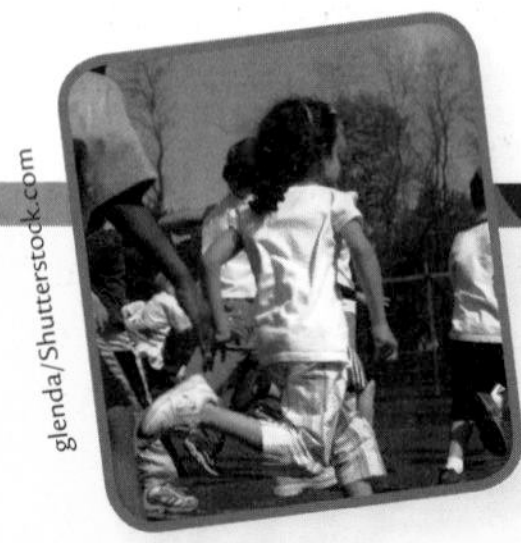
glenda/Shutterstock.com

Case Scenario 9.1

The physical activity initiative is located in a small community within a larger municipal area. The school system is a focal point for the initiative, which plans to change elementary, middle school, and high school policies to include regular physical education every day for all children. The authors plan to align the curriculum with a community physical activity challenge that includes weekly newsletters, team goals, and weekly group feedback. By aligning it with the in-school curriculum, they hope to encourage families to engage in the challenge together. Finally, the authors are planning to work with the school district to allow the school physical activity facilities to be open to the community after hours.

STEP 1: ADOPTION

Because the goal is to make changes in six schools (in our fictional community, there are three elementary schools, two middle schools, and one high school), and attract all adults in our community to participate, it is important to monitor Adoption. The six schools have been identified as places where the initiative will be delivered, along with the local churches (four of them) and health care clinics (three of them) to help reach a broad audience of adults. The target community does have some differences: two of the elementary schools and one of the middle schools have approximately 90% of their students eligible for free or reduced-cost lunches, whereas the high school is having problems passing federal standardized testing and could lose some of its funding if things don't improve. Otherwise, the elementary schools are about the same size, as are the middle schools. As for clinics, one is a community health center that serves Medicaid-eligible patients exclusively. The other two are associated with the local hospital system. The churches are all about the same size, but one is Baptist, one is Mormon, one is Catholic, and one is Methodist. To keep things simple, the congregations of each of the churches have the same demographic and economic profiles.

The community group sends out invitations to each of the settings described earlier. The high school declines the invitation, as do the Catholic and Methodist churches. All the elementary and middle schools agree to participate. The community health center and one of the hospital-associated clinics also agrees to participate. The rate of Adoption can be calculated by setting type (*i.e.,* 50% of churches, 83% of schools, and 67% of the clinics) or overall (69%).

There is a pattern that seems to explain why some settings decline. The high school administrators and teachers are really focused on getting test scores up and feel any curricular changes that don't teach to the test are a bad idea. Both the Catholic and Methodist churches have just become involved in a breast cancer awareness initiative and feel they

Case Scenario 9.1 *continued*

can't participate in another activity at the same time. The clinic that declines has just lost two physicians to retirement and is overloaded with their current responsibilities. All of the declining settings have legitimate competing demands that put constraints on their ability to participate. Luckily for our initiative, the settings that provide services to the lower economic status members of the community do agree to participate, increasing the likelihood that we will not miss this health disparate population.

There are 10 physicians in each of the participating clinics, for a total of 20, and one physical education teacher (who will be responsible for the curricular changes) in each of the five schools. All of the teachers are on board and excited about the new curriculum (100% Adoption). Of the physicians, 80% agree to participate by promoting the physical activity challenge to patients who are not meeting the guidelines for physical activity and to do screenings for high-risk patients to determine the safety of participating. The four physicians who decline are older and have been practicing longer, on average, than those that choose to participate. For policy changes, the school district superintendent agrees to support the curricular changes and make the school gym available after hours.

STEP 2: REACH

To determine the total number of people who will be eligible for the intervention, a choice has to be made. For the present scenario, this could be the number of students in each of the participating schools, the congregation size of the participating churches, and the number of patients at each of the clinics. The problem is that the goal is to get the whole community active, whereas the churches and clinics are just a way to advertise and help recruit people as opposed to delivering the intervention. In addition, there is some likely overlap between the churchgoers and patients, which could add some overestimation error to the calculation of the denominator. In this scenario, the census numbers for adults and school-aged children in the community is the best denominator. Census data are also used to determine the racial/ethnic breakdown in the community, the prevalence of poverty, and other demographic information. Using this and the state reports for the proportion of people meeting recommendations for physical activity, the sample is able to be described very well. In the end, our denominator is 3000 children and 15,000 adults.

School-based curricular activities reach 2000 of the 3000 children (the 1000 missing are those in the high school). As the physical activity challenge approaches, materials are sent home with the children, physicians make referrals to it, and announcements are made at the churches and placed in the church bulletin. In addition, presentations are conducted at the churches, and potential participants are allowed to register on-site. Finally, ads appear in the local newspaper, and posters are hung all over the community.

Prior to launching the challenge, 3000 adults enroll. Eighty-five percent of the adult respondents are women, most have a child in one of the participating schools, and the average household income is slightly higher than what is seen in the census data. Latino and African American women are just as likely to participate as Caucasian women, but minority men are less likely than Caucasian men to participate. When evaluating the policy change of making the school facilities available in the evenings, nearly 300 men, balanced on race and ethnicity, are gathering regularly to play basketball. It is noted that the men who used the gyms live, on average, within four city blocks of the school. Based on these data, Reach can be reported based on children (67% proportional Reach), adults (22%), or both (29%). The researchers are quite successful in engaging people across different household incomes but are not very successful in getting a large proportion of men involved.

continued

Case Scenario 9.1 *continued*

STEP 3: IMPLEMENTATION

Recall the intervention components include the school physical education policy and curriculum; open access to school facilities after school; and the community-wide physical activity challenge, with weekly newsletters, team goal setting, and feedback. For the curriculum, physical education teachers are cooperative with the preparation for the challenge, but not with the delivery of the rest of the curriculum. On average, they deliver about 50% of the material. For the adult portion, the physical activity challenge is delivered just as intended, and 100% of the newsletters with feedback on goals are sent out each week. About 5% of the mailings are returned with incorrect address or return to sender marked on them, reducing the Implementation of this component to 95%. The implementation numbers for children and adults are not combined because the separate numbers may be better to use when testing for Effectiveness based on Implementation.

The costs of activities aren't really clear. There is some concern at the schools that the utility bills (*e.g.*, heat and lights) will go up because the school is open later, but the information is never gathered from the schools. The cost of the physical activity challenge materials, and staff time in delivering them, are tracked. Neither the physicians' nor pastors' time is included in the cost estimate because they donate their time and are not involved in delivering any of the intervention. The researchers consider tracking the time needed to recruit and to determine what the most efficient recruitment strategies are but decide this is outside of the intervention Implementation evaluation.

STEP 4: EFFECTIVENESS

The researchers identify a validated and objective audit tool to determine physical activity to assess student behavior before school, during physical education class, and after school. They also add some brief and validated self-report physical activity recalls to the children's school readiness package so they can return them on the first day of school and the researchers can send them out again during the last week of school. For parents in the challenge and men who are using the gym, we use brief, validated self-report measures of physical activity prior to the first time the participant engaged in the program or used the gym. Participants are asked to complete the CDC Healthy Days measure and a short demographic questionnaire. The challenge participants are asked to report their physical activity weekly, and for those that use the gym we assess physical activity every 6 months from their first day at the gym. On each of the follow-up assessments, participants are asked about any injuries that may have occurred as a result of increasing physical activity.

By the completion of the challenge, approximately 2000 people are still participating and do the post-program follow-up. Because more than 30% are missing at the end, those people's before-program data are copied and used as their follow-up, too. This ensures that the researchers don't overestimate Effectiveness by assuming that people who don't do the follow-up probably didn't change their physical activity. For the kids in the study, we get about 90% to complete the follow-up.

Adults have increased their physical activity by about 45 minutes per week on average, whereas children have increased by nearly 120 minutes per week on average due to the new policy for more physical education. Interestingly, adults who use the gymnasium have increased by 90 minutes per week and report using the gym three nights a week on average. When looking across subgroups, it seemed that the program works best for parents of children in the schools. Adults with lower household income are more likely to be successful than those with higher income. When we consider Implementation, students in schools with better Implementation are more successful at increasing physical activity.

Case Scenario 9.1 *continued*

STEP 5: MAINTENANCE

Individual Level

A year after the changes are first implemented at the schools, the students are still participating in more physical activity than they were prior to the policy and curriculum changes. Adults that participated in the physical activity challenge are still more active than before the program, but less active than they were immediately after the program. The adults who did not do the challenge but used the open gym space maintain their activity levels, likely due to the schools still being open in the evenings. Changes have been maintained better in boys than girls for the students, but better for women than men in the challenge.

Organizational Level

After the first year of the program, the researchers meet with the school superintendent, principals, physical education teachers, pastors, and representatives from each of the referring health care clinics. All enjoyed the initial year of delivery and are interested in trying a second year. There is a lot of talk of small changes to the program and promotion, but everyone is ready to sustain the initiative. The superintendent indicates that the access to schools after hours will be added to the school wellness policy, and he will monitor the schools to make sure they adhere to the policy.

TAKE-HOME MESSAGE

It is highlighted again, although it is thought that each RE-AIM dimension is important and valuable, they may not all be applicable in your context. Still, here are five take-home messages for you:

1. Pay attention to who is participating in your programs or who is reached by your policy and environmental changes, know their characteristics and where you have gaps in reaching the breadth of your target population.
2. Track how participants with different characteristics fair in your programs, determine who it is working for and, just as importantly, who it is not working for.
3. Reach and representativeness are often driven by adoption. If you only get settings that primarily provide services to higher economic status and fewer minority clients, then the likelihood that you will reach a full spectrum of your target population is very low.
4. Monitoring Implementation in an ongoing way to help you ensure your initiatives are being delivered as intended. But as adaptations are made (as they invariably will be), it can also let you know if adaptations influence effectiveness either positively or negatively.
5. Focusing on maintenance will let you know if your efforts lead to long-term changes and demonstrate the value of your programs to your target population.

Changing physical activity is a challenging endeavor, especially when considering the issues associated with implementing different strategies within real-world settings. This chapter intended to highlight five areas of consideration that, if addressed and evaluated, can improve your chances of having a large impact in your target population. It is likely that you have considered most of these areas in your work at one time or another, and that by providing this information in a systematic way, with step-by-step instructions and an example scenario, that you will be able to complete a RE-AIM evaluation of your activities.

REFERENCES

1. Almeida FA, Shetterly S, Smith-Ray RL, Estabrooks PA. Reach and effectiveness of a weight loss intervention in patients with prediabetes in Colorado. *Prev Chronic Dis* [Internet]. 2010 [cited 2010 Sept];7(5):A103. Available from: http://www.cdc.gov/pcd/issues/2010/sep/09_0204.htm.
2. Almeida FA, Smith-Ray RL, Van Den Berg R, et al. Utilizing a simple stimulus control strategy to increase physician referrals for physical activity promotion. *J Sport Exerc Psychol.* 2005;27(4):505–14.
3. Antikainen I, Ellis R. A RE-AIM evaluation of theory-based physical activity interventions. *J Sport Exerc Psychol.* 2011;33(2):198–214.
4. Belansky ES, Cutforth N, Delong E, et al. Early effects of the federally mandated Local Wellness Policy on school nutrition environments appear modest in Colorado's rural, low-income elementary schools. *J Am Diet Assoc* [Internet]. 2010 [cited Nov];110(11):1712–17. Available from: doi 10.1016/j.jada.2010.08.004.
5. Berwick DM. Disseminating innovations in health care. *JAMA* [Internet]. 2003 Apr 16 [cited 2011 Oct 10];289(15):1969–75. Available from: http://jama.ama-assn.org/content/289/15/1969.full.pdf doi 10.1001/jama.289.15.1969.
6. Brownson RC, Housemann RA, Brown DR, et al. Promoting physical activity in rural communities: Walking trail access, use, and effects. *Am J Prev Med* [Internet]. 2000 Mar 15 [cited 2011 Oct 10];18(3):235–41. Available from: http://www.sciencedirect.com/science/article/pii/S0749379799001658 doi 10.1016/S0749-3797(99)00165-8.
7. Burke SM, Carron AV, Eys MA, Estabrooks PA. Group versus individual approach? A meta-analysis of the effectiveness of interventions to promote physical activity. *Sport Exerc Psychol Rev* [Internet]. 2006 [cited 2011 Oct 10];1:16. Available from: http://spex.bps.org.uk/spex/publications/sepr.cfm.
8. Caperchione C, Coulson F. The WellingTONNE Challenge Toolkit: Using the RE-AIM framework to evaluate a community resource promoting healthy lifestyle behaviours. *Health Educ J* [Internet]. 2010 Mar [cited 2011 Oct 10];69(1):126–34. Available from: http:// hej.sagepub.com/content/69/1/126.full.pdf doi10.1177/0017896910363301.
9. Damschroder LJ, Aron DC, Keith RE, Kirsh SR, Alexander JA, Lowery JC. Fostering implementation of health services research findings into practice: A consolidated framework for advancing implementation science. *Implement Sci* [Internet]. 2009 Aug 7 [cited 2011 Oct 10];4:50. Available from: http://www.implementationscience.com/content/4/1/50 doi 10.1186/1748-5908-4-50.
10. Davis M, Baranowski T, Resnicow K, et al. Gimme 5 fruit and vegetables for fun and health: Process evaluation. *Health Educ Behav* [Internet]. 2000 Apr [cited 2011 Oct 10];27(2):167–76. Available from: http://heb.sagepub.com/content/27/2/167.long doi 10.1177/109019810002700203.
11. De Meij JSB, Chinapaw MJM, Kremers SPJ, Van der Wal MF, Jurg ME, Van Mechelen W. Promoting physical activity in children: The stepwise development of the primary school-based JUMP-in intervention applying the RE-AIM evaluation framework. *Br J Sports Med* [Internet]. 2008 Nov 19 [cited 2011 Oct 10];44(12):879-887. Available from: http:// http://bjsm.bmj.com/content/44/12/879.long doi 10.1136/bjsm.2008.053827.
12. Doerksen SE, Estabrooks PA. Brief fruit and vegetable messages integrated within a community physical activity program successfully change behaviour. *Int J Behav Nutr Phys Act* [Internet]. 2007 Apr 10 [cited 2011 Oct 10];4:12. Available from: http://www.ijbnpa.org/content/4/1/12 doi doi:10.1186/1479-5868-4-12.
13. Dunton GF, Lagloire R, Robertson T. Using the RE-AIM framework to evaluate the statewide dissemination of a school-based physical activity and nutrition curriculum: "Exercise Your Options." *Am J Health Promot* [Internet]. 2009 [cited 2009 Mar–Apr]; 23(4):229–32. Available from: http://www.ncbi.nlm.nih.gov/pmc/articles/PMC2657926/?tool=pubmed doi 10.4278/ajhp.071211129.
14. Dzewaltowski DA, Estabrooks PA, Klesges LM, Bull S, Glasgow RE. Behavior change intervention research in community settings: How generalizable are the results? *Health Promot Int* [Internet]. 2004 [cited 2011 Oct 10];19(2):235–45. Available from: http://heapro.oxfordjournals.org/content/19/2/235.full.pdf+html doi 10.1093/heapro/dah211.
15. Dzewaltowski DA, Estabrooks PA, Welk G, et al. Healthy youth places: A randomized controlled trial to determine the effectiveness of facilitating adult and youth leaders to promote physical activity and fruit and vegetable consumption in middle schools. *Health Educ Behav* [Internet]. 2009 June [cited 2011 Oct 10];36(3):583–600. Available from: http://heb.sagepub.com/content/36/3/583 doi: 10.1177/1090198108314619.
16. Eakin E, Reeves M, Lawler S, et al. Telephone counseling for physical activity and diet in primary care patients. *Am J Prev Med* [Internet]. 2008 Dec 5 [cited 2011 Oct 10];36(2):142–149. Available from: http://www.sciencedirect.com/science/article/pii/S0749379708008970 doi 10.1016/j.amepre.2008.09.042.
17. Eakin EG, Brown WJ, Marshall AL, Mummery K, Larsen E. Physical activity promotion in primary care: Bridging the gap between research and practice. *Am J Prev Med* [Internet]. 2004 [cited Nov];27(4):297–303. doi 10.1016/j.amepre.2004.07.012.
18. Eakin EG, Lawler SP, Vandelanotte C, Owen N. Telephone interventions for physical activity and dietary behavior change: A systematic review. *Am J Prev Med* [Internet]. 2007 May [cited 2011 Oct 10];32(5): 419–34 Available from: http://www.sciencedirect.com/science/article/pii/S0749379707000104 doi 10.1016/j.amepre.2007.01.004.

19. Estabrooks P, Bradshaw M, Fox E, Berg J, Dzewaltowski DA. The relationships between delivery agents' physical activity level and the likelihood of implementing a physical activity program. *Am J Health Promot* [Internet]. 2004 May–June [cited 2011 Oct 10];18(5):350–3. Available from: http://ajhpcontents.org/doi/abs/10.4278/0890-1171-18.5.350 doi10.4278/0890-1171-18.5.350.
20. Estabrooks PA, Bradshaw M, Dzewaltowski DA, Smith-Ray RL. Determining the impact of Walk Kansas: Applying a team-building approach to community physical activity promotion. *Ann Behav Med* [Internet]. 2008;36(1):1–12. Available from: http://www.springerlink.com/content/w21404885lwx3424/ doi 10.1007/s12160-008-9040-0.
21. Estabrooks PA, Dzewaltowski DA, Glasgow RE, Klesges LM. School-based health promotion: Issues related to translating research into practice. *J Sch Health*. 2002;73:7.
22. Estabrooks PA, Gyurcsik NC. Evaluating the impact of behavioral interventions that target physical activity: Issues of generalizability and public health. *Psychol Sport Exerc* [Internet]. 2003 Jan [cited 2011 October 10];4(1): 41–55. Available from: http://www.sciencedirect.com/science/article/pii/S146902920200016X doi: 10.1016/S1469-0292(02)00016-X.
23. Estabrooks PA, Shoup JA, Gattshall M, Dandamudi P, Shetterly S, Xu S. Automated telephone counseling for parents of overweight children: A randomized controlled trial. *Am J Prev Med* [Internet]. 2008 Dec 16 [cited 2011 October 10];36(1):35–42. Available from: http://www.sciencedirect.com/science/article/pii/S0749379708008374 doi 10.1016/j.amepre.2008.09.024.
24. Estabrooks PA, Smith-Ray RL, Almeida FA , et al. Move more: Translating efficacious physical activity intervention principles into effective clinical practice. *Int J Sport Exerc Psychol* [Internet]. 2011 May 20 [cited 2011 Oct 10];9(1):4–18. Available from: http://www.tandfonline.com/doi/abs/10.1080/1612197X.2011.563123#.UZt_UCs4XBI doi: 10.1080/1612197X.2011.563123
25. Estabrooks PA, Smith-Ray RL, Dzewaltowski DA, et al. Sustainability of evidence-based community-based physical activity programs for older adults: Lessons from Active for Life. *Transl Behav Med* [Internet]. 2011 [cited 2011 Oct 10];1:7. Available from: http://www.springerlink.com/index/370162N8282NL370.pdf doi 10.1007/s13142-011-0039-x.
26. Estabrooks PA, Wages JG, Chappell D, et al. Comparing evidence-based principles to evidence-based program: A test of research practice partnerships. *Ongoing Study.*
27. Fjeldsoe B, Neuhaus M, Winkler E, Eakin E. Systematic review of maintenance of behavior change following physical activity and dietary interventions. *Health Psychol* [Internet]. 2011 Jan [cited 2011 Oct 10];30(1):99–109. Available from: http:// psycnet.apa.org/journals/hea/30/1/99.pdf doi 10.1037/a0021974.
28. Gaglio B, Glasgow RE. Evaluation approaches for dissemination and implementation research. Chapter in R Brownson, G Colditz, E Proctor, editors. *Dissemination and Implementation Research in Health: Translating Science to Practice*, Oxford University Press. Forthcoming.
29. Garber CE, Blissmer B, Deschenes MR, et al. American College of Sports Medicine position stand. Quantity and quality of exercise for developing and maintaining cardiorespiratory, musculoskeletal, and neuromotor fitness in apparently healthy adults: Guidance for prescribing exercise. *Med Sci Sports Exerc* [Internet]. 2011 Jul [cited 2011 Oct 10];43(7):1334–59. Available from: http://www.aliceveneto.com/1/upload/quantity_and_quality_of_exercise_for_developing.26_1_.pdf doi10.1249/MSS.0b013e318213fefb.
30. Glasgow RE, Bull SS, Gillette C, Klesges LM, Dzewaltowski DA. Behavior change intervention research in healthcare settings: A review of recent reports with emphasis on external validity. *Am J Prev Med* [Internet]. 2002 Jul [cited 2011 Oct 10];23(1):62–69. Available from: http://www.sciencedirect.com/science/article/pii/S0749379702004373 doi 10.1016/S0749-3797(02)00437-3.
31. Glasgow RE, Vogt TM, Boles SM. Evaluating the public health impact of health promotion interventions: The RE-AIM framework. *Am J Public Health* [Internet]. 1999 Sept [Cited 2011 October 10];89(9):1322–27. Available from: http://ajph.aphapublications.org/doi/abs/10.2105/AJPH.89.9.1322 doi10.2105/AJPH.89.9.1322.
32. Godin G, Jobin J, Bouillon J. Assessment of leisure time exercise behavior by self-report: A concurrent validity study. *Can J Public Health*. 1986;77(5):359–62.
33. Jenkins A, Christensen H, Walker JG, Dear K. The effectiveness of distance interventions for increasing physical activity: A review. *Am J Health Promot* [Internet]. 2009 [cited Nov–Dec];24(2):102–17. Available from: http://ajhpcontents.org/doi/abs/10.4278/ajhp.0801158 doi 10.42 7H/n}bp. OHO 1158.
34. Jilcott S, Ammerman A, Sommers J, Glasgow RE. Applying the RE-AIM framework to assess the public health impact of policy change. *Ann Behav Med* [Internet]. 2007 [cited 2011 Oct 10];34(2): 105–14. Available from: http://www.springerlink.com/content/840wu11643867432/ doi 10.1007/BF02872666.
35. Kahn EB, Ramsey LT, Brownson RC, et al. The effectiveness of interventions to increase physical activity– A systematic review. *Am J Prev Med* [Internet]. 2002 [cited 2002 May];22 Suppl 4:73–107. Available from: http://www.thecommunityguide.org/pa/pa-ajpm-evrev.pdf doi 10.1016/S0749-3797(02)00434-8.
36. Katula JA, Kritchevsky SB, Guralnik JM, et al. Lifestyle Interventions and Independence for Elders pilot study: Recruitment and baseline characteristics. *J Am Geriatr Soc* [Internet]. 2007 May [cited 2011 Oct 10];55(5):674-683. Available from: http://www.thelifestudy.org/docs/Published_Version_JGS_1136.PDF doi 10.1111/j.1532-5415.2007.01136.x.

37. King DK, Glasgow RE, Leeman-Castillo B. Reaiming RE-AIM: Using the model to plan, implement, and evaluate the effects of environmental change approaches to enhancing population health. *Am J Public Health* [Internet]. 2010 Sep 23 [cited 2011 Oct 10];100(11):2076-2084. Available from: http://ajph.aphapublications.org/doi/full/10.2105/AJPH.2009.190959doi10.2105/AJPH.2009.190959.
38. Klesges LM, Estabrooks PA, Dzewaltowski DA, Bull SS, Glasgow RE. Beginning with the application in mind: Designing and planning health behavior change interventions to enhance dissemination. *Ann Behav Med* [Internet]. 2005 Apr [cited 2011 October 10];29 Suppl:66–75. doi 10.1207/s15324796abm2902s_10.
39. Lee RE, McGinnis KA, Sallis JF, Castro CM, Chen AH, Hickmann SA. Active vs. passive methods of recruiting ethnic minority women to a health promotion program. *Ann Behav Med* [Internet]. 1997 [cited 1997];19(4):378–84. Available from: http://www.springerlink.com/content/d14423u68018j275/ doi 10.1007/BF02895157.
40. Lee RE, Medina AV, Mama SK, et al. Health is power: An ecological, theory-based health intervention for women of color. *Contemp Clin Trials* [Internet]. 2011 Jul 18 [cited 2011 Oct 10];32(6):916–23. Available from: http://www.sciencedirect.com/science/article/pii/S1551714411001820 doi10.1016/j.cct.2011.07.008.
41. McKenzie R, Naccarella L, Thompson C. Well for Life: Evaluation and policy implications of a health promotion initiative for frail older people in aged care settings. *Australas J Ageing* [Internet]. 2007 [cited Aug 6];26(3):135–40. doi 10.1111/j.1741-6612.2007.00238.x.
42. Mielenz T, Jackson E, Currey S, DeVellis R, Callahan LF. Psychometric properties of the Centers for Disease Control and Prevention Health-Related Quality of Life (CDC HRQOL) items in adults with arthritis. *Health Qual Life Outcomes*[Internet]. 2006 Sep 24 [cited 2011 Oct 10];4:66–73. Available from: http://www.ncbi.nlm.nih.gov/pmc/articles/PMC1609101/?tool=pubmed doi10.1186/1477-7525-4-66.
43. Rogers EM. Diffusion of preventive innovations. *Addict Behav* [Internet]. 2002 Nov–Dec [cited 2011 Oct 10];27(6):989–93. Available from: http://www.sciencedirect.com/science/article/pii/S0306460302003003 doi 10.1016/S0306-4603(02)00300-3.
44. Sallis JF, Cervero RB, Ascher W, Henderson KA, Kraft MK, Kerr J. An ecological approach to creating active living communities. *Annu Rev Public Health* [Internet]. 2006 [cited Apr];27:297–322. doi 10.1146/annurev.publhealth.27.021405.102100.
45. Schwartz MB, Lund AE, Grow HM, et al. A comprehensive coding system to measure the quality of school wellness policies. *J Am Diet Assoc*[Internet]. 2009 Jul [cited 2011 Oct 10];109(7):1256–62. Available from: http://citeseerx.ist.psu.edu/viewdoc/download?doi=10.1.1.175.4297&rep=rep1&type=pdf doi 10.1016/j.jada.2009.04.008.
46. Shoup JA, Gattshall M, Dandamudi P, Estabrooks P. Physical activity, quality of life, and weight status in overweight children. *Qual Life Res* [Internet]. 2008 [cited 2011 Oct 10];17(3):407–12. Available from: http://www.springerlink.com/index/95925t0328786v55.pdf doi 10.1007/s11136-008-9312-y.
47. Van Acker R, De Bourdeaudhuij I, De Cocker K, Klesges LM, Cardon G. The impact of disseminating the whole-community project '10,000 Steps': A RE-AIM analysis. BMC Public Health [Internet]. 2011 Jan 4 [cited 2011 Oct 10];11. Available from: http://www.biomedcentral.com/1471-2458/11/3 doi:10.1186/1471-2458-11-3.
48. van den Berg MH, Schoones JW, Vlieland T. Internet-based physical activity interventions: A systematic review of the literature. *J Med Internet Res* [Internet]. 2007 [cited Sept 30];9(3):44. Available from: http://www.jmir.org/2007/3/e26/ doi 10.2196/jmir.9.3.e26.
49. Wages JG, Jackson SF, Bradshaw MH, Chang M, Estabrooks PA. Different strategies contribute to community physical activity program participation in rural versus metropolitan settings. *Am J Health Promot* [Internet]. 2010 [cited Sept–Oct];25(1):36–39. doi 10.4278/ajhp.080729-ARB-143.
50. Wang G, Macera CA, Scudder-Soucie B, Schmid T, Pratt M, Buchner D. A cost-benefit analysis of physical activity using bike/pedestrian trails. *Health Promot Pract* [Internet]. 2005 [cited 2005 Apr];6(2):174–79. doi 10.1177/1524839903260687.
51. White SM, McAuley E, Estabrooks PA, Courneya KS. Translating physical activity interventions for breast cancer survivors into practice: An evaluation of randomized controlled trials. *Ann Behav Med* [Internet]. 2009 Mar 3 [cited 2011 Oct 10];37(1):10–19. Available from: www.springerlink.com/index/784r6j0r2u225423.pdf doi 10.1007/s12160-009-9084-9.
52. Wing RR, Jeffery RW, Pronk N, Hellerstedt WL. Effects of a personal trainer and financial incentives on exercise adherence in overweight women in a behavioral weight loss program. *Obes Res.* 1996;4(5):457–62.
53. Wing RR, Papandonatos G, Fava JL, et al. Maintaining large weight losses: The role of behavioral and psychological factors. *J Consult Clin Psychol* [Internet]. 2008 [cited Dec];76(6):1015–21. doi 10.1037/a0014159.

CHAPTER 10

Professional Practice and Practical Tips for the Application of Behavioral Strategies for the Physical Activity Practitioner

Carol Ewing Garber and Kimberly Samlut Perez

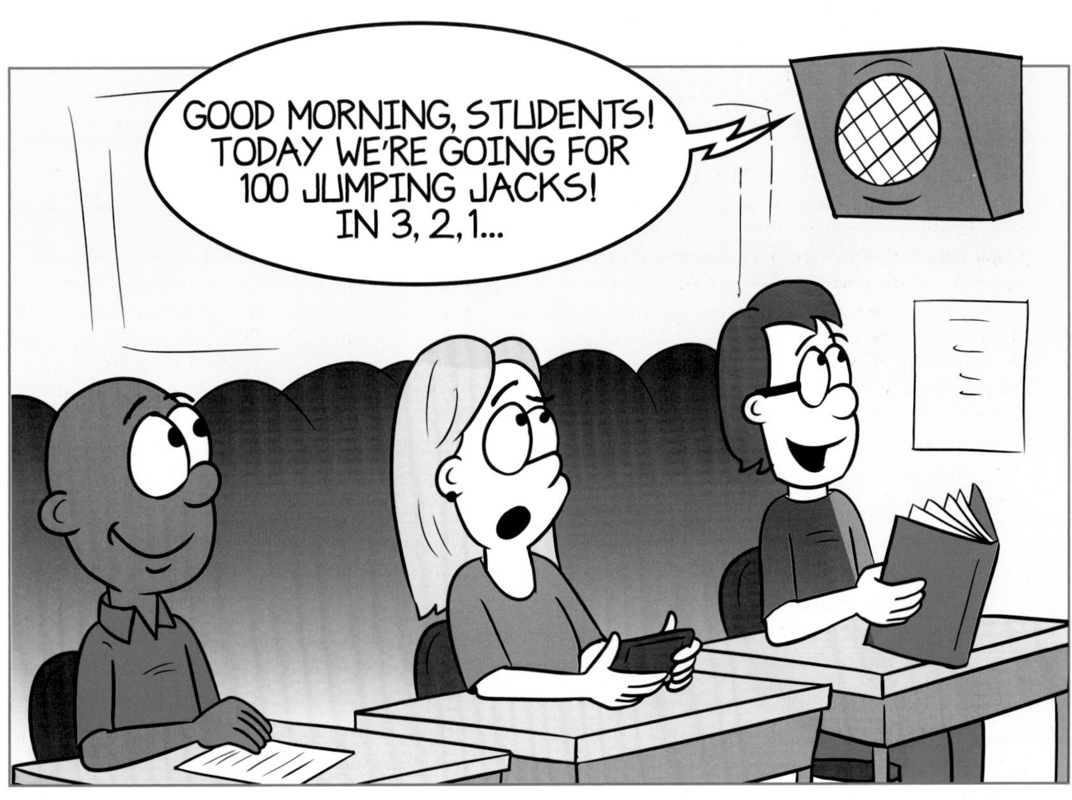
GOOD MORNING, STUDENTS!
TODAY WE'RE GOING FOR
100 JUMPING JACKS!
IN 3, 2, 1...

CONCEPT OVERVIEW

Physical activity behavior change may be influenced by the health and fitness professional's experience, competence, and personal characteristics (2,4). The health and fitness professional must take time to acquire and sharpen his or her counseling, communications, and professional skills and personal attributes in order to facilitate physical activity behavior change. This chapter will focus on the practical applications of professional skills, behaviors, and other factors that can facilitate or impede behavior change.

Health and fitness professionals work in many different settings that include—but are not limited to—fitness centers, community centers and nonprofits, worksites, and a variety of clinical settings. As a result, the scope of practice for the health and fitness practitioner is broad and there may be considerable variability in the professional standards of practice. The reader is referred to the *American College of Sports Medicine Guidelines* for more details about the scope of practice of various health and fitness professionals (1). However, there is foundational knowledge, skills, and professional behaviors shared among health and fitness professionals that apply across the broad array of settings and professional practice. This chapter will provide specific examples of behaviors, communication techniques, and program design guidelines that the practitioner can put into practice in nearly any setting.

COMMUNICATIONS

Verbal and Nonverbal Communications

The most successful professionals are aware of the importance of verbal and nonverbal communications in their interactions with their clients, colleagues, and potential clients. Encounters should begin with a friendly greeting accompanied with a smile, and eye-to-eye contact. Handshaking is customary in many settings, but some people prefer not to shake hands due to concerns about health, religion, or other reasons. Therefore, the health and fitness professional may want to allow the client to make the first move for a handshake, and take the cue from the client. When shaking hands, it is important to have a firm—but not too firm—handgrip, make direct eye contact, and say something like, "Nice to meet you, Mr. Jones."

When conversing, the face and both shoulders should be squared toward the client (or colleague), at the same time making regular eye contact. If seated, sit at or below the level of the client with a forward posture, thus sending the message that the professional is entirely focused on the client. The voice should be in a modulated tone that is audible to the client. The voice should be neither too loud nor too soft, and words should be clearly annunciated at a moderate speed to facilitate hearing and understanding of the information conveyed. Nonverbal indicators of active attention such as head nodding, judicious note taking, and hand gestures can add to the quality of these encounters.

The health and fitness professional's job is to educate, motivate, and promote physical activity and health behavior change. Verbal communication skills are at the core of the practice. Whether on the telephone or in person, what is said and how it is verbalized will affect how the client learns, receives information, accepts feedback, and, ultimately, may influence their willingness to change behavior. The first rule for effective verbal communication is that the practitioner must be committed to communicating effectively, and make efforts to do so with each client and colleague.

Verbal communications are best when adjusted according to a client's needs, capacity, and level of understanding. It is always important to remember that individualization is key. Speaking clearly and audibly in a pleasant tone and avoiding excessive slang increases the quality of the interaction and enhances professional impression. Short silent pauses that can be used to gather thoughts are perfectly acceptable and allow the client time to think about what has been said or to speak. Words and statements that may be viewed as derogatory or harassing in any way need to be avoided at all times. For example, commenting on a person's clothing or physical appearance may be perceived as sexual harassment. Comments about an ethnic, racial, or religious group, sexual orientation, body habits, or disabling condition can be perceived as derogatory. It is helpful for all health and fitness professionals to undergo formal training in sexual harassment and cultural sensitivity to enhance their effectiveness in working with diverse populations, and to increase awareness about how communications may be perceived negatively.

Telephone and Electronic Communications

Following up after a session in the early phases of a training program (or at any time there may be major changes or concerns) can do a lot to facilitate the development of rapport with the client, to provide social support, and to promote behavior change. A telephone call made to the client 24–48 hours after the first session can be very helpful. This allows the health and fitness professional an opportunity to check in with a client to assess how they have responded to training, see if they are experiencing any problems related to the exercise session, and to ask for feedback. This can also be done via e-mail depending on the client's preferences. Many clients may prefer electronic communications. The use of e-mail, text messaging, video conferencing, Web sites, and social media can be effective for promoting physical activity behavior change (3). It may also be beneficial from both a time management and record keeping perspective, and to maintain and provide social support and an open line of communication with clients.

If e-mail is the preferred method indicated by a client, it is important to include a clearly identified subject line to distinguish the source of the e-mail. For example, the subject line may include your name and title, such as "From Susan C., Personal Trainer, follow-up on session." It is particularly important when contacting a first-time client that the subject line clearly identifies who the e-mail is from and its purpose. Also, the body of the e-mail should include a brief introduction and the reasons for your communication (see Case Scenario 10.1 for an example).

Pavel Ignatov/Shutterstock.com

Case Scenario 10.1

INITIAL COMMUNICATIONS WITH THE CLIENT

Sam is a certified personal trainer at a local health club, making first contact with a potential new client, Mr. Jones, who has signed up for personal training services as part of his new membership. Sam has left several voicemail messages for Mr. Jones, but he has not received a call back. Sam notices in Mr. Jones membership application that he prefers receiving e-mail communications rather than phone calls. He also notes that Mr. Jones is a 62-year-old man who is a high-level executive at a major company, so he knows that Mr. Jones likely gets many e-mails each day and his may not be noticed. To increase the likelihood that Mr. Jones will read his e-mail, Sam starts his

continued

Case Scenario 10.1 *continued*

e-mail with a descriptive subject line. He then considers his e-mail content to ensure it is short and to the point, as is appropriate for e-mail communications. He also incorporates behavioral principles into his communications, drawing from the 5 A's counseling scheme and health behavior theories as discussed in previous chapters.

Sam writes his e-mail:

Subject Line: Your request for Personal Training Sessions at ExerClub

Dear Mr. Jones,

You have requested personal training at ExerClub. I would like to schedule a time to speak with you to gather some information so you can get started. Please let me know when it may be convenient for you to schedule a phone call. I have availability at many times during the day and evening and on weekends, so I can work around your schedule.

You can reach me on my cell phone, by e-mail, or by texting. I am looking forward to working with you to achieve your exercise goals.

Sincerely,

Sam Spencer, B.S. CPT
Personal Trainer, ExerClub
Cell (Voice and Text): 212-444-4444
E-mail: SSpencer@ExerClub.com

Mr. Jones responds to Sam's e-mail with a text asking him to call on Thursday at 8am. Sam replies by text:

Mr. Jones-Will call you Thurs. March 7 @ 8am @ 212-666-6666. Let me know if another number is better. Sam Spencer, ExerClub

Sam calls Mr. Jones at the appointed time:

Hello, Mr. Jones. This is Sam Spencer, the personal trainer at ExerClub. Is this time still okay to talk? Great! I am calling today to learn a little more about you so I can help you achieve your exercise goals. This will take about five minutes. Does this fit with your schedule today? Okay, great! Can you tell me a little about why you decided to start exercising?... I see... You have noticed you are often tired and you would like to increase your stamina. An exercise program can often help people feel more energetic. With most of my clients, we meet once or twice per week for 30–45 minutes to start, but we can meet more or less frequently depending on your preferences. I imagine you have a very busy schedule, so what do you think will work for you?... Twice per week sounds like a reasonable place to start—we can always revise this as needed.

To get started, we will need to schedule a visit to get more information about your health, exercise preferences, and to do some tests to evaluate your fitness so I can recommend a program that best fits your needs. After that, we can set up your training sessions. This first visit will take about 1 hour. Would you like to schedule that now?... Okay, how about Tues March 12 at 7am? Perfect! In the meantime, there are some information forms I can send you to fill out to save time during your visit. I can send them in the mail or by e-mail. Which do you prefer?... Okay, I will send them in the mail... Let me confirm your address... Thank you, Mr. Jones.

I look forward to meeting you on March 15 at 7am at ExerClub at Broadway and East 57th Street in Manhattan. I will send an electronic calendar request to your e-mail so you can easily put this into your calendar. I will also text or e-mail a reminder the day before. Do you have a preference? Okay, I will text you a reminder. Do you have any questions?... Thanks for your time, Mr. Jones... Goodbye.

It is important to remember that e-mails are generally not encrypted and are not secure. Employers and other individuals can access information sent via e-mail, text, or electronic chat, therefore these modes of communications are not appropriate for discussing or collecting personal and sensitive information. The practitioner and client must understand this limitation. The use of social networks, Web sites, chat rooms, videoconferencing, and blogs can be a valuable platform for exchanging information and ideas with clients or other professionals. These modes can be helpful in monitoring progress, problem solving, providing social support, and as a resource for general educational material about exercise and health topics, highlighting special events and resources for physical activity, program schedules, and the like.

TEACHING AND LEARNING

The practice context of the health and fitness professional involves the use of various behavioral and teaching strategies that are individualized to meet the client's learning style and personal preferences. To be effective, behavior change and learning theories should form the basis of the instructional methods and behavioral strategies employed. Effective teaching involves the combination of demonstration, visual observation, verbal explanations, and feedback (Figure 10.1). One of the most common forms of instruction involves the instructor demonstrating and explaining an exercise, followed by the client performing the exercise while the instructor observes and provides feedback. Table 10.1 provides some tips for teaching an exercise.

TABLE 10.1 Points Included in Teaching an Exercise

Introduce the exercise using a simple name.

Explain why the exercise is part of the program (*i.e.,* its benefits).

Compare the exercise to a familiar activity or an easy action verb.

> Example: "The first exercise we are beginning with today is a stationary lunge. This exercise is great for strengthening the muscles of the hip and the knee. You can think of this exercise as being like the squats we did on Monday, but this time our legs are staggered in front of each other instead of being next to each other so that the forward leg is doing the majority of the work."

Cue the exercise using as few words as possible, while demonstrating it so the client is receiving both verbal and visual cues. The key to effective cueing (without over-cueing) is using concise action words that are easy to follow.

Demonstrate the exercise while making eye contact.

Highlight any moves that you want them to think about by using action verbs or metaphors—it is always more effective to tell them what to do as opposed to what not to do.

> Example: While demonstrating the exercise, and using fingers to point to the areas that are being referred to, "As you can see, the forward foot is completely on the ground, hips are level, spine should remain tall reaching to the top of the head, and shoulders are squared toward the front. While maintaining a tall spine, begin by lowering the hips to the ground and then pushing back up. You can adjust your feet as necessary to make you feel more stable."

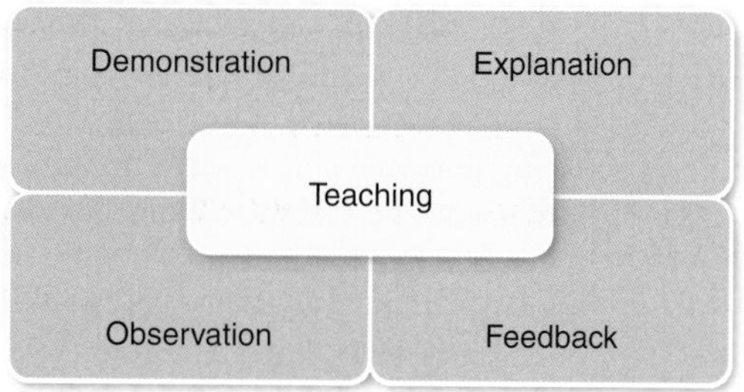

FIGURE 10.1. Components of teaching physical activities and exercise. (© Carol Ewing Garber, Ph.D., 2012. Used with permission.)

THE ENVIRONMENT

To facilitate physical activity behavior change, the physical environment in which counseling, testing, and training takes place should be pleasant, safe, and comfortable. This can be easily accomplished by maintaining a neat and clean facility that is free of clutter and physical hazards. For evaluation and counseling sessions, it is important that there is privacy and that the area is free from distractions. There may be a need for a noise canceling device to minimize the possibility of transfer of sensitive and personal information to others. Appropriate accommodations for persons with disability are made, to ensure accessibility of services to all.

STEP-BY-STEP: PREPARATION AND FOLLOW-UP FOR CLIENT SESSIONS

Being fully prepared for each encounter with a client—whether an intake, counseling, testing, or training session—is imperative, and will go a long way in facilitating the client's behavioral change and attainment of personal goals. With a busy schedule, it is often easy to underestimate the time needed for preparation, rely on previous experiences, or provide "cookie cutter" sessions for all clients, but this will not yield optimal results. Tailoring exercise counseling and training sessions based on the individual's characteristics is an effective strategy in facilitating physical activity behavior change (2). In addition, being unprepared can result in serious errors that could jeopardize client health or safety.

Thorough preparation for a session includes a review of the client's available records, such as current and past medical history and physical activity behavior and performance during previous training sessions. The review allows the health and fitness professional to thoughtfully consider how to approach the client, ensure that the session is tailored appropriately to the client's needs and readiness to change physical activity, and to maximize safety. Incorporating current information from credible sources is key for effective professional practice. However, being aware of recent news or magazine articles about exercise and being able to discuss these with the client can provide excellent opportunities for dialog and education.

Whenever possible, it is important to coordinate efforts with other health professionals such as the primary care physician, physical therapist, or dietician who may be working with the client. This helps ensure that all will be providing consistent advice and coordinated services, which will maximize the benefits to the client and reduce confusion that may interfere with behavior change. Each of these things can be done well before the client comes to his or her visit with the health and fitness professional, with prompt follow-up after the client's visit as needed.

STEP-BY-STEP: EXERCISE PROGRAMMING AND TESTING

Components of a Physical Activity Counseling Session

A physical activity counseling session is best conducted with open-ended questions designed to engage the client and health and fitness professional in an open dialogue. This fosters a highly interactive environment for developing the individualized physical activity program. The open-ended approach encourages the client to reveal true feelings, concerns, and relevant information because it helps to develop a "safe space" where the client feels comfortable and may be more willing to share personal information. There are many theoretical frameworks that can be applied to the counseling session, and the health and fitness professional is advised to develop one that fits the environment, time constraints, and clientele. However, there are elements that are commonly incorporated into every counseling session, depending on the theoretical model being applied. These include:

1. Clearly stating the purpose of the session
2. Assessment of the client's readiness to change behavior
3. Providing specific recommendations or advice to the client based on their responses, health status, sociodemographic considerations, environment, and physical activity goals
4. Summarizing the plans developed and ensuring client understanding
5. Setting up a time line and mode for following up (see Figure 10.2)

The most information is often obtained from the client by asking open-ended questions, but there is a place for polar (*i.e.*, "yes or no" questions) and objective questions, which are more specific in the responses expected. Table 10.2 presents a framework for asking effective questions.

Try to learn as much as you can from the client. This is an opportunity to create an open dialogue, set the framework for future meetings, and assist in developing an individualized program. In asking effective open-ended questions during the counseling session, the practitioner is using the client-centered skill of motivational interviewing. Motivational interviewing allows for two major achievements: one for the practitioner and the other for the client. For the practitioner, allowing the client to speak freely about their barriers, concerns, fears, likes, dislikes, etc., will provide much insight into the client's preferences, personality, and relapse risks, and it will facilitate the development of an individualized program. In other words, the health and fitness professional can utilize that information to develop an effective program that the client will enjoy and to which they may be able to adhere. The major achievement for the client is that they can make personal discoveries about their lifestyle, which further allows the client to develop tools and strategies to successfully manage a physical activity program. This interactive process also promotes a sense of shared teamwork and support to achieve the client's goals. Remember, this does not happen after one session; this give-and-take discussion is an ongoing process. It takes

Step 1
Clearly state the purpose of the session

Step 2
Assess the client's readiness to change behavior

Step 3
Provide specific recommendations or advice to the client

Step 4
Summarize the plans developed and ensure client understanding

Step 5
Set up a time line and mode for following up

FIGURE 10.2. Typical elements of a counseling session. (© Carol Ewing Garber, Ph.D., 2012. Used with permission.)

TABLE 10.2 Generating Effective Questions

Polar Question	Objective Question	Open-Ended Question
Do you enjoy exercising?	When you exercise would you say you prefer high-intensity activities or moderate-intensity activities?	What are some of the high-intensity activities you enjoy doing?
Do you smoke or have you quit smoking within the last year?	Around what time last year did you quit smoking?	That is great that you have not smoked in over 10 months. What changes have you noticed since you stopped?
Are you interested in gaining or losing weight?	What would you describe your ideal weight to be? In other words, what weight do you think will make you feel comfortable?	What factors do you feel may have contributed to your weight gain?

Note: Questions asked during the initial interview are often done as a follow-up to preparticipation paperwork that has previously been administered, thus using polar questions may be repetitious and unnecessary. Notice that open-ended questions often begin with a paraphrase of the response to the previous objective question.

work, time, and patience to make lifestyle and behavior changes. Plans and approaches often need to be modified due to changing circumstances, experiences, and attitudes.

Review of Health Status

As recommended by ACSM, a thorough review of health status is important as part of the initial intake of the client, with updates being part of regular visits. The reader is referred to Chapter 2 and the *American College of Sports Medicine Guidelines* for more information and tools for this purpose (1). Health information is important not only for client safety, but also to tailor the physical activity program to accommodate limitations imposed by an acute or chronic health condition.

REVIEW OF PHYSICAL ACTIVITY AND EXERCISE BEHAVIOR

Understanding the client's current and past physical activity behavior is crucial when formulating a new or revised program of exercise, as noted in Chapter 2. There are many available physical activity questionnaires or tools such as pedometers that can be used to assess and monitor physical activity and exercise behavior. From a behavioral standpoint, learning about the individual's perceptions and attitudes about previous, current, and future experiences is key to facilitating physical activity behavior change. Also of importance is the understanding of other cognitive, social, environmental, and psychological factors that can affect exercise preferences and behavior, such as self-efficacy, cultural norms, and neighborhood environment. While somewhat time consuming, a thorough understanding of these individual, social, and environmental factors will help the health and fitness professional develop an exercise program that is uniquely tailored to the individual, and increase the likelihood of adoption and adherence to exercise and physical activity. Table 10.3 presents tips for conducting a screening and initial counseling session.

TABLE 10.3 Tips for the Physical Activity Intake/Screening Session

Greet the client. Call the person "Mr./Ms. ___________." Then ask the client by what name they want to be called. This shows respect for the client and also helps confirm that you are speaking with the correct person.

Introduce yourself.

Example: "I am John, the Exercise Physiologist at the Excel Fitness Center."

Introduce the purpose of today's visit.

Example: "I am a certified personal trainer, and today I want to learn more about you so I can provide the best program for you."

Try to make the client feel comfortable. Sit at the same level or lower than the client—never stand or sit towering over the person.

Sit in a way that welcomes conversation. Make eye contact, lean forward, look interested in the client.

Speak clearly and slowly, and look at the client to see if they understand. Consider that the client may have a hearing or language difference that they are reluctant to reveal to you.

Use open-ended questions to start out.

Examples:
"How are you feeling today?"
"Can you tell me why you are here today?"
"Have you done any exercise before?"

Clarify and get more information. Clarify any answers that you don't understand or may be conflicting with other statements/information the client has given you. Ask for more detail about something that might be important (*i.e.,* chest discomfort).

Use reflective responses that repeat what the client said.

Example: "You mentioned that you have some pain in your right knee. Can you tell me more about that? What does it feel like? When does it hurt?"

Validate concerns that the client mentions.

Examples:
"It is intimidating to come to a fitness center for the first time."
"You seem worried that you will have trouble exercising because you aren't athletic."

Ask the client what they think the problem is concerning their health or fitness.

Examples:
"What do you think about your exercise habits right now?"
"What is your major health issue?"

Respond appropriately if the client avoids talking about something or seems anxious or uncomfortable about something.

Examples:
"Many people are worried about going to the gym because they are worried about their appearance."
"Many people are afraid to go to the gym because they might not know what to do. Has this happened to you?"

Sum up your take of what the client has told you.

Example: "Mr. Jones, I want to make sure that I understand correctly what you have told me... [repeat what they have said in your own words]."

continued

TABLE 10.3 Tips for the Physical Activity Intake/Screening Session (*Continued*)

Ask specific questions about the client's current and past health—relevant to your client's needs and fitness setting. Complete details on health screening are found in reference (1) (American College of Sports Medicine, 2013).

Example: "Now Mr./Ms. Jones, I need to ask you a few questions about your health, because your health can affect the types of exercise you can do safely."

The information to be gathered generally includes:

- History of current illness
- Past medical history
- Current medications (name, dose, purpose)—include over-the-counter medications and vitamins
- Allergies
- Risk factors for cardiovascular disease
- Alcohol or drug use
- Symptoms of angina pectoris, claudication, shortness of breath
- Any discomfort/pain related to exertion
- Sleep habits
- Psychosocial (*e.g.,* living situation, occupational status, education)

Ask directly if you want to know something. Clients often expect you to uncover problems and won't necessarily volunteer information.

Ask the client if there is anything that they are concerned about.

Example: "Is there anything we have not discussed that you would like to talk about?"

Ask the client if they have any questions.

End by summarizing the session, thanking the client, and letting the client know what to expect next.

Constantly repeat yourself while working with clients; one never knows whether the information relayed is being understood or if the client is attending to your message. For example, a client may not remember an instruction to keep their forward knee above their foot while performing a static lunge, or that a stretch should be held for 10–30 seconds.

A professional and nonjudgmental approach is helpful when inquiring about current and past exercise behavior. This helps maintain open lines of communication, allows for more frank dialogue between the professional and the client, and increases the likelihood that the client will feel comfortable in truthfully revealing their behavior and feelings about their exercise experiences, and—most importantly for continued exercise—they will continue to keep their appointments and return e-mails and phone calls. This openness will help the health and fitness professional and the client work through problems and barriers that are encountered by the client in their quest to be a regular exerciser. It is helpful for the health and fitness professional to be accepting that not all people like to exercise, and that many find exercise to be difficult or unpleasant and have concerns about their abilities to be physically active.

When obtaining a physical activity history, first explain what is meant by physical activity and exercise, as the client may lack a clear and comprehensive understanding. An inventory of all physical activity behavior, including activities of daily living, occupational and transportation physical activities, and exercise, is helpful because it gives information that will assist in fitness assessments and exercise prescription, but it may also offer clues as to an approach to take in developing a program. For example, if someone says they "hate to exercise" but "love to dance," consider suggesting a program that involves dance-like activities. In addition to learning about what and where exercise is being done—or has been done in the past—ask specifically about the client's exercise likes and dislikes.

Understanding these likes and dislikes will help in developing a program that is pleasant and enjoyable as possible for the client, improving the likelihood of exercise adoption and adherence. Knowledge about previous injuries and physical activity limitations is also helpful from both the health and behavioral perspective. For example, if someone had a previous knee injury, exercises that may aggravate the injury and cause pain can be avoided. On the other hand, exercising painful arthritic joints may be beneficial, so the client will need to be instructed about when and how to exercise through pain and when pain signals to them "stop exercising." Educate clients to be aware of the need to push themselves, while at the same time recognizing their limits. Since painful or unpleasant exercise reduces enjoyment, it will also be important to identify markers of improvement so the client can monitor the benefits of exercise, even if there may be some discomfort associated with it.

The social, occupational, and cultural environment of the client is also important from a behavior change perspective. Asking questions about occupation, living situation, and community are helpful in tailoring the program to the individual, and increasing the likelihood of their being able to start and maintain a regular program of physical activity. For example, the busy executive may have significant time limitations or limitations imposed by frequent travel, while the parents of young children may have to obtain childcare so they can exercise. Some religious and cultural groups may prohibit co-ed exercise situations, or may mandate dress that may make some types of exercise difficult. Some cultural groups may not be supportive of exercise or certain types of exercise, and this can vary by gender. Perceived neighborhood safety, community exercise resources, and climate are also considerations. Addressing these barriers to exercise can help ensure the development of an exercise program that the individual is able to do on a regular basis.

The development of an exercise program should be highly interactive, with active involvement of the client in the process to ensure buy-in and commitment and a program that best meets their needs and preferences. Before implementing the program, re-check with the client to see that it seems reasonable to them and it is consistent with their wishes. As part of the process, plan for potential barriers that may arise and address the probability of regression (missing sessions, not adhering to the program), and emphasize that the plan is a guide that can be adjusted as needed.

Counseling for Follow-up Testing and Referrals

If problems arise, it may be necessary to consider referrals to health care professionals for further evaluation or treatment before starting or resuming exercise. While the need for medical clearance or medical treatment can present a barrier for starting or changing an exercise program, this should be done as indicated according to *American College of Sports Medicine Guidelines* (1). The health and fitness professional can provide an easy-to-use form that clearly and concisely outlines the health concern and the specific questions that the health and fitness professional wants to be addressed. This can help the physician or other health professional to quickly and easily respond during the office visit. It is important to avoid unduly alarming the client when a potential health issue is uncovered, but at the same time the seriousness of the situation should be made clear. For example, if during the visit, the client's blood pressure is elevated on multiple measurements, mention this matter-of-factly to the client, without minimizing the import of the problem—*e.g.,* "Ms. Smith, your blood pressure seems a bit high today. Have you ever been told your blood pressure is high before? It may just be that you are in an unfamiliar situation, which can raise your blood pressure, but I think it would be a good idea to follow up with your doctor, just to be sure. I can fax this information to your doctor and you can follow up with a phone call, or, if you prefer, I can write down your blood pressure readings and you can make an appointment with your doctor."

When conducting fitness tests, make sure to explain fully to the client what the tests are and why they are being done. This is part of the consent process, which should go well beyond providing the client with a piece of paper and asking them to sign it. Rather, a full verbal explanation of the tests, risks, benefits, and alternatives to testing should be given, followed by an opportunity for the client to ask and have answers provided to all questions. It is important to ensure that the client understands that they may decline to take any of the tests, or to stop testing at any time. If any of the tests are mandatory according to the fitness center policy, this should be clearly communicated as well.

The Exercise Training Session

During the exercise training session, the focus is on teaching exercise skills and techniques and monitoring the client during exercise. What is unique about the health and fitness professional's role is the power to influence and heighten the sense of accomplishment by teaching and providing feedback. Verbal and nonverbal communication techniques are employed during exercise training sessions to motivate and encourage the client. During the initial phases of an exercise program, what motivates a person to return may be the hope of experiencing benefits and a sense of accomplishment from completing the exercises. Later on, the client may notice physical and mental changes such as better fitting clothing and feeling more energetic, and these provide further positive reinforcements. The health and fitness professional can assist the client in becoming more aware of their body and being able to notice subtle changes more readily. Incorporating self-monitoring data collection methods to demonstrate accomplishment or improvement such as logs, accumulation of distances or time, pedometer counts and other self-monitoring devices, and apps or online tools can also be helpful and effective monitoring methods that can facilitate physical activity behavior change (2).

TAKE-HOME MESSAGE

The health and fitness professional can do much to promote and facilitate physical activity behavior change in a client. Professional appearance, behavior, and communications of the health and fitness professional are keys to success, as is maintaining high standards of professional practice that is current and up to date. Employing teaching and health behavior change techniques based on theoretical constructs enhances client behavior change and physical activity adoption and adherence. Ethical considerations such as confidentiality and adhering to professional ethical standards are inherent in the practice of the health and fitness professional. In addition, cultural sensitivity, avoiding potentially derogatory speech and behaviors, and respectful and appropriate touching are also integral to the practice of the health and fitness professional.

REFERENCES

1. American College of Sports Medicine. *ACSM's guidelines for exercise testing and prescription*. 9th ed. Philadelphia (PA): Lippincott Williams & Wilkins; 2014.
2. Garber CE, Blissmer B, Deschenes MR, et al. Quantity and quality of exercise for developing and maintaining cardiorespiratory, musculoskeletal, and neuromotor fitness in apparently healthy adults: Guidance for prescribing exercise. *Med Sci Sports Exerc*. 2011;43(7):1334–59.
3. Marcus BH, Williams DM, Dubbert PM, et al. Physical activity intervention studies: What we know and what we need to know: A scientific statement from the American Heart Association Council on nutrition, physical activity, and metabolism (Subcommittee on Physical Activity); Council on Cardiovascular Disease in the Young; and the Interdisciplinary Working Group on Quality of Care and Outcomes Research. *Circulation*. 2006;114(24):2739–52.
4. Seguin RA, Economos CD, Palombo R, Hyatt R, Kuder J, Nelson ME. Strength training and older women: A cross-sectional study examining factors related to exercise adherence. *J Aging Phys Act*. 2010; 18(2):201–18.

Index

Note: Page numbers followed by *f* indicate figures; those followed by *t* indicate tables.

D

E

I

L

M

Q

R

T